CROSS-CULTURAL PERSPECTIVES IN MEDICAL ETHICS

Second Edition

Edited by

Robert M. Veatch

The Kennedy Institute of Ethics
Georgetown University

JONES AND BARTLETT PUBLISHERS

Sudbury, Massachusetts

BOSTON   TORONTO   LONDON   SINGAPORE

World Headquarters
Jones and Bartlett Publishers
40 Tall Pine Drive
Sudbury, MA 01776
978-443-5000
info@jbpub.com
www.jbpub.com

Jones and Bartlett Publishers
International
Barb House, Barb Mews
London W6 7PA
UK

Production Credits

Acquisitions Editor: Suzanne Jeans
Associate Editor: Amy Austin
Senior Production Editor: Lianne Ames
Manufacturing Buyer: Therese Bräuer
Design and Editorial Production Service: Thompson Steele, Inc.
Cover Design: Anne Spencer
Printing and Binding: Malloy Lithographing
Cover Printing: Malloy Lithographing

Library of Congress Cataloging-in-Publication Data

Cross-cultural perspectives in medical ethics / [edited by] Robert M. Veatch.—2nd ed.
    p. cm.
  Includes bibliographical references and index.
  ISBN 0-7637-1332-5
    1. Medical Ethics—Cross-cultural studies. 2. Medical ethics. I. Title: Cross cultural perspectives in medical ethics. II. Veatch, Robert M.

R725.5 .C76 2000
174'.2—dc21   99-089318

Printed in the United States
04 03 02 01 00   10 9 8 7 6 5 4 3 2 1

CONTENTS

CHAPTER 5 **Medical Ethical Theories Outside Western
Culture   217**

——— Acknowledgments ———

Chapter 1

"The Hippocratic Oath: Text, Translation, and Interpretation" abridged with permission from Edelstein, Ludwig. *The Hippocratic Oath: Text, Translation and Interpretation.* Baltimore/London, The Johns Hopkins University Press, 1943, pp. 1–64.

"Declaration of Geneva" by the World Medical Association. Copyright 1986, World Medical Association. Reprinted with permission of the World Medical Association.

"The Florence Nightingale Pledge" reprinted from "Editorial Comment." *The American Journal of Nursing* 11 (May 1911):596.

"Solemn Oath of a Physician of Russia" *Kennedy Institute of Ethics Journal* 3(4, 1993):419. ©1993. Johns Hopkins University Press.

Chapter 2

"The Oath According to Hippocrates In So Far as a Christian May Swear It" reprinted from W. H. S. Jones. *The Doctor's Oath: An Essay in the History Of Medicine.* Cambridge: At The University Press, 1924.

"Medical Ethics" extracted from Percival, Thomas. *Medical Ethics; Or, a Code of Institutes and Precepts, Adapted to the Professional Conduct of Physicians and Surgeons; to Which Is Added an Appendix; Containing a Discourse on Hospital Duties; [by Rev. Thomas Bassnett Percival, LL.B.] and Notes and Illustrations.* Manchester: Printed by S. Russell, for J. Johnson, St. Paul's Church Yard, and R. Bicherstaff, Strand, London, 1803.

"Principles of Medical Ethics (1957)" reprinted with permission from the American Medical Association.

"Toward an Expanded Medical Ethics: The Hippocratic Ethic Revisited" reprinted by permission from Pellegrino, Edmund D. "Toward an Expanded Medical Ethics: The Hippocratic Ethic Revisited." In *Hippocrates Revisited: A Search for Meaning,* edited by Roger J. Bulger. New York: Medcom Press, 1973, pp. 133–147.

"Principles of Medical Ethics (1980)" reprinted with permission from *Code of Medical Ethics.* American Medical Association, copyright © 1998.

CHAPTER 3

"Oath of Asaph" from "Oath of Asaph" translation by Dr. Suessman Muntner. In Tendler, M. D., (ed.). *Medical Ethics: A Compendium of Jewish Moral, Ethical and Religious Principles in Medical Practice*, fifth edition. New York: Committee of Religious Affairs, Federation of Jewish Philanthropies of New York, Inc., 1975. Used with permission from the Committee of Religious Affairs, United Jewish Appeal, Federation of Jewish Philanthropies of New York, Inc.

"A Comparison of the Oaths of Hippocrates and Asaph" from Glick, Shimon. "A Comparison of the Oaths of Hippocrates and Asaph." *Koroth* 9 (No. 3–4, 1986):297-302. Used with permission from Dr. Samuel Kottek, History of Medicine Department, Israel Institute of the History of Medicine and Science.

"The Obligation to Heal in the Judaic Tradition" based on "Theological Considerations in the Care of Defective Newborns," by J. David Bleich. Reprinted in abridged form from Chester A. Swinyard, editor, *Decision Making and the Defective Newborn*, 1979, pp. 512–561 with permission from Charles C. Thomas, Publisher, Springfield, Illinois.

"Ethical and Religious Directives for Catholic Health Care Services" © 1995 by the United States Catholic Conference, Inc., Washington, D.C. Reprinted with permission. All Rights Reserved.

"The Patient as Person" by Ramsey, Paul. Excerpted with permission from *The Patient as Person*. New Haven, Connecticut: Yale University Press, 1970, pp. xi–xviii. Copyright 1970 Yale University.

"Within Shouting Distance: Paul Ramsey and Richard McCormick on Method" by Lisa S. Cahill. Shortened with permission from *Journal of Medicine and Philosophy* 4:398–417, December 1979, © 1979 by D. Reidel Publishing Co. Reprinted with permission of Kluwer Academic Publishers.

"Code, Covenant, Contract, or Philanthropy" by William F. May. Reprinted with permission from William F. May and the *Hastings Center Report* 5 (December 1975):29–38.

CHAPTER 4

"Just Doctoring: Medical Ethics in the Liberal State" reprinted from Brennan, Troyen A. *Just Doctoring: Medical Ethics in the Liberal State*. Berkeley: University of California Press, 1991, pp. 3–10, 48–53 with the permission of the Regents of the University of California and the University of California Press.

"Autonomy" from *Who Should Decide? Paternalism in Health Care* by James F. Childress. Copyright © 1982 by Oxford University Press, Inc. Used by permission of Oxford University Press, Inc.

"Canterbury v. Spence" extracted from Canterbury v. Spence, United States Court of Appeals, District of Columbia, 1972, 464 F.2d 772, 150 U.S.App.D.C. 263.

"Justice: A Philosophical Review" by Allen Buchanan. Reprinted with permission from D. Reidel Company from "Justice: A Philosophical Review." *Justice and Health Care*. Edited by Earl Shelp. Dordrecht, Holland: D. Reidel Publishing Company, 1981, pp. 3–21.

"Medical Care as a Right: A Refutation" by Sade, Robert M. Reprinted with permission from "Medical Care as a Right: A Refutation." *New England Journal of Medicine* 285 (1971):1288–1292.

"Securing Access to Health Care" excerpted from President's Commission for the Study of Ethical Problems in Medicine and Biomedical and Behavioral Research. *Securing Access to Health Care: A Report on the Ethical Implications of Differences in the Availability of Health Services*. Washington, D.C.: U.S. Government Printing Office, 1983.

"A Patient's Bill of Rights" Reprinted with permission of the American Hospital Association, copyright © 1992.

"Convention for Protection of Human Rights and Dignity of the Human Being with Regard to the Application of Biology and Biomedicine: Convention on Human Rights and Biomedicine" by the Council of Europe, "Convention for the Protection of Human Rights and Dignity of the Human Being with Regard to the Application of Biology and Medicine: Convention on Human Rights and Biomedicine." Strasbourg: Conseil de l'Europe, 1997.

"Consumer Bill of Rights and Responsibilities" Report to the President of the United States, Advisory Commission on Consumer Protection and Quality in the Health Care Industry, November 1997.

CHAPTER 5

"The Oath of Soviet Physicians" from "The Oath of Soviet Physicians." Zenonas Danilevicius, trans. *Journal of the American Medical Association* 217 (1971):834. Used with permission of the American Medical Association.

"Toward a Bioethics in Post-Communist Russia" from Tichtchenko, Pavel D., and Boris G. Yudin. "Toward a Bioethics in Post-Communist Russia." *Cambridge Quarterly of Healthcare Ethics* 4 (1992):295–303. Reprinted with the permission of Cambridge University Press.

"Islamic Code of Medical Professional Ethics" from Rahman, Abdul, C. Amine, and Ahmed Elkadi. "Islamic Code of Medical Professional Ethics." *Papers Presented to the First International Conference on Islamic Medicine Celebrating the Advent of the Fifteenth Century Hijri.* Kuwait Ministry of Health: Kuwait, 1981, with permission from the Kuwait Ministry of Health.

"Medical Ethics in India" by Desai, Prakash. "Medical Ethics in India." *Journal of Medicine and Philosophy* 13 (1988):231-55. Copyright © by The Journal of Medicine and Philosophy, Inc. Reprinted by permission.

"Oath of Initiation (Caraka Samhita)" Reprinted with permission from *Medical History* 14 (1970):195–96.

"The 17 Rules of Enjuin (For Disciples in Our School)" Excerpted from *Western Medical Pioneers in Feudal Japan,* by John Z. Bowers, reprinted with permission from The Johns Hopkins Press, 1970, pp. 8–10.

"Buddhism, Zen and Bioethics" from Nolan, Kathleen. "Buddhism, Zen, and Bioethics." *Bioethics Yearbook. Vol. 3, Theological Developments in Bioethics 1990–1992.* Edited by Andrew B. Lustig, Baruch A. Brody, H. Tristram Engelhardt, Laurence B. McCullough, et al. Dordrecht: Kluwer Academic Publishers, 1993, pp. 185–216. Reprinted with permission.

"Medicine—the Art of Humaneness: On Ethics of Traditional Chinese Medicine" from Qiu, Ren-Zong. "Medicine—The Art of Humaneness: On Ethics of Traditional Chinese Medicine." *Journal of Medicine and Philosophy* 13 (1988):277-300. Copyright © by The Journal of Medicine and Philosophy, Inc. Reprinted by permission.

"Sun Szu-miao and the Origins of the Debate on Medical Ethics in China" from Unschuld, Paul U. *Medical Ethics in Imperial China: A Study in Historical Anthropology,* Berkeley, California: University of California Press, 1979, pp. 24–36. Reprinted by permission of the Regents of the University of California and the University of California Press.

"Medical Ethics and Chinese Culture" from Ren-Zong Qiu, "Medical Ethics and Chinese Culture," in Transcultural Dimensions in Medical Ethics, ed. Edmund Pellegrino, University Publishing, 1992, pp. 155–174.

"Health Ethics in Chinese Law" based on Sass, Hans-Martin. "Regulations on Criteria for Medical Ethics and Its Implementation." *Medizinische Materialien Heft* 43(June 1989):16–18, published by the Zentrum für Medizinisches Ethik, Bochum, Germany, and "Health Ethics in Chinese Law" by the People's Republic of China, National People's Congress. *The Journal of Medicine and Philosophy* 14 (No. 3, 1989):361–62. Copyright © by The Journal of Medicine and Philosophy, Inc. Reprinted by permission.

Chapter 6

"African Ethical Theory and the Four Principles" by Peter Kasenene. "African Ethical Theory and the Four Principles" In *Principles of Health Care Ethics.* Edited by Raanan Gillon. Principles of Health Care Ethics. New York: Wiley, 1994, pp. 183–92. Reproduced by permission of John Wiley & Sons Limited.

"Toward an African-American Perspective on Bioethics" from Dula, Annette. "Toward an African-American Perspective on Bioethics." *Journal of Health Care for the Poor and Underserved.* 2(2, 1991):259–269, copyright © by Sage Publications, Inc. Reprinted by permission of Sage Publications, Inc.

PREFACE

The renaissance in medical ethics of the past twenty years has provided dramatic cases involving dying patients, genetic manipulations, and allocation of scarce resources. It has also stimulated an interest in theories or systems of medical ethics. In *Medical Ethics*[1] I have attempted to provide one such systematic account. In doing so I became vividly aware of the rich and varied history of medical ethical systems and of the more systematic work on principles of normative ethics that underlie more specific and ad hoc stands taken on particular issues.

While Hippocrates, the Oath that bears his name, and the ethical principles of the American Medical Association have often been assumed to be the core of Western medical ethics, it is becoming increasingly clear that there are important alternatives to the Hippocratic system. They arise not only in the major Western religious traditions, each of which has what could be called a medical ethic of its own, but also in secular philosophical systems such as liberal political philosophy. They also arise in non-Western traditions including Marxism, Islam, and the major traditions of the East. Especially, when the first edition of this book was prepared, the foundational documents for these traditions often have existed only in obscure journals and out-of-print foreign sources. In the period since the publishing of the first edition, many more sources have become available, but many of them remain in print only in sources that are not easily accessible. My objective here has been to gather together these documents and combine them with a selection of readings that will introduce the key ethical principles of normative ethics and provide a brief example of how they can be applied to medical ethical issues. They are intended to provide the basic readings that will introduce the student of medical ethics—whether physician, college student, or interested lay person—to the fundamental concepts, principles, and categories underlying the major issues in medical ethics today. For the second edition, I have been able to replace earlier sources with newly appearing articles, some of which add greatly to the understanding of the particular tradition under consideration. Increasingly, the problem has not been finding a text dealing with the various traditions, but selecting which of several available best conveys the richness and uniqueness of the tradition being discussed.

The original manuscript for this volume included two additional entrees that I would very much have liked to present. They are both from the revised edition of the *Encyclopedia of Bioethics*, which is generally a wonderful source of high-quality writing on the various religious and cultural traditions. The article for the *Encyclopedia* by Allen Verhey on "Protestant Perspectives on Medical Ethics" and the one by Jose Mainetti entitled "Medical Ethics in Latin

America" both provide excellent accounts of their respective traditions. Unfortunately, the requested reprint fees would have made the cost of this volume prohibitive. The reader is encouraged to turn directly to the *Encyclopedia of Bioethics*, which is available in many libraries, for these important contributions.

This collection is very different from any reader on the issue of biomedical ethics existing today. It is designed for undergraduate, graduate, and professional school courses in medical and bioethics where the objective is to provide an understanding of alternative systems of medical ethics and to introduce systematically the basic principles of normative ethics. It can be used as a companion reader to *Medical Ethics*, but is designed to be a free-standing anthology. This text could not have been prepared and edited into its present form without the help of people who have provided careful and committed assistance in research and administration, especially David Singh, who provided extensive research assistance, and Julie Eddinger, who spent long hours in administrative assistance including preparation of the manuscript. To them I express my gratitude.

Note

[1] Veatch, Robert M., ed. *Medical Ethics*, Second Edition. Boston: Jones and Bartlett, 1997.

INTRODUCTION

Since about 1970 there has been an explosion of interest in medical ethics. Problems of abortion, genetic engineering, human experimentation, and euthanasia have forced medical professionals and lay people alike to rethink traditional medical solutions as they apply to current ethical problems. Many of the standard discussions of the problems confronting medical ethics have proceeded to explore the alternative positions, topic by topic, and the arguments supporting them. Typical books have included chapters on these issues as well as on allocation of scarce medical resources, informed consent, psychiatric ethics, confidentiality, and the ethics of preventive medicine.

The problem with this approach is that as soon as one probes any one of these topics, one encounters more basic philosophical questions, questions that usually cut across the controversies surrounding any of these topics. For example, deciding whether to tell a dying patient the traumatic news of her impending death raises the question of whether the ethical goal is to avoid her psychological suffering or to honor her right to the truth. But that is precisely the issue underlying many conflicts over informed consent in human experimentation. Similar conflicts between choosing a course that avoids suffering and a course that honors someone's purported basic rights arise in problems of determining whether to abort a genetically afflicted fetus, choosing how to allocate scarce beds in intensive care units, and deciding whether to keep medical records confidential.

Anyone who must face these difficult questions in medical ethics is working, at least implicitly, from within a framework. What is needed is a more systematic framework from which these problems may be approached. Our preexisting ethical frameworks deal with normative questions—such as what principles or norms are relevant and whether morality can be reduced to rules. They also deal with basic issues such as the meaning of ethical terms and how moral claims are justified. When our frameworks are systematic, coherent, and consistent, they might be termed theories. Theories include answers to such questions as the relation of doing good to avoiding harm, the relation of the individual to society, and the relation of claims of rights to the production of good consequences, and so forth.

Western physicians and many lay people have traditionally thought of the Hippocratic Oath as the starting point of thinking about medical ethics. The Oath and the tradition growing out of the Hippocratic ethical writings, in fact, do provide one more or less systematic approach to medical ethics. The core principle, that the physician should do what he or she thinks benefits the patient, is stated twice in the Oath, and at least until recently, has been widely accepted by physicians in the Hippocratic tradition since the time of the Oath's writing.

The Hippocratic tradition, however, is not the only more or less systematic way of thinking about problems in medical ethics. Many religious traditions have medical ethical traditions of their own, and they may differ significantly from the Hippocratic tradition. These religious traditions have developed their medical ethical positions in varying degrees. In fact, the Hippocratic tradition could be thought of as an alternative religious tradition in conflict with the major religious systems of the world. The Hippocratic Oath had its origins in a quasi-religious Greek cult that probably had close connections with Pythagoreanism.

Likewise, various philosophical traditions have implications for medical ethics just as the religious systems do. We would expect to reach different positions on problems in medical ethics depending on whether we stand in the tradition of liberal political philosophy, Marxism, existentialism, or some other philosophical school.

This volume is a collection of the most significant writings on these more systematic approaches to medical ethics. The first chapter offers an exploration of the Hippocratic tradition beginning with the Oath itself and the most important twentieth century scholarly analysis of the Oath's origins and meaning. It also includes three explicit, modern adaptations of the Oath each of which attempts to place the Oath in a modern setting without making any substantive moral changes of major significance. These three come from surprisingly different sources: the World Medical Association, the profession of nursing, and the physicians of Post-Soviet Russia. While each makes modest accommodation to modern thought—removing references to the Greek gods, for instance—the core language is essentially unchanged.

The second chapter introduces several codifications that are still in the Hippocratic tradition, which, however, introduce several significant changes. For example, a medieval effort attempts to rewrite the Oath so it is suitable for the Christian physician—an adjustment that requires several substantive ethical changes in addition to the substitution of a reference to the Christian deity. Thomas Percival's late eighteenth century code, which was to become the foundation of modern Anglo-American medical ethics, reflects enlightenment moral philosophy at least as much as it does the Hippocratic ethic as does the 1957 version of the American Medical Association's Code of Ethics. These are followed by a thoughtful contribution by Edmund Pellegrino, who recognizes the need to modify the Hippocratic tradition to produce an ethic acceptable for the twentieth century. This chapter closes with the 1980 version of the AMA's code, a position that is significantly different from both Percival and the AMA's 1957 document, so different, in fact, that it is essentially no longer Hippocratic. It talks not only about physician duties to society (a perspective lacking in the Hippocratic Oath, but present in Percival and the early AMA codes), but also, for the first time in any document from a professional physician organization, of the *rights* of patients.

Chapter 3 moves to major Western religious alternatives, the ethical systems of Judaism, Catholicism, and Protestantism as they relate to medicine. Even the casual reader will see that one cannot subscribe fully to any of these major religious perspectives without standing in conflict with the Hippocratic ethic.

Chapter 4 turns to secular Western ethical systems: liberal political philosophy and the concepts of autonomy and justice—both of which are absent from the Hippocratic ethic. Their relation to the major Western religions is more complex, but particularly in the case of justice, the links between the secular and the religious ethics are quite close. Protestantism is sometimes seen as the precursor to the contemporary secular stress on autonomy, although that relationship is also controversial. It is here that the modern emphasis on rights is taken up, first in the more traditional emphasis on consent and the right not to be touched, and then in the more recent focus on the right of persons to access to health care and consumer rights.

Brief explorations of non-Western traditions are taken up in Chapter 5: the medical ethics of the Soviet and post-Soviet era in Eastern Europe as well as the traditions of Islam, Hinduism, Buddhism, and the Chinese viewpoints, both ancient and modern.

Finally, the second edition is able to draw on a literature that was not available when the first edition appeared ten years ago: the cultures of Africa and African-American medical ethics. When the first edition was written, I knew that there certainly were ethical perspectives in Africa and in non-Anglo subcultures in the United States even though no one had yet done enough serious analysis to give accounts of them. Fortunately, in the interim several wonderful articles have appeared making clearer the thinking of persons standing in these traditions. As I indicated in the preface, it was my intention to include similar writings on Latin American perspectives, but reprint fees made that impossible. I must simply refer the reader to the *Encyclopedia of Bioethics* and other sources that are becoming available. We now know that it would be a serious mistake to assume that these subcultures can be squeezed into the various secular and religious traditions even if some of their members simultaneously reflect some of the thought of secular liberal political philosophy, Roman Catholicism, or some of the other traditions taken up here.

Once one grasps the breadth of alternatives, it is natural to ask what might justify adoption of one of these positions. In fact, many persons may find themselves standing in more than one of these traditions simultaneously. One may be both a Jew and a physician. Another may be both a Catholic and a proponent of liberal political philosophy. The appropriate question is what it should take to justify one position or another. One soon discovers that the ancient codes such as the Hippocratic Oath differ in important details from more modern professional codifications such as the Principles of Ethics of the American Medical Association. More critically, it is not obvious that one should turn automatically to the codes of the medical profession. Particularly, if one is not a physician, one may be inclined toward some of the other traditions. What should happen, for instance, if the code of a religious group conflicts with that of a professional organization or national government? What is the ultimate standard for determining what is right conduct for health professionals and lay people in medicine? Who has the authority to articulate or establish a standard? Who should be the one to adjudicate moral disputes or discipline those who violate the accepted norms?

This outline of the kinds of problems that need to be addressed in any complete medical ethical position was first developed in my 1981 book entitled *A Theory of Medical Ethics.* They are also taken up in the textbook I edited entitled *Medical Ethics,* the second edition of which appeared in 1997. In *A Theory of Medical Ethics* I argue for a particular set of answers to the questions raised. That is not the task of the present volume, however. Its purpose is to provide a basis for the reader to see the radical differences in points of view and help the reader begin the process of forming his or her own ethic for medicine. In order to understand what the issues are and to begin to develop one's own positions on them, it is important to be exposed to many different points of view. This collection of articles is designed to provide those alternative points of view. It was originally developed as readings for a course on comparative medical ethical theories. It can be used either as a free-standing collection of the most significant writings on problems in systems of medical ethics, or in conjunction with *Medical Ethics* or some other systematic exploration of these ideas.

Robert M. Veatch
Washington, DC
October 1999

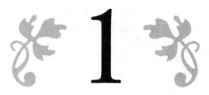

The

Hippocratic

Tradition

Introduction

By far the most significant ethical tradition in the medical ethics of Western physicians is that surrounding the Hippocratic Oath. This Hippocratic tradition began as a minority movement within Greek medicine, grounded in a group or school identified with a figure called Hippocrates. The Hippocratic group articulated important and novel positions placing medicine on a more empirical footing. A large collection of writings associated with this school have been brought together. They are collectively often referred to as the Hippocratic corpus. As with other ancient collections the content was not universally agreed upon. Many writings were clearly not by the historical figure, Hippocrates. They were written over several centuries.

Some of the writings in the collection have a particularly ethical content. The Hippocratic Oath is the most famous. It shows the clear marks of a cult or school. It contains an oath of secrecy as well as a code with a set of moral imperatives. The most famous of these imperatives could be called the Hippocratic principle, the notion that the physician ought to act so as to benefit the patient and keep the patient from harm according to the physician's ability and judgment.

The Oath contains some more esoteric provisions including a prohibition on "cutting for the stone," presumably kidney stone surgery. It contains a pledge of confidentiality committing the Hippocratic physician to refrain from disclosing "those things that ought not be spread abroad." While this implies that some things perhaps ought to be "spread abroad," it at least shows ancient roots for the notion of confidentiality in medical ethics. Extremely complex questions arise regarding the authorship, dating, meaning, and philosophical context of the Oath. In the opening essay, historian Ludwig Edelstein provides a plausible account of the origins of the Oath.

The Oath has gone through many revisions and updatings. Medieval Christians were aware of it. In fact some scholars have suggested that the Hippocratic perspective in Greek medical ethics emerged as dominant because of its compatibility with Judeo-Christian thought. On the other hand, there is very little evidence that early Christians accepted the Oath. There are extremely few references to Hippocrates in early Christian literature, and they tend to separate Christian medical ethics from Hippocratic. A medieval attempt to write a Christian version of the Oath contains many significant changes.

Regardless of its origin and compatibility with Judeo-Christianity, the Oath has been viewed by Western physicians as the source document of the essence of ethics for physicians. In 1948 the World Medical Association adopted the Declaration of Geneva, which is clearly a recasting of the Hippocratic Oath in modern language. The core Hippocratic principle is rendered, "The health of my patient will be my first consideration." The text of this declaration is the second selection in this chapter.

Various other professional organizations and other groups have attempted to write codes of ethics, pledges, or oaths that they think epitomize the essence of the ethics for the practice of their profession. Some of these are self-consciously patterned after the Hippocratic Oath just as the Declaration of Geneva was. This chapter includes two such paraphrases of the Oath as examples. In the next chapter we shall see that other organizations have placed themselves in the Hippocratic tradition, but have seen fit to make more substantive changes in the ethic of the Oath.

The Hippocratic Oath: Text, Translation, and Interpretation

Ludwig Edelstein

──────────INTRODUCTION TO READING──────────

The scholar who has contributed most to the modern understanding of the Hippocratic tradition is the medical historian Ludwig Edelstein. His essay, "The Hippocratic Oath," which was first published in 1943, helped generations of physicians, historians, and medical ethicists understand that the Hippocratic Oath is not a document that can be understood apart from its historical context. Edelstein applies the skills of the classicist to show that the Hippocratic Oath is quite different from many other Hippocratic writings. Also, it is written somewhat later than some of the other, more scientific treatises attributed to the historical figure Hippocrates; quite possibly, it dates from the fourth century BC. Edelstein argues that the Oath is best understood as a code reflecting the views of a minority group of physicians, probably of Pythagorean persuasion. Although other scholars have called into question some of the details of Edelstein's interpretation, the main points are widely accepted today. A much shortened version of Edelstein's essay is reprinted here without the extensive references that include detailed comparisons of ancient and modern texts.

Oath

I swear by Apollo Physician and Asclepius and Hygieia and Panaceia and all the gods and goddesses, making them my witnesses, that I will fulfill according to my ability and judgment this oath and this covenant:

To hold him who has taught me this art as equal to my parents and to live my life in partnership with him, and if he is in need of money to give him a share of mine, and to regard his offspring as equal to my brothers in male lineage and to teach them this art—if they desire to learn it—without fee and covenant; to give a share of precepts and oral instruction and all the other learning to my sons and to the sons of him who has instructed me and to pupils who have signed the covenant and have taken an oath according to the medical law, but to no one else.

I will apply dietetic measures for the benefit of the sick according to my ability and judgment; I will keep them from harm and injustice.

I will neither give a deadly drug to anybody if asked for it, nor will I make a suggestion to this effect. Similarly I will not give to a woman an abortive remedy. In purity and holiness I will guard my life and my art.

I will not use the knife, not even on sufferers from stone, but will withdraw in favor of such men as are engaged in this work.

Whatever houses I may visit, I will come for the benefit of the sick, remaining free of all intentional injustice, of all mischief and in particular of sexual relations with both female and male persons, be they free or slaves.

What I may see or hear in the course of the treatment or even outside of the treatment in regard to the life of men, which on no account one must spread abroad, I will keep to myself holding such things shameful to be spoken about.

If I fulfill this oath and do not violate it, may it be granted to me to enjoy life and art, being honored with fame among all men for all time to come; if I transgress it and swear falsely, may the opposite of all this be my lot.

Interpretation

The Hippocratic Oath clearly falls into two parts. The first specifies the duties of the pupil toward his teacher and his teacher's family and the pupil's obligations in transmitting medical knowledge. The second gives a number of rules to be observed in the treatment of diseases, a short summary of medical ethics as it were. Most scholars consider these two sections to be only superficially connected or at least determined by different moral standards. Be this as it may, the two parts certainly diverge in their subject matter, and, for the purpose of analyzing their content, it is advantageous first to discuss them separately and then to ask how they are related to each other. Again for the sake of convenience, I shall deal with the so-called ethical code first, the main question being whether the historical setting in which these rules of conduct were conceived can be ferreted out.

Unfortunately, most of the statements contained in the document are worded in rather general terms; they are vague in their commending of justice, of purity and holiness, concepts which in themselves do not imply any distinct meaning but may be understood in various ways. Yet there are two stipulations that have a more definite character and seem to point to the basic beliefs underlying the whole program which is here evolved: the rules concerning the application of poison and of abortive remedies. Their interpretation should therefore provide a clue for a historical identification of the views embodied in the Oath of Hippocrates.

I.   The Ethical Code

A.   Rules Concerning Poison and Abortion.   "I will neither give a deadly drug to anybody if asked for it, nor will I make a suggestion to this effect. Similarly I will not give to a woman an abortive remedy. In purity and holiness I will guard my life and my art."-such is the vow made. It concerns the physician not so much in his capacity as the healer of diseases but rather in that of the pharmacist who is in possession of the drugs which he prescribes. Poison is a drug and so is the pessary. The physician agrees not to deliver either one to his patient. The term used on both instances is the same; just as he will not *give* the pessary to a woman who comes to seek his help, he will not *give* to anyone who is under his care.

Why regulations concerning cases of abortion are introduced into the document is immediately understandable. Under ancient conditions the physician was often presented with the problem as to whether he should give an abortive remedy. But what about the physician's supplying poison? Did he so frequently have occasion to give poison that it seemed worthwhile to ordain what he should do in such instances? What exactly is the situation referred to in the Oath?

All modern interpreters assume that the interdiction of the supplying of poisons means that the physician is charged not to assist his patient in a suicide which he might contemplate. Some interpreters claim that here the physician is also, or even primarily, asked to refrain from any criminal attempt on his patient's life. Cases of poisoning, they say, were very frequent in antiquity; the law, though of course it threatened punishment for murder, was of little avail because the lack of proper scientific methods made it impossible to ascertain whether poison had been administered or not. As a means of strengthening civil jurisdiction, therefore, a clause was introduced into the ancient medical code which today would be entirely out of place. There is no evidence, however, that the Oath refers to anybody except patient and physician. The words in question, then, can mean only that the doctor promises not to supply his patient with poison if asked by him to do so nor to suggest that he take it. It is the prevention of suicide, not of murder that is here implied.

But was suicide an instance to be reckoned with in medical practice? Could the doctor ever advise such an act to his patient? In antiquity this was indeed the case. If the sick felt that their pains had become intolerable, if no help could be expected, they often put an end to their own lives. This fact is repeatedly attested and not only in general terms; even the diseases are specified which in the opinion of the ancients gave justification for a voluntary death. Moreover, the taking of poison was the most usual means of committing suicide, and the patient was likely to demand the poison from his physician who was in possession of deadly drugs and knew those which brought about an easy and painless end. On the other hand, such a resolution naturally was not taken without due deliberation, except perhaps in a few cases of great distress or mental strain. The sick wished to be sure that further treatment would be of no avail, and to render this verdict was the physician's task. The patient, therefore, consulted with him, or urged his friends to speak to the doctor. If the latter, in such a consultation, confirmed the seriousness or hopelessness of the case, he suggested directly or indirectly that the patient commit suicide.

Of course, I do not mean to claim that everybody whose illness had become desperate thought of ending his own life. Even if human aid was no longer effectual, recourse to the gods was still possible, and men did seek succor in the sanctuaries; even if the pain was excruciating and relief was to be had neither from human nor from divine physicians, men could, and did go on living in spite of all their suffering. Yet the fact remains that throughout antiquity many people preferred voluntary death to endless agony. This form of "euthanasia" was an everyday reality. Consequently it is quite understandable that the Oath deals with the attitude which the physician should take in regard to the possible suicide of his patient. From a practical point of view it was no less important to tell the ancient doctor what to do when faced with such a situation than it was to advise him about cases of abortion.

The relevance of the "pharmacological rules" for a medical oath having been established, one may now ask why the Oath forbids the physician to assist in suicide or in abortion. Apparently these prohibitions did not echo the general feeling of the public. Suicide was not censured in antiquity. Abortion was practiced in Greek times no less than in the Roman era, and it was resorted to without scruple. Small wonder! In a world in which it was held justifiable to expose children immediately after birth, it would hardly seem objectionable to destroy the embryo. Why then should the physician not give a helping hand to those of his patients who wanted to end their own lives or to those who did not wish to have offspring?

For a moment one might harbor the idea that the interdiction of poison and of abortive remedies was simply the outgrowth of medical ethics. After all, medicine is the art of healing, of preserving life. Should the physician assist in bringing about death? I do not propose to discuss this issue in general terms. It suffices here to state that in antiquity many physicians actually gave their patients the poison for which they were asked. Apparently *qua* physicians they felt no compunction about doing so. Although in later centuries some refused to participate in an attempt on men's lives, because, as they said, it was unfitting for their sect "to be responsible for anyone's death or destruction," it is not reported that they ever employed the same reasoning in cases of self-murder. As for abortions, many physicians prescribed and gave abortive remedies. Medical writings of all periods mention the means for the destruction of the embryo and the occasions where they are to be employed. In later centuries some physicians rejected abortion under all circumstances; they supported their decision with a reference to the prohibition in the Hippocratic Oath and added that it was the duty of the doctor to preserve the products of nature. Soranus, the greatest of the ancient gynecologists, had little patience with these colleagues of his. In agreement with many other physicians he contended that it was necessary to think of the life of the mother first, and he resorted to abortion whenever it seemed necessary, much as he deprecated it if performed for no other reason than the wish to preserve beauty or to hide the consequences of adultery. In short, the strict attitude upheld by the Oath was not uncontested even from the medical point of view. In antiquity it was not generally considered a violation of medical ethics to do what the Oath forbade. An ancient doctor who accepted the rules laid down by "Hippocrates" was by no means in agreement with the opinion of all his fellow physicians; on the contrary, he adhered to a dogma which was much stricter than that embraced by many, if not by most of his colleagues. Simple reflection on the duties of the physician, on the task of medicine alone, under these circumstances, can hardly have led to the formulation and adoption of the "pharmacological stipulations."

In my opinion, the Oath itself points to other, more fundamental considerations that must have been instrumental in outlining the prohibitions under discussion. For the physician, when forswearing the use of poison and of abortive remedies, adds: "In purity and in holiness I will guard my life and my art." It might be possible to construe purity as a quality insisted upon by the craftsman who is conscious of the obligations of his art. The demand for holiness, however, can hardly be understood as resulting from practical thinking or technical responsibility. Holiness belongs to another realm of values and is indicative of standards of a different, a more elevated character.

Yet certainly not such purity and holiness are meant as might accrue to men from obedience to civil law or common religion. Ancient jurisdiction did not discriminate against suicide; it did not attach any disgrace to it, provided that there was sufficient reason for such an act. And self-murder as a relief from illness was regarded as justifiable, so much so that in some states it was an institution duty legalized by the authorities. Nor did Greek or Roman law protect the unborn child. If, in certain cities, abortion was prosecuted, it was because the father's right to his offspring had been violated by the mother's action. Ancient religion did not proscribe suicide. It did not know of any eternal punishment for those who voluntarily ended their lives. Likewise it remained indifferent to foeticide. Its tenets did not include the dogma of an immortal soul for which men must render account to their creator. Law and religion then left the physician free to do whatever seemed best to him.

From all these considerations it follows that a specific philosophical conviction must have dictated the rules laid down in the Oath. Is it possible to determine this particular philosophy? To take the problem of suicide first: Platonists, Cynics and Stoics can be eliminated at once. They held suicide permissible for the diseased. Some of these philosophers even extolled such an act as the greatest triumph of men over fate. Aristotle, on the other hand, claimed that it was cowardly to give in to bodily pain, and Epicurus admonished men not to be subdued by illness. But does that mean that the Oath is determined by Aristotelian or Epicurean ideas? I shall not insist that it is hard to imagine a physician resisting the adjurations of his patients if he has nothing but Aristotle's or Epicurus' exhortations to courage to quote to them and to himself. It is more important to stress the fact that the Aristotelian and Epicurean opposition to suicide did not involve moral censure. If men decided to take their lives, they were within their rights as sovereign masters of themselves. The Aristotelian and Epicurean schools condoned suicide. Later on the Aristotelians even gave up their leader's teaching, and under the onslaught of the Stoic attack withdrew their disapproval of self-murder. At any rate, Aristotelianism and Epicureanism do not explain a rejection of suicide which apparently is based on a moral creed and a belief in the divine.

Pythagoreanism, then, remains the only philosophical dogma that can possibly account for the attitude advocated in the Hippocratic Oath. For indeed among all Greek thinkers the Pythagoreans alone outlawed suicide and did so without qualification. The Platonic Socrates can adduce no other witness than the Pythagorean Philolaus for the view that men, whatever their fate, are not allowed to take their own lives. And even in later centuries the Pythagorean school is the only one represented as absolutely opposed to suicide. Moreover, for the Pythagorean, suicide was a sin against God who had allocated to man his position in life as a post to be held and to be defended. Punishment threatened those who did not obey the divine command to live; it was considered neither lawful nor holy to seek release, "to bestow this blessing upon oneself." Any physician who accepts such a dogma naturally must abstain from assisting in suicide or even from suggesting it. Otherwise he would be guilty of a crime, he no less than his patient, and in this moral and religious conviction the doctor can well find the courage to remain deaf to his patient's insistence, to his sufferings, and even to the clamor of the world which disagrees almost unanimously with the stand taken by him. It seems safe to state this much: the fact that in the Hippocratic Oath the physician is enjoined to refrain from aiding or advising suicide points to an influence of Pythagorean doctrines.

In my opinion the same can be asserted of the rule forbidding abortion and rejecting it without qualification. Most of the Greek philosophers even commended abortion.

It was different with the Pythagoreans. They held that the embryo was an animate being from the moment of conception. That they did so is expressly attested by a writer of the third century AD. The same can be concluded from the Pythagorean system of physiology as it was outlined in the Hellenistic period by Alexander Polyhistor: the germ is a clot of brain containing hot vapors within it, and soul and sensation are supposed to originate from this vapor. Similar views were previously accepted by Philolaus in the fourth century BC. Consequently, for the Pythagoreans, abortion, whenever practiced, meant destruction of a living being. Granted that the righteousness of abortion depends on whether the embryo is animate or not, the Pythagoreans could not but reject abortion unconditionally.

Furthermore, abortion was irreconcilable with their ethical beliefs no less than with their scientific views. In their ascetic rigorism, in their strictness concerning sexual matters and regarding matrimony in particular, they went further than any other sect. They banned extra-marital relations. Even in matrimony coitus was held justifiable only for the purpose of producing offspring. Besides, children to them were more than future members of a community or citizens of a state. It was considered man's duty to beget children so as to leave behind in his own place another worshiper of the gods. With such convictions how could the Pythagoreans ever allow abortive remedies to be applied? How could they fail to condemn practices of this kind, so common among their compatriots?

It stands to reason, then, that the Hippocratic Oath, in its abortion-clause no less than in its prohibition of suicide, echoes Pythagorean doctrines. In no other stratum of Greek opinion were such views held or proposed in the same spirit of uncompromising austerity. When the physician, after having forsworn ever to give poison or abortive remedies, adds: "in purity and holiness I will guard my life and my art," it must be the purity and holiness of the "Pythagorean way of life" to which he dedicates himself.

B. *The General Rules of the Ethical Code.* The question now arises whether what is true of certain of the ethical clauses of the Hippocratic Oath is true of all of them, in other words, whether the whole medical code is in agreement with Pythagorean philosophy. By this latter term I mean Pythagoreanism as it was understood in the fourth century BC. It is to this form of the dogma that the rules discussed so far were related, and it seems fair to assume that the rest of the stipulations, if at all influenced by Pythagorean thinking, correspond to the same concept of Pythagoreanism. At any rate, wherever I shall speak of Pythagorean doctrines without qualification, it is neither the teachings of the "historical" Pythagoras, nor those of the later so-called Neo-Pythagoreans which I have in mind, but rather those theories and beliefs which writers of the fourth century BC, men like Plato, Aristotle and their pupils attributed to Pythagoras and his followers.

1. *The Tripartite Division of Medicine.* To start, then, with the analysis of that section of the ethical code which deals with the treatment of diseases proper: here mention is made of diet, drugs and cutting. In a more technical language, medicine is viewed as comprising dietetics, pharmacology and surgery. Consequently those matters are discussed which seem most important for the attitude of the physician within these three departments of his art. Now a division of medicine into the branches is not unusual and in itself is not indicative of any particular medical or philosophical school. But, according to Aristoxenus, the Pythagoreans were among those who accepted this particular classification of medicine; moreover, the sequence of the various parts of the healing art in the Pythagorean doctrine is the same as it is in the Hippocratic Oath, dietetics coming first, pharmacology next, surgery last.

a. DIETETIC MEANS. In detail, the physician is asked to use dietetic means to the advantage of his patients as his judgment and capacity permit; moreover he is enjoined to keep them from mischief and injustice. That the doctor's dietetic prescriptions should be given to help the patient is an obvious truth. It is the goal of all good craftsmanship to seek the best for the object with which the craftsman is concerned. Every ancient physician would have subscribed to such a formulation. It suffices to say that the Pythagorean physicians did not feel differently, for this school acknowledged the useful and the advantageous as second among the aims of human endeavor.

But what exactly is meant by the promise to keep the patient from mischief and injustice? Can this really imply, as some scholars have suggested, that the physician shall enforce his treatment even against the resistance or indifference of his patient's family? It is true, interference of others may occur and the physician may have to contend with it, but this happens rarely, too seldom indeed to have been considered in the medical code. Moreover, while mischief may be done to the sick by his friends, why should this danger be any greater in regard to the dietetic treatment of diseases for which case alone mention is made of it, than it would be in regard to everything else the physician may prescribe or do? No, it can scarcely be protection from the wrong done by others that the physician vows to give to his patients. But since it can neither be protection from the wrong which he himself may do, one must conclude that he promises to guard his patients against the evil which they may suffer through themselves. That men by nature are liable to inflict upon themselves injustice and mischief, and that this tendency becomes apparent in all matters concerned with their regimen, this is indeed an axiom of Pythagorean dietetics.

The Pythagoreans defined all bodily appetites as propensities of the soul, as a craving for the presence or absence of certain things. Most of these appetites they considered as acquired or created by men themselves, and therefore they thought human desires were to be watched closely and to be scrutinized severely. As a natural process they acknowledged only that the body should take in an appropriate amount of food and should be cleansed again appropriately after it had been filled. To overload oneself with superfluous food and drink was regarded as an acquired inclination of the soul.

But unfortunately all bodily passions have the tendency to increase indefinitely. Of themselves they become "idle, irreverent, harmful and licentious," as one can readily see in those who are in the position to live according to their wishes. In order to live right from early youth on, one must learn to hold in contempt those things that are "idle and superfluous." It is necessary, therefore, to select the nourishment of the body with great caution, to determine its quality and quantity most carefully, a supreme wisdom entrusted to the physicians.

This is the Pythagorean doctrine concerning the regimen of the healthy. It is clear, I think, that in such a theory bodily and psychic factors are blended in a peculiar way. At the same time there is a moral element involved: unhealthy desire is uncontrolled desire; a decision is to be made between those appetites which ought to be satisfied and those which ought to be disregarded. Moreover, the Pythagorean teaching, in a strange manner, insists on negative instances. Not that alone which one does is important; that which one does not do, or is not allowed to do, carries just as much consequence. Right living is brought about not only, not even primarily, through positive actions, but rather through avoidance of those steps that are dangerous, through the repression of insatiable desires which if left to themselves would cause damage.

The same consideration for body and soul, the same combination of precepts and prohibitions seems to be characteristic of the Pythagorean treatment of diseases. Most illnesses, in the opinion of these philosophers, are due to opulent living; too much food is consumed which cannot be digested properly, and thus extravagance destroys the body, just as it destroys wealth. If health, the retention of the form, changes into disease, the destruction of the form, the body needs purification through medicine, just as the sick soul needs purification through music. The physician in such a case must give assistance by changing the patient's regimen. He must use dietetical means, as the Hippocratic Oath says. In choosing them he will be intent on his patient's benefit according to the best of his judgment and ability. Whatever he prescribes, as a true follower of Pythagoras he will remember one fundamental truth: everything that is given to the body creates a certain disposition of the soul. Men in general, though they are aware of the fact that some things, such as wine, may suddenly bring about a striking change in a person's behavior, do not apprehend that every kind of food or drink causes a certain mental habit, slight as the variations may be. But the physician knows that his art primarily consists in this knowledge. Consequently, he must see to it that the soul of the sick, through a wrong diet, does not fall into "idle, irreverent, harmful and licentious passions." Since he acts according to this principle when assisting the healthy, he must certainly do likewise when treating the sick. Or in the words of the Hippocratic Oath: the physician must protect his patient from the mischief and injustice which he may inflict upon himself if his diet is not properly chosen. He must be a physician of the soul no less than of the body; he must not overlook the moral implications of his actions, nor even the negative indices to be watched; for the regimen followed by a person concerns both his bodily and his psychic constitution.

The rules concerning dietetics, then, agree with Pythagoreanism, in fact they acquire meaning only if seen in the light of Pythagorean teaching. That the pharmacological precepts, the stipulations concerning poison and abortion, are Pythagorean in origin has already been demonstrated. It remains to be shown that the laws laid down for surgery, too, are most easily understandable on the theory that they are founded in Pythagorean doctrine.

b. SURGERY. The physician vows: "I will not use the knife either on sufferers from stone, but I will give place to such as are craftsmen therein"; this at least is the most common rendering of the words in question. Supposing that it be correct, what should be the reason for the prohibition here pronounced? The treatment of stone-diseases by operation, in Greek medicine, seems to have been an old-established procedure; at any rate, since the rise of Alexandrian medicine, such an operation was performed throughout the centuries. Why then is it forbidden in the Oath?

The words must mean what in the opinion of all early interpreters they seemed to mean: lithotomy is here excluded because the performance of operations is held to be incompatible with the physician's craft, and by the one example given the Oath intends to exclude surgery in general from the field of the physician. It is possible that originally more operations were named as forbidden, that these references are missing only in the preserved text. But such a hypothesis cannot be verified. It is more probable, however, that the statement as it stands is intact but in itself carries broader implications. For instead of translating "I will not use the knife either on sufferers from stone," it is equally well possible to translate "I will not use the knife, not even on sufferers from stone." This would signify that the physician directly renounces operative surgery altogether. He will not resort to it even in the case of that disease which more than any other, according to the testimony of the ancients, drove men to suicide. The prohibition could not be formulated in more emphatic and solemn words.

Whatever rendering is chosen, the statement under discussion enjoins a separation of medicine and surgery. Driven back to this interpretation which no doubt is drastically at variance with reality, one feels almost inclined to say with Littre that such an explanation must be rejected, and that consequently the motive for the interdiction of lithotomy in the Oath remains obscure. It is likewise true, however, that one medical sect valued surgery less highly than dietetics and pharmacology, I mean the Pythagorean physicians. As Aristoxenus says, they believed "most of all" in dietetics; they applied poultices more liberally than did their predecessors, but "thought less" of the efficacy of drugs; "they believed least of all using the knife and in cauterizing." In other words, according to Aristoxenus, the Pythagoreans attributed different values to the various branches of medicine, and in their classification operative surgery together with cauterization was ranked lowest. If one remembers that in Aristoxenus' opinion the Pythagoreans explained most diseases as the result of unreasonable living, one is at first inclined to conclude that they were the more appropriate means of treatment. Still this can hardly be the whole truth. For Plato in the *Timaeus*, when outlining the Pythagorean treatment of diseases, does not mention cutting or cauterizing at all, though he agrees with Aristoxenus in placing the importance of pharmacology after that of dietetics. Evidently, then there must have been Pythagoreans who refused to apply any surgical means of treatment which were otherwise so universally used in Greek medicine. This inference from the Platonic *Timaeus* seems quite certain though no express statement to this effect is preserved.

It is most likely that Aristoxenus' report is one of his typical attempts to reconcile the rigorous Pythagorean attitude with the demands of common sense and the exigencies of daily life: such compromises he introduces in many instances where other sources attest the uncompromising attitude of the Pythagoreans. Seen from this angle, the stipulation of the Oath appears as another compromise, more lenient and at the same time more rigid than that reported by Aristoxenus: the use of cauterization obviously is allowed, operative surgery is completely eliminated. On the other hand, the Pythagorean physician will allow others to help his patient in his extremity. The stipulation against operating is valid only for him who has dedicated himself to a holy life. The Pythagoreans recognized that men in general could not observe any elaborate rules of purity; in this fact they say no argument against that which they considered right for themselves. To give place to another craftsman, especially in such instances where the patient might fall prey to a sinful temptation, certainly was a duty demanded by philanthropy, by commiseration with those who suffered.

But why should the Pythagorean have avoided the use of the knife? The answer can only be conjecture: he who believed that bloody sacrifices should not be offered to the gods and saw in them a defilement of divine purity could well believe that he himself would be defiled in his purity and holiness by using the knife in bloody operations. However that may be, it is only in connection with Pythagorean medicine that the injunction of the Hippocratic Oath, according to which operative surgery was forbidden to the physician, acquires any meaning and plausibility at all. The rules given in regard to surgery no less than those concerning dietetics and pharmacology are Pythagorean in character.

2. *Two General Provisions.* Those stipulations of the Oath which deal with the medical treatment proper are finally followed by two or more general provisions bearing on medical ethics in the strict sense of the word. The behavior of the physician toward his patient and the patient's family is regulated; reticence is imposed upon him in regard to whatever he may see or hear. Is it really true that in non-medical literature no parallels can be found to these postulates? In my opinion, these ethical rules, too, in their specific wording are understandable only in connection with Pythagorean doctrine.

a. REFRAINING FROM INJUSTICE AND MISCHIEF. As for the first vow, he who swears the Oath promises to come, into whatever house he enters, to help the sick, refraining from injustice and mischief, especially from all sexual incontinence. That the physician should act for the sole purpose of assisting his patient, is a demand that seems self-evident. It certainly is as compatible with any ethical standard to which a doctor may subscribe, as it is with Pythagorean ethics. It may seem equally natural that the physician is bidden to refrain from all injustice and mischief. Yet, the appropriateness of the statement does not imply that it is not in need of further explanation, be it in regard to its meaning or its motivation. Those who believe that only medical parallels can be adduced for the stipulation of the Oath point to seemingly similar utterances in one of the so-called Hippocratic writings, the book "On the Physician." Here it is stated that in his relations with the sick the doctor ought to be just, for the patients have no small dealings with their physician. They put themselves into his hands, and the physician comes in contact with women and maidens and with very precious possessions indeed; so toward all these self-control should be used. I do not wish to raise the issue, whether justice is here commended for utilitarian rather than moral reasons. Nor do I emphasize the fact that only if it had a moral bent could this assertion be likened to the Oath. In refutation of the argument of modern interpreters it is enough to say that the parallel referred to is by far less comprehensive and less rigorous than the statement which it is supposed to explain. The Oath, unlike the Hippocratic treatise "On the Physician," does not speak only of the avoidance of injustice, it also excludes mischief. Moreover, the oath enjoins continence in regard to women and men alike; it stresses that the same continence must be observed toward free-born people and slaves, features that are entirely missing in the other passage. A more satisfactory interpretation of the words in question, therefore, must be sought.

Now a plea for justice and continence may of course be derived from many ancient philosophical systems. As for justice, the Platonists and the Aristotelians praised its dignity no less than did the Pythagoreans. But so much it is safe to claim: that the physician is required to abstain from all intentional injustice and mischief—such a formulation savors of the famous Pythagorean sayings by which injustice and mischief are proscribed, even if committed against animals and plants. And, indeed, to blend the concept of justice with that of forbearance is characteristic of the Pythagoreans. They abhorred violence; only if provoked by injustice would they resort to force. In recoiling from aggression the asceticism of Pythagorean ethics culminated. Moreover, the consequences drawn in the Oath from the ethical standards there imposed are in strict keeping with those principles which the Pythagoreans enforced upon their followers. Their views on sexual matters were severer than those of all other ancient philosophers. They alone judged sexual relations in terms of justice, meaning thereby not that which is forbidden or allowed by law: for the husband to be unfaithful to his wife was considered to be unjust toward her. The Pythagoreans upheld the equality of men and women. They alone condemned sodomy. Besides, in the performance of moral duties, they did not discriminate between social ranks. In that respect free-born people and slaves, for the Pythagoreans, were on equal footing. Everything, then, that the Oath stipulates in regard to sexual continence agrees with tenets of Pythagorean ethics, in fact with the ideals of these philosophers alone.

Finally, as a Pythagorean postulate the clause takes on a peculiar significance for the physician. It is justice first of all that is required from him. This virtue, to the average people, meant to live in accordance with the laws of the state. To Plato, wherever he does not speak of justice in his own peculiar usage as the perfect working of the human soul in all its functions, justice was mainly a civic virtue. Aristotle tried to establish justice as a political virtue, and as one that applies to contracts and dealings in the law-courts. All these aspects are also inherent in the Pythagorean concept of justice, and they certainly are of some concern for the physician. While in his direct dealing with men, in his personal contact with them and their households, it may be of less importance whether generally speaking he is a law-abiding citizen, it makes a great difference indeed, whether he is an honest man or not. It is in this sense that even the author of the Hippocratic book "On the Physician" counsels the doctor not to infringe upon the possessions of others with whom he is doing business. But such justice, essential as it may be for good morals, is not all that the Pythagorean ideal of justice implies. To the adherents of this dogma, justice was the social virtue par excellence. As Aristoxenus reports, they believed that "in any relation with others" some kind of justice is involved. "In all intercourse" it is possible to take "a well-timed and ill-timed attitude." In order to do what is proper, one must differentiate according to circumstances. Speech and actions necessarily vary depending on the particular situation and the persons concerned. From the right decision result timeliness, appropriateness, and fitness of behavior, and it is justice that reveals itself in good manners. Interpreted in the light of Pythagorean teaching, then, the recommendation of justice epitomizes all duties of the physician toward his patient in the contacts of daily life, all he should do or say in the course of his practice; it gives the rules of medical deportment in a nutshell.

b. THE PROMISE OF SILENCE. Last but not least: The promise of silence. The physician accepts the obligation to keep to himself all that he sees or hears during the treatment; he also swears not to divulge whatever comes to his knowledge outside of his medical activity in the life of men. The latter phrase in particular has always seemed strange. It is so far-reaching in scope that it can hardly be explained by professional considerations alone. To be sure, other medical writings also advise the physician to be reticent. The motive in doing so is the concern for the physician's renommée which might suffer if he is a prattler. But the Oath demands silence in regard to that "which on no account one must spread abroad." It insists on secrecy not as precaution but as a duty. In the same way silence about things which are not to be communicated to others was considered a moral obligation by the Pythagoreans. They did not tell everything to everybody. They did not indiscriminately impart their knowledge to others. They expected the scientist to be reticent and ready to listen. Certainly if the doctor who promises not to talk about anything that he may see or hear is to be placed in any philosophical school, it must be the Pythagorean.

To sum up the results of the analysis of the ethical code: the provisions concerning the application of poison and of abortive remedies, in their inflexibility, intimated that the second part of the Oath is influenced by Pythagorean ideas. The interpretation of the other medical and ethical stipulations showed that they, too, are tinged by Pythagorean theories. All statements can be understood only, or at any rate they can be understood best, as adaptations of Pythagorean teaching to the specific task of the physician. Even from a formal point of view, these rules are reminiscent of Pythagoreanism: just as in the Oath the doctor is told what to do and what not to do. Far from being the expression of the common Greek attitude toward medicine or of the natural duties of the physician, the ethical code rather reflects opinions which were peculiarly those of a small and isolated group.

II. The Covenant

The ethical code by the acceptance of which the physician gives a higher sanction to his practical endeavor is preceded by a solemn agreement concerning medical education. The pupil promises to regard his teacher as equal to his parents, to share his life with him, to support him with money if he should be in need of it. Next he vows to hold his teacher's children as equals to his brothers and to teach them the art without fee and covenant if they should wish to learn it. Finally he takes upon himself the obligation to impart precepts, oral instruction and all the other learning to his own sons, to those of his teacher and to pupils who have signed the covenant and have taken an oath according to the medical law, to all these, but to no one else.

Whatever the precise purport of the single terms and phrases used in this covenant, so much is immediately clear in regard to its general meaning and is commonly admitted: the teacher here is made the adopted father of the pupil, the teacher's family becomes the pupil's adopted family. In other words, the covenant establishes between teacher and pupil the closest and most sacred relationship that can be imagined between men, and it does so for no other apparent reason than that the pupil is being instructed in the art.

In explaining this stipulation modern interpreters usually allege that in Greece, in early centuries, medicine like all the other arts was passed on from father to son in closed family guilds. When at a certain time these organizations began to receive outsiders in to their midst, they are said to have demanded from them full participation in the responsibilities of the "real" children. Consequently those who wished to be admitted to all the privileges and rights of the family had to become its members through adoption. The Hippocratic covenant, then, it is claimed, is an engagement which was signed by newcomers joining one of the medical families, and it was probably the family of the Asclepiads in which this formula held good.

The evidence for such a theory, in my opinion, is insufficient. Galen is the only ancient author who asserts that the Asclepiads, after having been for generations the sole possessors of medicine, later shared their knowledge with people not belonging to their clan. And even he says that these outsiders were men whom the family esteemed "on account of their virtue"; he does not contend that they were made members of the family or forced to accept any obligations. It is hardly by chance, therefore, that Galen himself does not refer to the Hippocratic Oath as bearing out the truth of his story. In any case, his words cannot be adduced as corroborative proof for the assumptions of modern scholars. Nor does it increase the strength of the modern argument if Galen's testimony is combined with that of Plato, according to whom "physicians taught their sons medicine and . . . Hippocrates taught outside pupils for a fee." Though Plato says this, it still does not follow that the outsiders became the adopted children of their masters. On the contrary, who will believe that the young Athenian aristocrat Hippocrates of whom Plato speaks would have considered paying a fee to the great Hippocrates for instruction, had that meant that he should enter the family of the Coan physician!

There is one particular historical setting, however, one particular province of Greek pedagogics where a counterpart of the Hippocratic covenant can be found: the Pythagoreans of the fourth century apparently were wont to honor those by whom they had been instructed as their fathers by adoption. So Epaminondas is said to have done; and in Epaminondas' time it was told of Pythagoras himself that he had revered his teacher as a son reveres his father. If the Hippocratic covenant is viewed against the background of such testimony, the specific form in which the pupil is here bound to his teacher is no longer an unexplainable and isolated phenomenon. Compared with Pythagorean concepts of teaching and learning as they were evolved in the fourth century BC, the vow of the medical student assumes definite historical meaning.

This result seems to imply that the covenant as a whole must be influenced by Pythagorean philosophy. The agreement between the Hippocratic treatise and the Pythagorean reports concerns so unusual a circumstance that they are most unlikely to be independent of each other. Nor is it probable that the Pythagoreans derived their pattern of instruction from a medical manifesto that in the range of medical education and indeed of general education is without parallel. Nevertheless one should hesitate to claim Pythagorean origin for the covenant by reason of one feature only, even if it be the main feature of this document. But as matters stand, all the other demands enjoined upon the pupil may likewise by explained only in connection with Pythagorean views and customs, or at least they are compatible with them.

To take those duties first which the pupil acknowledged in regard to his mentor: he is asked to share his life with his teacher and to support him with money if need be. That the Pythagorean pupil shared his money with his teacher if necessary, one may readily believe. To support his father was the son's duty, even according to common law. This obligation was the more binding for the Pythagorean, who was taught to honor his parents above all others. But the Pythagorean also came to his teacher's assistance in all the vicissitudes of life, wherever and whenever he was needed: he tended him in illness; he procured burial for him. All this is admiringly reported of Pythagoras himself. The Pythagorean pupil was indeed supposed to share his life with his master, as the son does with his father. He did much more than advance money to him in case of an emergency.

Next, the Hippocratic covenant admonishes the pupil to regard his teacher's offspring as his brothers, and without fee and covenant to teach them his art if they wish to learn it. That the teacher's children should be the pupil's brothers naturally follows from the fact that the disciple acknowledges his master as his father. Thus the teacher's sons and his pupils become one flesh and blood. But the preference shown for the interest of the members of the family, the unselfishness commended in the relationship to them, the confidence put in their reliability without any insistence on formal guarantees—all these features are characteristic of Pythagorean ethics. The Pythagoreans were admonished to turn to their brothers first, and to make friends with them before all others outside the family. Moreover, all Pythagoreans considered themselves brothers and were believed, like brothers, to have divided their earthly goods among themselves. Their unquestioned belief in their brothers' trustworthiness did not falter even in the face of death. Under these circumstances, how could the Pythagorean do other than teach his adopted brothers without fee the knowledge which he had acquired? What assurances could he expect or ask of them before he instructed them in the art that he had learned from their father?

Finally, the fact that in the Hippocratic covenant teaching is divided into precepts, oral instruction and the other learning, is best understood as a Pythagorean classification. The precepts of Pythagoras, handed down from one generation to the other, were greatly renowned throughout the centuries. "Oral instruction" and "learning" were the two categories under which Aristoxenus listed all that was "taught and said" in Pythagorean circles, and all that the members of the school tried "to learn and remember." That knowledge, according to the covenant, is to be imparted to a closed circle of selected people alone, most assuredly is in agreement with those principles on which the transmission of Pythagorean doctrine was based. The Pythagoreans differed from all other philosophical sects in that they did not divulge their teaching to everybody. They carefully examined those who wished to join them. It is attested even that they exacted an oath from the pupil who was to be admitted, just as the Hippocratic treatise speaks of outsiders who sign the covenant and take an oath before they are allowed to participate in the course of studies.

To sum up: not only the main feature of the covenant, the father-son relationship between teacher and pupil but also all the detailed stipulations concerning the duties of the pupil can be paralleled by doctrines peculiar to the followers of Pythagoras. If related to Pythagoreanism, the specific formulas used in the covenant acquire meaning and definiteness. What otherwise appears exaggerated, or strange, or even fictitious, thus becomes the adequate expression of a real situation. Since the rules proposed show no affinity with any other Greek educational theory or practice, it seems permissible to claim that the Hippocratic covenant is inspired by Pythagorean doctrine.

III. The Unity of the Document

Covenant and ethical code, the two parts of which the so-called Hippocratic Oath consists, in the preserved text form a unity. Without any marked transition the first section is followed by the second. Is there any reason for believing that the two have not always belonged together?

It seems certain that the obligations laid down in the covenant and in the ethical code are assumed by the physician simultaneously, that is, at the moment of his entering the medical profession as a practitioner in his own right. The promise to help the teacher and the stipulation concerning the teaching to be given to others point to the fact that he who takes the Oath has become an independent craftsman. In the same way the rules regarding the practitioner's behavior are best understandable if imposed upon the doctor who is now starting out on his career. For as long as the pupil is still under the supervision of his teacher, his actions of necessity are regulated by his master's orders. In short, covenant and ethical code are signed together, not by the beginner but rather by the student who has completed his course.

Moreover the two parts are a spiritual unity. For it is not true, contrary to what is sometimes claimed, that the covenant exhibits a realistic business attitude, whereas the ethical code is determined by a lofty and exalted standard of conduct. The agreement concerning teaching and the rules of professional behavior both reflect the same idealistic outlook on human affairs, they are steeped in Pythagorean doctrine. The same can be said of the preamble and the peroration by which the document is introduced and concluded as one coherent formula.

At this point, I think, I can say without hesitation that the so-called Oath of Hippocrates is a document uniformly conceived and thoroughly saturated with Pythagorean philosophy. In spirit and in letter, in form and content, it is a Pythagorean manifesto. The main features of the Oath are understandable only in connection with Pythagoreanism; all its details are in complete agreement with this system of thought. If only one or another characteristic had been uncovered, one might consider the coincidence fortuitous. Since the concord is complete, and since there is no counterinstance of any other influence, all indications point to the conclusion that the Oath is a Pythagorean document.

IV. Date and Purpose of the Oath

The origin of the Hippocratic Oath having been established, it should now be possible to determine the time when the Oath was written and the purpose for which it was intended. What answers regarding these questions are to be deduced from the analysis of the document?

As for the date, it seems one must conclude that the Oath was not composed before the fourth century BC. All the doctrines followed in the treatise are characteristic of Pythagoreanism as it was envisaged in the fourth century BC. It is most probable even that the Oath was outlined only in the second half or toward the end of the fourth century for the greater part of the parallels adduced are taken from the works of pupils of Aristotle.

Two of the main provisions of the Oath are connected with theories that are attributed either directly or indirectly to Philolaus, a contemporary of Plato. This makes the turn of the fifth to the fourth century the *terminus post quem* for the composition of the Oath. Moreover, even if one or another ethical precept ascribed to the Pythagoreans by Aristoxenus and accepted in the Hippocratic Oath was held also by older Pythagoreans, the whole program of instruction envisaged in the Oath in conformity with the Pythagorean model is characteristic of fourth century Pythagoreanism; for it presupposes the destruction of the Pythagorean society in the last decades of the fifth century. As Aristoxenus related, it was after the uprising in Italy that Lysis went to Thebes where he taught Epaminondas and was revered by him as his adopted father. In a letter ascribed to him, Lysis protests against those who after the dissolution of the society made the Pythagorean dogma available to everybody. Pythagoras himself, Lysis asserts, had charged his daughter never to give his writings to those "outside of the house." Whether this letter is genuine or not, it must have been for some such reasons that Lysis bound Epaminondas to himself as his adopted son. This afforded the only solution which made it possible to initiate outsiders into the Pythagorean doctrine, and yet to keep it a secret, a "family secret," as is also the intention of the Oath. But such a relationship between teacher and pupil could be instituted only after the disappearance of the great fraternity that had existed before. Only at that moment did the transmission of the Pythagorean doctrine become the concern of the individual Pythagorean; in earlier times it had been promoted by the society itself. The Hippocratic Oath, which calls the teacher the adopted father of the pupil, can hardly have been composed, therefore, before the fourth century BC.

Nor is it likely that the document is of later origin. In the fourth century BC Pythagoreanism reached the peak of its importance. Its influence gradually began to wane from the beginning of the Hellenistic period. When in the first century BC the Pythagorean system was revived and again became a potent factor in philosophical speculation, it took on traits very different from those which are characteristic of the earlier dogma and the prescripts of the Oath. Moreover, in Alexandria medical ethics was integrated into the teaching of the medical sects. Closely connected as these newly established schools were with philosophy, Pythagoreanism played no part in their teaching. A direct influence of Pythagorean philosophy on medicine, however, is not probable.

Yet in the fourth century BC the Hippocratic Oath in every respect was a timely manifesto. It stands to reason, then, that it was in the fourth century BC that Pythagorean philosophy led to the formulation of the Hippocratic Oath. Does this imply that the document must have been outlined by a philosopher rather than by a physician? Not at all. The Hippocratic Oath is a program of medical ethics, and there is no reason to question that it was composed by a doctor. But ancient physicians often belonged to philosophical schools or studied with philosophers. The Pythagorean teaching aroused considerable interest among the physicians of the fourth century. It is quite possible that a physician, strongly impressed by what he had learned from the Pythagoreans either through personal contact or through books, conceived this medical code in conformity with Pythagorean ideals.

V. Conclusion

The so-called Hippocratic Oath has always been regarded as a message of timeless validity. From the interpretation given it follows that the document originated in a group representing a small segment of Greek opinion. That the Oath at first was not accepted by all ancient physicians is certain. Medical writings, from the time of Hippocrates down to that of Galen, give evidence of the violation of almost every one of its injunctions. This is true not only in regard to the general rules concerning helpfulness, continence and secrecy. Such deviations one would naturally expect. But for centuries ancient physicians, in opposition to the demands made in the Oath, put poison in the hands of those among their patients who intended to commit suicide; they administered abortive remedies; they practiced surgery.

At the end of antiquity a decided change took place. Medical practice began to conform to that state of affairs which the Oath had envisaged. Surgery was separated from general practice. Resistance against suicide, against abortion, became common. Now the Oath began to be popular. It circulated in various forms adapted to the varying circumstances and purposes of the centuries. Generally considered the work of the great Hippocrates, its study became part of the medical curriculum. The commentators supposed that the master had written the Oath as the first of all his books and made it incumbent on the beginner to read this treatise first.

Small wonder! A new religion arose that changed the very foundations of ancient civilization. Yet, Pythagoreanism seemed to bridge the gulf between heathendom and the new belief. Christianity found itself in agreement with the principles of Pythagorean ethics, its concepts of holiness and purity, justice and forbearance. The Pythagorean god who forbade suicide to men, his creatures, was also the God of the Jews and the Christians. As early as in the "Teaching of the Twelve Apostles" the command was given: "Thou shalt not use philtres; thou shalt not procure abortion; nor commit infanticide." Even the Church Fathers abounded in praise of the high-mindedness of Hippocrates and his regulations for the practice of medicine.

As time went on, the Hippocratic Oath became the nucleus of all medical ethics. In all countries, in all epochs in which monotheism, in its purely religious or in its more secularized form, was the accepted creed, the Hippocratic Oath was applauded as the embodiment of truth. Not only Jews and Christians, but the Arabs, the mediaeval doctors, men of the Renaissance, scientists of the Enlightenment, and scholars of the nineteenth century embraced the ideals of the Oath. I am not qualified to outline the successive stages of this historical process. But I venture to suggest that he who undertakes to study this development will find it better understandable if he realizes that the Hippocratic Oath is a Pythagorean manifesto and not the expression of an absolute standard of medical conduct.

Declaration of Geneva

The World Medical Association

─────────────INTRODUCTION TO READING─────────────

The Hippocratic Oath is only the first of a long line of codes and oaths adopted by Western physicians. The Declaration of Geneva, which is written to be a modern version of the Hippocratic Oath by the World Medical Association, shows a quite conscious connection to the Oath. The Declaration of Geneva is explicit in its commitment that the first duty of the physician is the health of the patient. Certain changes are reflected in the modernization in addition to the removal of the obvious references to the Greek deities. The commitment to keeping the knowledge of medicine secret has been dropped; confidentiality seems more bluntly protected without exception; the prohibition on giving abortive pessaries was (after considerable dispute) softened to a commitment to respect life from the moment of conception; and the prohibition on surgery for stones has been dropped. Still, the Declaration is very much in the Hippocratic tradition.

At the time of being admitted as a Member of the Medical Profession:

I SOLEMNLY PLEDGE myself to consecrate my life to the service of humanity.

I WILL GIVE to my teachers the respect and gratitude which is their due;

I WILL PRACTICE my profession with conscience and dignity;

THE HEALTH OF MY PATIENT will be my first consideration;

I WILL RESPECT the secrets which are confided in me;

I WILL MAINTAIN by all the means in my power, the honor and the noble traditions of the medical profession;

MY COLLEAGUES will be my brothers;

I WILL NOT PERMIT considerations of religion, nationality, race, party politics or social standing to intervene between my duty and my patient;

I WILL MAINTAIN the utmost respect for human life, from the time of conception; even under threat, I will not use my medical knowledge, contrary to the laws of humanity;

I MAKE THESE PROMISES solemnly, freely and upon my honor.

The Florence Nightingale Pledge

————————————INTRODUCTION TO READING————————————

The Florence Nightingale Pledge was written over 100 years ago, but not by Florence Nightingale herself. Rather, it was written in her honor to represent, "the highest type of nurse and ideal." The oath was prepared in 1893 by a committee led by one Lystra Eggert Gretter, the superintendent of nursing at the Farrand Training School in Detroit. Clearly, it was modeled after the Hippocratic Oath. Indeed, with the exception of the first and last sentences, the Florence Nightingale oath closely parallels the Hippocratic Oath. It treats the issues of confidentiality and avoiding harm to patients identically, often using the same phrases. At one time, the oath was recited by graduating nurses. Today it is considered to be something of an anachronism primarily because of its antiquated presentation of the physician-nurse relationship. Despite this, however, the oath has endured the historical currents of nursing.

I solemnly pledge myself before God and presence of this assembly, to pass my life in purity and to practise my profession faithfully. I will abstain from whatever is deleterious and mischievous and will not take or knowingly administer any harmful drug. I will do all in my power to elevate the standard of my profession, and will hold in confidence all personal matters committed to my keeping, and family affairs coming to my knowledge in the practice of my calling. With loyalty will I endeavor to aid the physician in his work and devote myself to the welfare of those committed to my care.

Solemn Oath of a Physician of Russia

────────────INTRODUCTION TO READING────────────

During the period of the Soviet Union, an Oath existed for Soviet physicians that had a decidedly non-Hippocratic character. Soon after the collapse of the Union, however, the Russian physicians desired to replace that Soviet oath with one more committed to the welfare of individual patients and less oriented to the interests of the state. A group headed by Yu.P. Lisizyn, a member of the Russian Academy of Medicine, produced a new oath. It was originally published in Meditsinskaya Gazeta (No. 44, S June 1992). The Oath has been approved by the Minister of Health and the Minister of Higher Education of the Russian Federation and has been taken by the graduating classes of Moscow Medical University since that time. A comparison with the Hippocratic Oath makes clear that the authors used that ancient physician's oath as their model. The references to the Greek gods and goddesses is gone, but the pledge of loyalty is retained almost verbatim. So is the promise not to convey medical precepts to nonphysicians. The central Hippocratic pledge to work for the benefit of the sick according to the physician's ability and judgment is likewise repeated word for word from the Hippocratic text. The text retains the prohibition on giving a deadly drug, the slightly ambiguous promise of confidentiality, and the concluding appeal to reward or punishment depending on whether the oath is kept.

In the presence of my Teachers and colleagues in the great science of doctoring, accepting with deep gratitude the rights of a physician granted to me

I SOLEMNLY PROMISE:

- to regard him who has taught me the art of doctoring as equal to my parents and to help him in his affairs and if he is in need;

- to impart any precepts, oral instruction, and all other learning to my pupils who are bound by the obligation of medical law but to no one else;

- I will conduct my life and my art purely and chastely, being charitable and not causing people harm;

- I will never deny medical assistance to anyone and will render it with equal diligence and patience to a patient of any means, nationality, religion, and conviction;

- no matter what house I may enter, I will go there for the benefit of the patient, remaining free of all intentional injustice and mischief, especially sexual relations;

- to prescribe dietetic measures and medical treatment for the patient's benefit according to my abilities and judgment, refraining from causing them any harm or injustice;

- I will never use my knowledge and skill to the detriment of anyone's health, even my enemy's;

- I will never give anyone a fatal drug if asked nor show ways to carry out such intentions;

- whatever I may see and hear during treatment or outside of treatment concerning a person's life, which should not be divulged, I will keep to myself, regarding such matters as secret;

- I promise to continue my study of the art of doctoring and do everything in my power to promote its advancement, reporting all my discoveries to the scientific world;

- I promise not to engage in the manufacture or sale of secret remedies;

- I promise to be just to my fellow doctors and not to insult their persons; however, if it is required for the benefit of a patient, I will speak the truth openly and impartially;

- in important cases I promise to seek the advice of doctors who are more versed and experienced than I; when I myself am summoned for consultation, I will acknowledge their merit and efforts according to my conscience.

If I fulfill this Oath without violating it, let me be given happiness in my life and art. If I transgress it and give a false Oath, let the opposite be my lot.

—Translated by Podovalenko Larisa Yurievna and Chris Speckhard

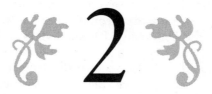

Modifying

the

Hippocratic Tradition

Introduction

It is widely assumed that since the time of Hippocrates all physicians have considered the Hippocratic Oath to be the definitive summary of their ethical responsibilities. That, however, is not the case. In ancient Greece the Hippocratic tradition represented only one school of medicine, and it was a minority tradition even then. As we shall see in the following chapter, Judaism and Christianity each had its own tradition of medical ethics. There is no evidence that ancient Christian physicians took the Oath seriously, at least in the first eight or nine centuries of the common era.

A Christian form of the Oath appeared in the Middle Ages. The oldest existing manuscript dates from the tenth or eleventh century, but the origin of a Christian form of the oath is probably much earlier.[1] It is sometimes interpreted as evidence that, at least by this time, Christian physicians accepted the Oath. This was, after all, about the time that ancient Greek and Roman culture was being rediscovered. Even if in an earlier time ancient Christians were consciously thinking of themselves as set apart from the Greco-Roman culture, by this period the two cultures were being amalgamated. Others, however, point to the rather substantial changes in the Christian version of the Oath, changes readily apparent in the first selection of this chapter.

By the eighteenth century, the medical education was taking its modern form. Particularly, at the University of Edinburgh, a modern medical ethics was emerging. It was aware of the Hippocratic ethical tradition, but makes no direct use of the Oath. The respect shown the Hippocratic writings by the physicians of the day implies that they were not consciously rejecting Hippocrates. On the other hand, there is little evidence that physicians of the day were schooled in the Hippocratic Oath. The language of the medical ethics of the day is, for the most part, not inconsistent with the Hippocratic ideal, but it is much more closely reflective of the utilitarian philosophers of the Scottish enlightenment, of David Hume, Adam Smith, and Thomas Reid. While the Hippocratic tradition focused on benefits for the individual patient, the medical ethics beginning in this period, while still focusing on benefits and harms, opens up more to concern about the welfare of the community and others who are not directly in a patient/physician relation. The excerpt from Thomas Percival's *Medical Ethics* reflects this more social perspective. At the same time, the ethics that we are dubbing "neo-Hippocratic" do not move beyond consideration of benefits and harms. They do not assume a more deontological perspective as the traditions in succeeding chapters do. They also continue to reflect the work of physicians self-consciously writing for professional organizations or groups. This is still the ethic of physician collectives, not that of the broader society.

When the AMA was founded in 1847, one of its first tasks was the adoption of a code of ethics. It was borrowed, in part, from Percival's *Medical Ethics*. Other portions were adapted from the American physician/statesman, Benjamin Rush, one of the signers of the Declaration of Independence. He studied medicine at the University of Edinburgh. Although the writers for the AMA make no direct mention of Hippocrates, they are still very much within the Hippocratic tradition, focusing, as Percival did, on the moral relations of the physician with the community as well as the individual. In 1957 a major revision of its principles of medical ethics was adopted. It changed the form of the ethical code from a long, detailed series of injunctions to a brief set of principles, but it continues to make explicit the physician's obligation and commitment to the community. Still, service to the patient and promotion of patient-well-being were central to this version of the AMA's principles. The paternalism of the Hippocratic tradition still prevails. Little, if any, moral weight is given to matters other than the physician's judgment of what will benefit the patient.

By this period, the Hippocratic ethic was beginning to be called into question in a number of ways. It focused almost exclusively on the welfare of individual patients. The physician in the oath was seen as dealing with individual, isolated patients. In reality, medicine was becoming a much more complex, social, institutional entity with hospitals, and eventually group practices, health-care teams, complex insurance mechanisms, and critical resource-allocation problems. The isolated individual doctor-patient relationship was becoming a thing of the past. Furthermore, patients and lay people generally were more educated. Patients were beginning to insist on a more active role in decision making and shaping of the moral norms for the physician-patient relationship. The very idea that ethics was simply a matter of producing benefits and avoiding harms was challenged by those in ethical traditions deemed more "deontological," that is, more oriented to duties and rights that are not determined solely by the consequences of actions. Edmund Pellegrino is one of the first to sense the trends that call into question the ancient ethic of the Hippocratic tradition. Without quite completely breaking with the Hippocratic tradition, he calls for a very substantial updating of it.

By 1980, tension had grown even greater. Broader cultural influences made the 1957 principles sound dated, especially the use of masculine pronouns. More fundamental changes in ethical theory were brewing. For the first time in the history of organized Western medicine, there was discussion of "rights," rather than simply "benefits and harms." Compassion and respect for human dignity were identified as the virtues of the physician rather than the more traditional virtues of purity and holiness, as expressed in the Hippocratic Oath, or more paternalistic early AMA codes.

Note

1. Jones, W. H. S. *The Doctor's Oath: An Essay in the History of Medicine.* Cambridge: At The University Press, 1924, pp. 4, 55.

The Oath According to Hippocrates
In So Far as a Christian May Swear It

———————————INTRODUCTION TO READING———————————

The role of the Hippocratic Oath in early Christian culture is very difficult to determine. While some older analyses have assumed that the Oath was used by Christians from soon after Christianity's founding,[1] there is very little evidence of its use among Christians, at least for the first eight centuries. Only two mentions of it appear in existing writings of the ancient Christian fathers, and both clearly distinguish the duties of Christian physicians from those of the Oath. By the tenth or eleventh century, a Christian form of the Oath existed, which may have had much earlier precursors. While some would take its existence as evidence of support for the Hippocratic tradition in medieval Christianity, others would point to the number of significant changes that had to be made as evidence that ethics for Christian physicians was substantially different from that of the pagan Hippocratic tradition.[2] In addition to the obvious dropping of the references to the Greek gods and goddesses, the Christian form omits the pledge of secrecy, the commitment to special treatment of teachers and their sons, a stronger, more inclusive prohibition on abortion, and the omission of the pagan prohibition on surgery. Whether these changes signal a break with the pagan version or an attempt by physicians who are not theologically sophisticated to harmonize Christian and Hippocratic traditions is, perhaps, a matter of opinion. Sure, however, the differences are dramatic.

Notes

1. Jones, W. H. S. *The Doctor's Oath: An Essay in the History of Medicine.* Cambridge: At The University Press, 1924, pp. 4, 55.

2. Veatch, Robert M., and Carol G. Mason. "Hippocratic vs. Judeo-Christian Medical Ethics: Principles in Conflict." *The Journal of Religious Ethics* 15 (Spring 1987):86–105.

Blessed be God the Father of our Lord Jesus Christ, who is blessed for ever and ever; I lie not.

I will bring no stain upon the learning of the medical art. Neither will I give poison to anybody though asked to do so, nor will I suggest such a plan. Similarly I will not give treatment to women to cause abortion, treatment neither from above nor from below. But I will teach this art, to those who require to learn it, without grudging and without an indenture. I will use treatment to help the sick according to my ability and judgment. And in purity and in holiness I will guard my art. Into whatsoever houses I enter, I will do so to help the sick, keeping myself free from all wrongdoing, intentional or unintentional, tending to death or to injury, and from fornication with bond or free, man or woman. Whatsoever in the course of practice I see or hear (or outside my practice in social intercourse) that ought not to be published abroad, I will not divulge, but consider such things to be holy secrets. Now if I keep this oath and break it not, may God be my helper in my life and art, and may I be honoured among all men for all time. If I keep faith, well; but if I forswear myself may the opposite befall me.

Medical Ethics; Or a Code of Institutes and Precepts, Adapted to the *Professional Conduct* of Physicians and Surgeons

Thomas Percival

──────────────INTRODUCTION TO READING──────────────

Modern Anglo-American professional medical ethics has its roots in the Scottish enlightenment of the late eighteenth century. Faculty and students of the medical school at the University of Edinburgh in close conversation with philosophers, theologians, and other humanists of the day generated a literature on the moral duties of the physician. This litera- ture, which directly shapes American medical ethics of the nineteenth century, stands in the tradition of Hippocrates in that it is generated by medical professionals and reiterates the Hippocratic claim that the physi- cian should work for the benefit of the patient.

The authors, however, make almost no explicit acknowledgment of the Hippocratic Oath. They do not consciously reject it, but don't explicitly quote it or use its language the way the Declaration of Geneva, the Florence Nightingale Pledge, or the Russian Oath do. Rather they reflect the consequentialist ethics of the day, expressing morality in terms of benefit and harm. To the extent they go beyond the concepts of the Oath, they move in the direction of the social utilitarians, bringing into consider- ation the more social concerns of providing care for the working classes and recognizing responsibility to the society as well as the individual patient.

In the excerpt that follows taken from Manchester physician Thomas Percival's *Medical Ethics,* the Hippocratic virtues of purity and holiness are replaced by those of the British gentleman, including the "virtue" of *condescension* understood as a willingness to "get down" to the level of the less educated patient. Percival also makes clear that he is concerned about societal interests and the allocation of resources to the poor as well as more traditional Hippocratic commitment to the individual patient. He makes clear, however, that he retains the paternalism of the Hippocratic tradition regarding withholding of information from the patient to protect the patient from the distress of bad medical news.

Percival, a physician in Manchester, England, in the last half of the eighteenth century, was asked to draw up a "scheme of professional conduct relative to hospitals and other medical charities," in part, to respond to tensions generated at the Manchester Infirmary. The original work was published in 1794. A revised edition, from which the following selection is taken, appeared in 1803. The concern about these tensions among physicians (who were said to practice "physic" or what we today might call "internal medicine"), surgeons (who were considered practitioners of a separate craft just emerging into professional status), and apothecaries and the proper division of labor (and fees) among them is apparent in the text.

The first chapter focuses on the hospital, where poorer patients would more likely be seen. Similar principles for private patients are articulated in the second chapter. He is committed to fair treatment of the poor and lower fees than for the rich, but not to letting the patient choose his or her own physician, which would be too much of a burden. The patient's case should not be discussed with colleagues in front of the patient, and physicians should not speak critically of the work of colleagues in the patient's presence unless all other means of addressing the concern have been pursued. He is committed to confidentiality, and females should be treated with "delicacy." New remedies should be tried, but only after consultation with colleagues. No consent from patients is envisioned, either for routine therapy or experiments. Percival is clearly moving beyond the focus on the interests of the individual patient, suggesting systematic data gathering for what might now be called public health and research purposes. In the final section presented here, he also clearly moves beyond the paternalism of the Hippocratic tradition that easily justifies dishonesty to patients in order to maintain their hope. Here Percival goes through intricate mental gymnastics to affirm the importance of truthfulness to patients while recognizing that in some exceptional cases humane deception of the patient may be necessary.

Chapter 1 of Professional Conduct, Relative to Hospitals, or Other Medical Charities

I. Hospital physicians and surgeons should minister to the sick, with due impressions of the importance of their office; reflecting that the ease, the health, and the lives of those committed to their charge depend on their skill, attention, and fidelity. They should study, also, in their deportment, so to unite *tenderness* with *steadiness*, and *condescension* with *authority*, as to inspire the minds of their patients with gratitude, respect, and confidence.

II. The *choice* of a *physician* or *surgeon* cannot be allowed to hospital patients, consistently with the regular and established succession of medical attendance. Yet personal confidence is not less important to the comfort and relief of the sick-poor, than of the rich under similar circumstances: And it would be equally just and humane, to enquire into and to indulge their partialities, by occasionally calling into consultation the favourite practitioner. The rectitude and wisdom of this conduct will be still more apparent, when it is recollected that patients in hospitals not unfrequently request their discharge, on a deceitful plea of having received relief; and afterwards procure another recommendation, that they may be admitted under the physician or surgeon of their choice. Such practices involve in them a degree of falsehood [sic]; produce unnecessary trouble; and may be the occasion of irreparable loss of time in the treatment of diseases.

III. The *feelings* and *emotions* of the patients, under critical circumstances, require to be known and to be attended to, no less than the symptoms of their diseases. Thus, extreme *timidity*, with respect to venœsection, contraindicates its use, in certain cases and constitutions. Even the *prejudices* of the sick are not to be contemned, or opposed with harshness. For though silenced by authority, they will operate secretly and forcibly on the mind, creating fear, anxiety, and watchfulness.

IV. As misapprehension may magnify real evils, or create imaginary ones, no *discussion* concerning the nature of the case should be entered into before the patients, either with the house surgeon, the pupils of the hospitals, or any medical visitor.

V. In the large wards of an infirmary the patients should be interrogated concerning their complaints, in a *tone* of *voice* which cannot be *overheard*. *Secrecy*, also, when required by peculiar circumstances, should be strictly observed. And females should always be treated with the most scrupulous *delicacy*. To neglect or to sport with their feelings is cruelty; and every wound thus inflicted tends to produce a callousness of mind, a contempt of decorum, and an insensibility to modesty and virtue. Let these considerations be forcibly and repeatedly urged on the hospital pupils.

VI. The *moral* and *religious influence* of sickness is so favourable to the best interests of men and of society, that it is justly regarded as an important object in the establishment of every hospital. The *institutions* for promoting it should, therefore, be encouraged by the physicians and surgeons, whenever seasonable opportunities occur. And by pointing out these to the officiating clergyman, the sacred offices will be performed with propriety, discrimination, and greater certainty of success. The character of a physician is usually remote either from superstition or enthusiasm: And the aid, which he is now exhorted to give, will tend to their exclusion from the sick wards of the hospital, where their effects have often been known to be not only baneful, but even fatal.

VII. It is one of the circumstances which softens the lot of the poor, that they are exempt from the solicitudes attendant on the disposal of property. Yet there are exceptions to this observation: And it may be necessary that an hospital patient, on the bed of sickness and death, should be reminded, by some friendly monitor, of the importance of a *last will* and *testament* to his wife, children, or relatives, who, otherwise, might be deprived of his effects, of his expected prize money, or of some future residuary legacy. This kind office will be best performed by the house-surgeon, whose frequent attendance on the sick diminishes their reserve, and entitles him to their familiar confidence. And he will doubtless regard the performance of it as a duty. For whatever is right to be done, and cannot by another be so well done, has the full force of moral and personal obligation.

VIII. he physicians and surgeons should not suffer themselves to be restrained, by par simonious considerations, from prescribing *wine*, and *drugs* even of *high price*, when required in diseases of extraordinary malignity and danger. The efficacy of every medicine is proportionate to its purity and goodness; and on the degree of these properties, *cæteris paribus*, both the cure of the sick, and the speediness of its accomplishment must depend. But when drugs of inferior quality are employed, it is requisite to administer them in larger doses, and to continue the use of them a longer period of time; circumstances which, probably, more than counterbalance any savings in their original price. If the case, however, were far otherwise, no œconomy, of a fatal tendency, ought to be admitted into institutions, founded on principles of the purest beneficence, and which, in this age and country, when well conducted, can never want contributions adequate to their liberal support.

IX. The medical gentlemen of every charitable institution are, in some degree, responsible for, and the guardians of, the honour of each other. No physician or surgeon, therefore, should *reveal* occurrences in the hospital, which may injure the reputation of any one of his colleagues; except under the restriction contained in the succeeding article.

X. No *professional charge* should be made by a physician or surgeon, either publicly or privately, against any associate, without previously laying the complaint before the gentlemen of the faculty belonging to the institution, that they may judge concerning the reasonableness of its grounds, and the measures to be adopted.

XI. A proper *discrimination* being established in all hospitals between the *medical* and *chirurgical cases*, it should be faithfully adhered to, by the physicians and surgeons, on the admission of patients.

XII. Whenever cases occur, attended with circumstances not heretofore observed, or in which the ordinary modes of practice have been attempted without success, it is for the public good, and in an especial degree advantageous to the poor (who, being the most numerous class of society, are the greatest beneficiaries of the healing art) that *new remedies* and *new methods* of *chirurgical treatment* should be devised. But in the accomplishment of this salutary purpose, the gentlemen of the faculty should be scrupulously and conscientiously governed by sound reason, just analogy, or well authenticated facts. And no such trials should be instituted, without a previous consultation of the physicians or surgeons, according to the nature of the case.

XIII. To advance professional improvement, a friendly and unreserved *intercourse* should subsist between the gentlemen of the faculty, with a free communication of whatever is extraordinary or interesting in the course of their hospital practice. And an *account* of every *case* or *operation*, which is rare, curious, or instructive, should be drawn up by the physician or surgeon, to whose charge it devolves, and entered in a register kept for the purpose, but open only to the physicians and surgeons of the charity.

XIV. *Hospital registers* usually contain only a simple report of the number of patients admitted and discharged. By adopting a more comprehensive plan, they might be rendered subservient to medical science, and beneficial to mankind.

...

XVII. The establishment of a *committee* of the *gentlemen* of the *faculty*, to be held monthly, would tend to facilitate this interesting investigation, and to accomplish the most important objects of it. By the free communication of remarks, various improvements would be suggested; by the regular discussion of them, they would be reduced to a definite and consistent form; and by the authority of united suffrages, they would have full influence over the governors of the charity. The exertions of individuals, however benevolent or judicious, often give rise to jealousy; are opposed by those who have not been consulted; and prove inefficient by wanting the collective energy of numbers.

XVIII. The harmonious intercourse, which has been recommended to the gentlemen of the faculty, will naturally produce *frequent consultations*, viz. of the physicians on medical cases, of the surgeons on chirurgical cases, and of both united in cases of a compound nature, which falling under the department of each, may admit of elucidation by the reciprocal aid of the two professions.

XIX. In consultations on medical cases, the junior physician present should *deliver* his *opinion* first, and the others in the progressive order of their seniority. The same order should be observed in chirurgical cases; and a majority should be decisive in both: But if the numbers be equal, the decision should rest with the physician or surgeon, under whose care the patient is placed. No decision, however, should restrain the acting practitioner from making such variations in the mode of treatment, as future contingencies [sic] may require, or a farther insight into the nature of the disorder may show to be expedient.

...

Chapter 11 of Professional Conduct in Private, or General Practice

I. The *moral rules of conduct*, prescribed towards hospital patients, should be fully adopted in private or general practice. Every case, committed to the charge of a physician or surgeon, should be treated with attention, steadiness, and humanity: Reasonable indulgence should be granted to the mental imbecility and caprices of the sick: Secrecy, and delicacy when required by peculiar circumstances, should be strictly observed. And the familiar and confidential intercourse, to which the faculty are admitted in their professional visits, should be used with discretion, and with the most scrupulous regard to fidelity and honour.

II. The strictest *temperance* should be deemed incumbent on the faculty; as the practice both of physic and surgery at all times requires the exercise of a clear and vigorous understanding: And on emergencies, for which no professional man should be unprepared, a steady hand, an acute eye, and an unclouded head, may be essential to the well being, and even to the life, of a fellow-creature.

...

III. A physician should not be forward to make gloomy prognostications; because they savour of empiricism, by magnifying the importance of his services in the treatment or cure of the disease. But he should not fail, on proper occasions, to give to the friends of the patient, timely notice of danger, when it really occurs, and even to the patient himself, if absolutely necessary. This office, however, is so peculiarly alarming, when executed by him, that it ought to be declined, whenever it can be assigned to any other person of sufficient judgment and delicacy. For the physician should be the minister of hope and comfort to the sick; that by such cordials to the drooping spirit, he may smooth the bed of death; revive expiring life; and counteract the depressing influence of those maladies, which rob the philosopher of fortitude, and the Christian of consolation.

IV. *Officious interference*, in a case under the charge of another, should be carefully avoided. No meddling inquiries should be made concerning the patient; no unnecessary hints given, relative to the nature or treatment of his disorder; nor any selfish conduct pursued, that may directly or indirectly tend to diminish the trust reposed in the physician or surgeon employed. Yet though the character of a professional busy-body, whether from thoughtlessness or craft, is highly reprehensible, there are occasions which not only justify but require a spirited interposition. When artful ignorance grossly imposes on credulity; when neglect puts to hazard an important life; or rashness threatens it with still more imminent danger; a medical neighbour, friend, or relative, apprized of such facts will justly regard his interference as a duty. But he ought to be careful that the information, on which he acts, is well founded; that his motives are pure and honourable; and that his judgment of the measures pursued is built on experience and practical knowledge, not on speculative or theoretical differences of opinion. The particular circumstances of the case will suggest the most proper mode of conduct. In general, however, a personal and confidential application to the gentlemen of the faculty concerned, should be the first step taken, and afterwards, if necessary, the transaction may be communicated to the patient or to his family.

V. When a physician or surgeon is called to a patient, who has been before under the care of another gentleman of the faculty, a consultation with him should be even proposed, though he may have discontinued his visits: His practice, also, should be treated with candour, and justified, so far as probity and truth will permit. For the want of success in the primary treatment of a case, is no impeachment of professional skill or knowledge; and it often serves to throw light on the nature of a disease, and to suggest to the subsequent practitioner more appropriate means of relief.

VII. *Consultations* should be *promoted*, in difficult or protracted cases, as they give rise to confidence, energy, and more enlarged views in practice. On such occasions no rivalship or jealousy should be indulged: Candour, probity, and all due respect should be exercised towards the physician or surgeon first engaged: And as he may be presumed to be best acquainted with the patient and with his family, he should deliver all the medical directions agreed upon, though he may not have precedency in seniority or rank. It should be the province, however, of the senior physician, first to propose the necessary questions to the sick, but without excluding his associate from the privilege of making farther enquiries, to satisfy himself, or to elucidate the case.

...

XIII. *Visits* to the sick should not be *unseasonably repeated;* because, when too frequent, they tend to diminish the authority of the physician, to produce instability in his practice, and to give rise to such occasional indulgences, as are subversive of all medical regimen.

Sir William Temple has asserted, that "an honest physician is excused for leaving his patient, when he finds the disease growing desperate, and can, by his attendance, expect only to receive his fees, without any hopes or appearance of deserving them." But this allegation is not well founded: For the offices of a physician may continue to be highly useful to the patient, and comforting to the relatives around him, even in the last period of a fatal malady; by obviating despair, by alleviating pain, and by soothing mental anguish. To decline attendance, under such circumstances, would be sacrificing, to fanciful delicacy and mistaken liberality, that moral duty which is independent of, and far superior to, all pecuniary appreciation.

XIV. Whenever a physician or surgeon *officiates* for another, who is sick or absent, during any considerable length of time, he should receive the fees accruing from such additional practice: But if this fraternal act be of short duration, it should be gratuitously performed; with an observance always of the utmost delicacy towards the interest and character of the professional gentleman, previously connected with the family.

XV. Some general rule should be adopted, by the faculty, in every town, relative to the *pecuniary acknowledgments* of their patients; and it should be deemed a point of honour to adhere to this rule, with as much steadiness, as varying circumstances will admit. For it is obvious that an average fee, as suited to the general rank of patients, must be an inadequate gratuity from the rich, who often require attendance not absolutely necessary; and yet too large to be expected from that class of citizens, who would feel a reluctance in calling for assistance, without making some decent and satisfactory retribution.

But in the consideration of fees, let it ever be remembered, that though mean ones from the affluent are both unjust and degrading, yet the characteristical beneficence of the profession is inconsistent with sordid views, and avaricious rapacity. To a young physician, it is of great importance to have clear and definite ideas of the ends of his profession; of the means for their attainment; and of the comparative value and dignity of each. Wealth, rank, and independence, with all the benefits resulting from them, are the primary ends which he holds in view; and they are interesting, wise, and laudable. But knowledge, benevolence, and active virtue, the means to be adopted in their acquisition, are of still higher estimation. And he has the privilege and felicity of practising an art, even more intrinsically excellent in its mediate than in its ultimate objects. The former, therefore, have a claim to uniform pre-eminence.

XVI. All members of the profession, including apothecaries as well as physicians and surgeons, together with their wives and children, should be attended *gratuitously* by any one or more of the faculty, residing near them, whose assistance may be required. For as solicitude obscures the judgment, and is accompanied with timidity and irresolution, medical men, under the pressure of sickness, either as affecting themselves or their families, are peculiarly dependent upon each other. But visits should not be obtruded officiously; as such unasked civility may give rise to embarrassment, or interfere with that choice, on which confidence depends.

...

XXI. The use of *quack medicines* should be discouraged by the faculty, as disgraceful to the profession, injurious to health, and often destructive even of life. Patients, however, under lingering disorders, are sometimes obstinately bent on having recourse to such as they see advertised, or hear recommended, with a boldness and confidence, which no intelligent physician dares to adopt with respect to the means that he prescribes. In these cases, some indulgence seems to be required to a credulity that is insurmountable: And the patient should neither incur the displeasure of the physician, nor be entirely deserted by him. He may be apprized of the fallacy of his expectations, whilst assured, at the same time, that diligent attention should be paid to the process of the experiment he is so unadvisedly making on himself, and the consequent mischiefs, if any, obviated as timely as possible. Certain active preparations, the nature, composition, and effects of which are well known, ought not to be proscribed as quack medicines.

XXII. No physician or surgeon should dispense a secret *nostrum*, whether it be his invention, or exclusive property. For if it be of real efficacy, the concealment of it is inconsistent with beneficence and professional liberality. And if mystery alone give it value and importance, such craft implies either disgraceful ignorance, or fraudulent avarice.

XXV. A wealthy physician should not give advice *gratis* to the affluent; because it is an injury to his professional brethren. The office of physician can never be supported but as a lucrative one; and it is defrauding, in some degree, the common funds for its support, when fees are dispensed with, which might justly be claimed.

Note **VII.** *Chap.* **II.** *Sect.* **III.** "**A physician should be the minister of hope and comfort to the sick.**" Mr. Gisborne, in one of his interesting letters to me on the subject of Medical Ethics, suggests, that it would be adviseable to add, *as far as truth and sincerity will admit.* "I know very well," says he, "that the sentence, as it now stands, conveys to you, and was meant by you to convey to others, the same sentiment which it would express after the proposed addition. But if I am not mistaken in my idea, that, there are few professional temptations to which medical men are more liable, and frequently from the very best principles, than that of unintentionally using language to the patient and his friends, more encouraging than sincerity would vindicate, on cool reflection; it may be right scrupulously to guard the avenues against such an error."

In the *Enquiry into the Duties of Men*, the same excellent moralist thus delivers his sentiments more at large. "A professional writer, speaking, in a work already quoted,[1] respecting the performance of surgical operations in hospitals, remarks, that it may be a salutary, as well as an humane act, in the attending physician, occasionally to assure the patient that every thing goes on well, *if that declaration can be made with truth.* This restriction, so properly applied to the case in question, may with equal propriety be extended universally to the conduct of a physician, when superintending operations performed, not by the hand of a surgeon, but by nature and medicine. Humanity, we admit, and the welfare of the sick man commonly require, that his drooping spirits should be revived by every encouragement and hope, which can honestly be suggested to him. But truth and conscience forbid the physician to cheer him by giving promises, or raising expectations, which are known, or intended to be, delusive. The physician may not be bound, unless expressly called upon, invariably to divulge, at any specific time, his opinion concerning the uncertainty or danger of the case: but he is invariably bound never to represent the uncertainty or danger as less than he actually believes it to be; and whenever he conveys, directly or indirectly, to the patient or to his family, any impression to that effect, though he may be misled by mistaken tenderness, he is guilty of positive falsehood. He is at liberty to say little; but let that little be true. St. Paul's direction, *not to do evil, that good may come*, is clear, positive, and universal."[2]

Whether this subject be viewed as regarding general morality, or professional duty, it is of high importance; and we may justly presume, that it involves considerable difficulty and intricacy, because opposite opinions have been advanced upon it by very distinguished writers. THE ANCIENTS, though sublime in the abstract representations of virtue, are seldom precise and definite in the detail of rules for its observance. Yet in some instances they extend their precepts to particular cases: And Cicero, in the Third Book of his Offices, expressly admits of limitations to the absolute and immutable obligation of fidelity and truth.

The maxim of the poet, also, may be adduced as intended to be comprehensive of the moral laws, by which human conduct is to be governed:

Sunt certi denique fines,
Quos ultrá citráque nequit consistere rectum.[†]

The early FATHERS of the Christian church, Origen, Clement, Tertullian, Lactantius, Chrysostom, and various others, till the period of St. Augustine, were latitudinarians on this point. But the holy father last mentioned, if I mistake not, in the warmth of his zeal, declared that he would not utter a lie, though he were assured of gaining Heaven by it. In this declaration there is a fallacy, by which Augustine probably imposed upon himself. For a lie is always understood to consist in a *criminal* breach of truth, and therefore under no circumstances can be justified. It is alleged, however, that falsehood may lose the essence of lying, and become even praise-worthy, when the adherence to truth is incompatible with the practice of some other virtue of still higher obligation. This opinion almost the whole body of CIVILIANS adopt, with full confidence of its rectitude.

···

Every practitioner must find himself occasionally in circumstances of very delicate embarrassment, with respect to the contending obligations of veracity and professional duty: And when such trials occur, it will behove him to act on fixed principles of rectitude, derived from previous information, and serious reflection. Perhaps the following brief considerations, by which I have conscientiously endeavoured to govern my own conduct, may afford some aid to his decision.

Moral truth, in a professional view, has two references; one to the party to whom it is delivered, and another to the individual by whom it is uttered. In the first, it is a *relative duty*, constituting a branch of justice; and may be properly regulated by the divine rule of equity prescribed by our Saviour, to *do unto others, as we would*, all circumstances duly weighed, *they should do unto us*. In the second, it is a *personal* duty, regarding solely the sincerity, the purity, and the probity of the physician himself. To a patient, therefore, perhaps the father of a numerous family, or one whose life is of the highest importance to the community, who makes enquiries which, if faithfully answered, might prove fatal to him, it would be a gross and unfeeling wrong to reveal the truth. His right to it is suspended, and even annihilated; because its beneficial nature being reversed, it would be deeply injurious to himself, to his family, and to the public: And he has the strongest claim, from the trust reposed in his physician, as well as from the common principles of humanity, to be guarded against whatever would be detrimental to him. In such a situation, therefore, the only point at issue is, whether the practitioner shall sacrifice that delicate sense of veracity, which is so ornamental to, and indeed forms a characteristic excellence of the virtuous man, to this claim of professional justice and social duty. Under such a painful conflict of obligations, a wise and good man must be governed by those which are the most imperious; and will therefore generously relinquish every consideration, referable only to himself. Let him be careful, however, not to do this, but in cases of real emergency, which happily seldom occur; and to guard his mind sedulously against the injury it may sustain by such violations of the native love of truth.

Notes

1. Percival's Medical Ethics. Chap. 1.
2. Duties of men, vol. II. p. 148.
† Horat. Sat. Lib. I. Sat. I. 106.

Principles of Medical Ethics (1957)

American Medical Association

──────────────INTRODUCTION TO READING──────────────

The American Medical Association, at its first meetings in Philadelphia in 1847, adopted a long statement on ethics. It was drawn in part from the document written by Thomas Percival in the 1790s (published in 1803) as part of the adjudication of a dispute among physicians, surgeons, and apothecaries. Several revisions of the AMA's statements on ethics were adopted over the years. In 1957 the AMA adopted a new set of principles expressed in a shorter, more abstract form. One of the themes that begins to emerge in the early codes of Percival and becomes more apparent in the AMA codes is the tension between the duty of the physician to the patient and the social duty the physician may owe to the society. This theme, totally absent from the original Hippocratic Oath, is already present in Percival's writing and becomes a more critical issue in the versions of the AMA's codes written in the twentieth century. This is particularly apparent in the tenth principle of the 1957 version of the AMA Principles, but also in the references to service to humanity and commitment to the public. For example, in this code confidences may be broken not only to benefit the patient, but also to benefit the community.

Preamble

These principles are intended to aid physicians individually and collectively in maintaining a high level of ethical conduct. They are not laws but standards by which a physician may determine the propriety of his conduct in his relationship with patients, with colleagues, with members of allied professions, and with the public.

Section 1

The principle objective of the medical profession is to render service to humanity with full respect for the dignity of man. Physicians should merit the confidence of patients entrusted to their care, rendering to each a full measure of service and devotion.

Section 2

Physicians should strive continually to improve medical knowledge and skill, and should make available to their patients and colleagues the benefits of their professional attainments.

Section 3

A physician should practice a method of healing founded on a scientific basis; and he should not voluntarily associate professionally with anyone who violates this principle.

Section 4

The medical profession should safeguard the public and itself against physicians deficient in moral character or professional competence. Physicians should observe all laws, uphold the dignity and honor of the profession and accept its self-imposed disciplines. They should expose, without hesitation, illegal or unethical conduct of fellow members of the profession.

Section 5

A physician may choose whom he will serve. In an emergency, however, he should render service to the best of his ability. Having undertaken the care of a patient, he may not neglect him; and unless he has been discharged he may discontinue his services only after giving adequate notice. He should not solicit patients.

Section 6

A physician should not dispose of his services under terms or conditions which tend to interfere with or impair the free and complete exercise of his medical judgment and skill or tend to cause a deterioration of the quality of medical care.

Section 7

In the practice of medicine a physician should limit the source of his professional income to medical services actually rendered by him, or under his supervision, to his patients. His fee should be commensurate with the services rendered and the patient's ability to pay. He should neither pay nor receive a commission for referral of patients. Drugs, remedies or appliances may be dispensed or supplied by the physician provided it is in the best interest of the patient.

Section 8

A physician should seek consultation upon request; in doubtful or difficult cases; or whenever it appears that the quality of medical service may be enhanced thereby.

Section 9

A physician may not reveal confidences entrusted to him in the course of medical attendance, or the deficiencies he may observe in the character of patients, unless he is required to do so by law or unless it becomes necessary in order to protect the welfare of the individual or of the community.

Section 10

The honored ideals of the medical profession imply that the responsibilities of the physician extend not only to the individual, but also to society where these responsibilities deserve his interest and participation in activities which have the purpose of improving both the health and the well-being of the individual and the community.

Toward an Expanded Medical Ethics: The Hippocratic Ethic Revisited

Edmund D. Pellegrino

──────────INTRODUCTION TO READING──────────

By the 1970s, the problems with the Hippocratic tradition manifest in the Hippocratic Oath and the Declaration of Geneva began to become more and more severe. Edmund Pellegrino, a physician and medical humanist at Georgetown University, exposes these problems in his essay "Toward an Expanded Medical Ethics: The Hippocratic Ethic Revisited." He emphasizes the problems with the exclusive focus on the individual that we have already seen in Percival and the AMA's modification of the Hippocratic tradition. He also points out that this is only one of the potential problems with the Hippocratic tradition as received. He argues that in the modern world the patient increasingly is capable of and desires to participate in decisions. He warns the physician against assuming that his or her own judgments about what is beneficial will be shared by patients. He warns that the modern situation requires a more conscious theory of values and awareness of the possibility of conflicting values. Finally, he observes that medicine today is much more institutionalized than it was in the time of

Greek medicine. This means that new, more social ethical problems such as cost containment and competition for resources must be addressed, problems not in the consciousness of the Greek Hippocratic physician.

Custom without truth is but the seniority of error.
—*Saint Cyprian, Epistles LXXIV*

The good physician is by the nature of his vocation called to practice his art within a framework of high moral sensitivity. For two millennia this sensitivity was provided by the Oath and the other ethical writings of the Hippocratic corpus. No code has been more influential in heightening the moral reflexes of ordinary men. Every subsequent medical code is essentially a footnote to the Hippocratic precepts, which even to this day remain the paradigm of how the good physician should behave.

The Hippocratic ethic is marked by a unique combination of humanistic concern and practical wisdom admirably suited to the physician's tasks in society. In a simpler world, that ethic long sufficed to guide the physician in his service to patient and community. Today, the intersections of medicine with contemporary science, technology, social organization, and changed human values have revealed significant missing dimensions in the ancient ethic. The reverence we rightly accord the Hippocratic precepts must not obscure the need for a critical examination of their missing dimensions—those most pertinent for contemporary physicians and society. The need for expanding traditional medical ethics is already well-established. It was first underscored by the shocking revelations of the Nuremberg trials. A spate of new codes has appeared which attempt to deal more responsibly with the promise and the[1-3]

More recently, further ethical inquiries have been initiated to reflect the change in moral climate and medical attitudes toward abortion, population control, euthanasia, transplanting organs, and manipulating human behavior and genetic constitution.[1-5]

In actual fact, some of the major proscriptions of the Hippocratic Oath are already being consciously compromised: confidentiality can be violated under certain conditions of law and public safety; abortion is being legalized; dangerous drugs are used everywhere; and a conscious but controlled invasion of the patient's rights in human experimentation is now permitted.

This essay will examine some important dimensions of medical ethics not included in the Hippocratic ethic and, in some ways, even obscured by its too rigorous application. To be considered here are the ethics of participation, the questions raised by institutionalizing medical care, the need for an axiology of medical ethics, the changing ethics of competence, and the tensions between individual and social ethics.

An analysis of these questions will reveal the urgent need for expanding medical ethical concerns far beyond those traditionally observed. A deeper ethic of social and corporate responsibility is needed to guide the profession to levels of moral sensitivity more congruent with the expanded duties of the physician in contemporary culture.

The Hippocratic Ethic

The normative principles which constitute what may loosely be termed the Hippocratic ethic are contained in the Oath and the deontological books: *Law, Decorum, Precepts,* and *The Physician.* These treatises are of varied origin and combine behavioral imperatives derived from a variety of sources—the schools at Cos and Cnidus, intermingled with Pythagorean, Epicurean, and Stoic influences.[6-7]

The Oath[8] speaks of the relationships of the student and his teacher, advises the physician never to harm the patient, enjoins confidentiality, and proscribes abortion, euthanasia, and the use of the knife. It forbids sexual commerce with the women in the household of the homesick. The doctor is a member of a select brotherhood dedicated to the care of the sick, and his major reward is a good reputation.

Law discusses the qualities of mind and the diligence required of the prospective physician from early life.[9] *The Physician* emphasizes the need for dignified comportment, a healthy body, a grave and kind mien, and a regular life.[9(pp. 311-313)] In Decorum, we are shown the unique practical wisdom rooted in experience which is essential to good medicine and absent in the quack; proper comportment in the sick room dictates a reserved, authoritative, composed air; much practical advice is given on the arts and techniques of clinical medicine. [9(pp.279-301)] *Precepts* again warns against theorizing without facts, inveighs against quackery, urges consideration in setting fees, and encourages consultation in difficult cases.[8(pp. 313-333)]

Similar admonitions can be found scattered throughout the Hippocratic corpus, but it is these few brief ethical treatises which have formed the character of the physician for so many centuries. From them, we can extract what can loosely be called the Hippocratic ethic—a mixture of high ideals, common sense, and practical wisdom. A few principles of genuine ethics are often repeated and intermingled with etiquette and homespun advice of all sorts. The good physician emerges as an authoritative and competent practitioner, devoted to his patient's well-being. He is a benevolent and sole arbiter who knows what is best for the patient and makes all decisions for him.

There is in the Hippocratic corpus little explicit reference to the responsibilities of medicine as a corporate entity with responsibility for its members and duties to the greater human community. The ethic of the profession as a whole is assured largely by the moral behavior of its individual members. There is no explicit delineation of the corporate responsibility of physicians for one another's ethical behavior. On the whole, the need for maintaining competence is indirectly stated. There are, in short, few explicit recommendations about what we would today call "social ethics." These characteristics of the

Hippocratic ethic have been carried forward to our day. They are extended in the code of Thomas Percival, which formed the basis of the first code of ethics adopted by the American Medical Association in 1847.[10] They were sufficient for the less complex societies of the ancient and modern worlds but not for the contemporary twentieth-century experience. The Hippocratic norms can no longer be regarded as unchanging absolutes but as partial statements of ideals, in need of constant reevaluation, amplification, and evolution.

Without in any way denigrating the essential worth of the Hippocratic ethic, it is increasingly apparent that the ideas conveyed about the physician are simplistic and incomplete for today's needs. In some ways, it is even and antipathetic to the social and political spirit of our times. For example, the notion of the physician as a benevolent and paternalistic figure who decides all for the patient is inconsistent with today's educated public. It is surely incongruous in a democratic society in which the rights of self-determination are being assured by law. In a day when the remote effects of individual medical acts are so consequential, we cannot be satisfied with an ethic which is so inexplicit about social responsibilities. Nowhere in the Hippocratic Oath is the physician recognized as a member of a corporate entity which can accomplish good ends for man that are more than the sum of individual good acts. The necessity for a stringent ethic of competence and a new ethic of shared responsibility which flows from team and institutional medical care are understandably not addressed.

It is useful to examine some of these missing ethical dimensions as examples of the kind of organic development long overdue in professional medical ethical codes.

The Ethics of Participation

The central and most admirable feature of the Oath is the respect it inculcates for the patient. In the Oath, the doctor is pledged always to help the patient and keep him from harm. This duty is then exemplified by specific prohibitions against abortion, use of deadly drugs, surgery, breaches of confidence, and indulgence in sexual relations with members of the sick person's household. Elsewhere, in *The Physician, Decorum*, and *Precepts*, the physician is further enjoined to be humble, careful in observation, calm and sober in thought and speech. These admonitions have the same validity today that they had centuries ago and are still much in need of cultivation.

But in one of these same works, *Decorum*, we find an excellent example of how drastically the relationship between physician and patient has changed since Hippocrates' time. The doctor is advised to "Perform all things calmly and adroitly, concealing most things from the patient while you are attending him." A little further on, the physician is told to treat the patient with solicitude, "revealing nothing of the patient's present and future condition."[9(pp. 297, 299)] This advice is at variance with social and political trends and with the desires of most educated patients. It is still too often the modus operandi of physicians dreaming of a simpler world in which authority and paternalistic benevolence were the order of the day.

Indeed, a major criticism of physicians today centers on this very question of disclosure of essential information. Many educated patients feel frustrated in their desire to participate in decisions which affect them as intimately as medical decisions invariably do. The matter really turns on establishing new bases for the patient's trust. The knowledgeable patient can trust the physician only if he feels the latter is competent and uses that competence with integrity and for ends which have value for the patient. Today's educated patient wants to understand what the physician is doing, why he is doing it, what the alternatives may be, and what choices are open. In a democratic society, people expect the widest protection of their rights to self-determination. Hence, the contemporary patient has a right to know the decisions involved in managing his case.

When treatment is specific, with few choices open, the prognosis good, and side effects minimal, disclosing the essential information is an easy matter. Unfortunately, medicine frequently deals with indefinite diagnoses and nonspecific treatments of unspecific value. Several alternatives are usually open; prognosis may not be altered by treatment; side effects are often considerable and discomfort significant. The patient certainly has the right to know these data before therapeutic interventions are initiated. The Nuremberg Code and others were designed to protect the subject in the course of human experimentation by insisting on the right of informed and free consent. The same right should be guaranteed in the course of ordinary medical treatment as well.

So fundamental is this right of self-determination in a democratic society that to limit it, even in ordinary medical transactions, is to propagate an injustice. This is not to ignore the usual objections to disclosure: the fear of inducing anxiety in the patient, the inability of the sick patient to participate in the decision, the technical nature of medical knowledge, and the possibility of litigation. These objections deserve serious consideration but will, on close analysis, not justify concealment except under special circumstances. Obviously, the fear of indiscriminate disclosure cannot obfuscate the invasion of a right, even when concealment is in the interest of the patient.

Surely, the physician is expected by the patient and society to use disclosure prudently. For the very ill, the very anxious, the poorly educated, the too young, or the very old, he will permit himself varying degrees of disclosure. The modes of doing so must be adapted to the patient's educational level, psychologic responses, and physiologic state. It must be emphatically stated that the purpose of disclosure of alternatives, costs, and benefits in medical diagnosis and treatment is not to relieve the physician of the onus of decision or displace it on the patient. Rather, it permits the physician to function as the technical expert and adviser, inviting the patient's participation and understanding as aids in the acceptance of the decision and its consequences. This is the only basis for a mature, just, and understandable physician-patient relationship.

Deontologic versus Axiologic Ethics

The most important human reason for enabling the patient to participate in the decisions which affect him is to allow consideration of his personal values. Here, the Hippocratic tradition is explicitly lacking since its spirit is almost wholly deontological, that is, obligations are stated as absolutes without reference to any theory of values. Underlying value systems are not stated or discussed. The need for examining the intersection of values inherent in every medical transaction is unrecognized. The values of the physician or of medicine are assumed to prevail as absolutes, and an operational attitude of "noblesse oblige" is encouraged.

A deontologic ethic was not inappropriate for Greek medicine, which did not have to face so many complex and antithetical courses of action. But a relevant ethic for our times must be more axiologic than deontologic, that is, based in a more conscious theory of values. The values upon which any action is based are of enormous personal and social consequence. An analysis of conflicting values underlies the choice of a noxious treatment for a chronic illness, the question of prolonging life in an incurable disease, or setting priorities for using limited medical resources. Instead of absolute values, we deal more frequently with an intersection of several sets and subsets of values: those of the patient, the physician, sciences, and society. Which shall prevail when these values are in conflict? How do we decide?

The patient's values must be respected whenever possible and whenever they do not create injustice for others. The patient is free to delegate the decision to his physicians, but he must do this consciously and freely. To the extent that he is educated, responsible, and thoughtful, modern man will increasingly want the opportunity to examine relative values in each transaction. When the patient is unconscious or otherwise unable to participate, the physician or the family acts as his surrogate, charged as closely as possible to preserve his values.

The Hippocratic principle of *primum non nocere*, therefore, must be expanded to encompass the patient's value system if it is to have genuine meaning. To impose the doctor's value system is an intrusion on the patient; it may be harmful, unethical, and result in an error in diagnosis and treatment.

Disclosure is, therefore, a necessary condition if we really respect each patient as a unique being whose values, as a part of his person, are no more to be violated than his body. The deontologic thrust of traditional medical ethics is too restrictive in a time when the reexamination of all values is universal. It even defeats the very purposes of the traditional ethic, which are to preserve the integrity of the patient as a person.

Individual versus Social Ethics

Another notably unexplored area in the Hippocratic ethic is the social responsibility of the physician. Its emphasis on the welfare of the individual patient is exemplary, and this is firmly explicated in the Oath and elsewhere. Indeed, in *Precepts*, this respect for the individual patient is placed at the very heart of medicine: "Where there is love of one's fellow man, there is love of the Art."[8(p. 319)]

As Ford has shown, today too the physician's sense of responsibility is directed overwhelmingly toward his own patient.[11] This is one of the most admirable features of medicine, and it must always remain the central ethical imperative in medical transactions. But it must now be set in a context entirely alien to that in which ancient medicine was practiced. In earlier eras the remote effects of medical acts were of little concern, and the rights of the individual patient could be the exclusive and absolute base of the physician's actions. Today, the growing interdependence of all humans and the effectiveness of medical techniques have drastically altered the simplistic arrangements of traditional ethics. The aggregate effects of individual medical acts have already changed the ecology of man. Every death prevented or life prolonged alters the number, kind, and distribution of human beings. The resultant competition for living space, food, and conveniences already imperils our hope for a life of satisfaction for all mankind.

Even more vexing questions in social ethics are posed when we attempt to allocate our resources among the many new possibilities for good inherent in medical progress and technology. Do we pool our limited resources and manpower to apply curative medicine to all now deprived of it or continue to multiply the complexity of services for the privileged? Do we apply mass prophylaxis against streptococcal diseases, or repair damaged valves with expensive heart surgery after they are damaged? Is it preferable to change cultural patterns in favor of a more reasonable diet for Americans or develop better surgical techniques for unplugging fat-occluded coronary arteries? Every health planner and concerned public official has his own set of similar questions. It is clear that we cannot have all these things simultaneously.

This dimension of ethics becomes even more immediate when we inquire into the responsibility of medicine for meeting the urgent sociomedical needs of large segments of our population. Can we absolve ourselves from responsibility for deficiencies in distribution, quality, and accessibility of even ordinary medical care for the poor, the uneducated and the disenfranchised? Do we direct our health care system to the care of the young in ghettos and underdeveloped countries or to the affluent aged? Which course will make for a better world? These are vexing questions of the utmost social concern. Physicians have an ethical responsibility to raise these questions and, in answering them, to work with the community in ordering its priorities or make optimal use of available medical skills.

It is not enough to hope that the good of the community will grow fortuitously out of the summation of good acts of each physician for his own patients. Societies are necessary to insure enrichment of the life of each of their members. But they are more than the aggregate of persons within them. As T. S. Eliot puts it, "What life have you if you have not life together? There is no life that is not in community."[12]

Society supports the doctor in the expectation that he will direct himself to socially relevant health problems, not just those he finds interesting or remunerative. The commitment to social egalitarianism demands a greater sensitivity to social ethics than is to be found in traditional codes. Section ten of the American Medical Association Principles of Medical Ethics (1946) explicitly recognizes the profession's responsibility to society. But a more explicit analysis of the relationships of individual and social ethics should be undertaken. Medicine, which touches on the most human problems of both the individual and society, cannot serve man without attending to both his personal and communal needs.

The Hippocratic ethic and its later modifications were not required to confront such paradoxes. Today's conscientious physician is very much in need of an expanded ethic to cope with his double responsibility to the individual and to the community.

The Ethics of Institutionalized Medicine

The institutionalization of all aspects of medical care is an established fact. With increasing frequency, the personal contract inherent in patient care is made with institutions, groups of physicians, or teams of health professionals. The patient now often expects the institution or group to select his physician or consultant and to assume responsibility for the quality and quantity of care provided.

Within the institution itself, the health care team is essential to the practice of comprehensive medicine. Physicians and nonphysicians now cooperate in providing the spectrum of special services made possible by modern technology. The responsibility for even the most intimate care of the patient is shared. Some of the most important clinical decisions are made by team members who may have no personal contact at all with the patient. The team itself is not a stable entity of unchanging composition. Its membership changes in response to the patient's needs, and so may its leadership. Preserving the traditional rights of the patient, formerly vested in a single identifiable physician, is now sometimes spread anonymously over a group. Competence, confidentiality, integrity, and personal concern are far more difficult to assure with a group of diverse professionals enjoying variable degrees of personal contact with the patient.

No current code of ethics fully defines how the traditional rights of the medical transaction are to be protected when responsibility is diffused within a team and an institution. Clearly, no health profession can elaborate such a code of team ethics by itself. We need a new medical ethic which permits the cooperative definition of normative guides to protect the person of the patient served by a group, none of whose members may have sole responsibility for care. Laymen, too, must participate, since boards of trustees set the overall policies which affect patient care. Few trustees truly recognize that they are the ethical and legal surrogates of society for the patients who come to their institutions seeking help.

Thus, the most delicate of the physician's responsibilities, protecting the patient's welfare, must now be fulfilled in a new and complicated context. Instead of the familiar one-to-one unique relationship, the physician finds himself coordinator of a team, sharing with others some of the most sensitive areas of patient care. The physician is still bound to see that group assessment and management are rational, safe, and personalized. He must especially guard against the dehumanization so easily and inadvertently perpetrated by a group in the name of efficiency.

The doctor must acquire new attitudes. Since ancient times, he has been the sole dominant and authoritarian figure in the care of his patient. He has been supported in this position by traditional ethics. In the clinical emergency, his dominant role is still unchallenged, since he is well trained to make quick decisions in ambiguous situations. What he is not prepared for are the negotiations, analysis, and ultimate compromise fundamental to group efforts and essential in nonemergency situations. A whole new set of clinical perspectives must be introduced, perspectives difficult for the classically trained physician to accept, but necessary if the patient is to benefit from contemporary technology and organization of health care.

The Ethics of Competence

A central aim of the Oath and other ethical treatises is to protect the patient and the profession from quackery and incompetence. In the main, competence is assumed as basic fulfillment of the Hippocratic ideal of *primum non nocere.*

The Hippocratic works preach the wholly admirable common-sense ethos of the good artisan: careful work, maturation of skills, simplicity of approach, and knowledge of limitations. This was sound advice at a time when new discoveries were so often the product of speculation untainted by observation or experience. The speculative astringency of the Hippocratic ethic was a potent and necessary safeguard against the quackery of fanciful and dangerous "new" cures.

With the scientific era in medicine, the efficacy of new techniques and information in changing the natural history of disease was dramatically demonstrated. Today, the patient has a right to access to the vast stores of new knowledge useful to medicine. Failure of the physician to make this reservoir available and accessible is a moral failure. The ethos of the artisan, while still a necessary safeguard, is now far from being a sufficient one.

Maintaining competence today is a prime ethical challenge. Only the highest standard of initial and continuing professional proficiency is acceptable in a technological world. This imperative is now so essential a feature of the patient-physician transaction that the ancient mandate, "Do no harm," must be supplemented: "Do all things essential to optimal solution of the patient's problem." Anything less makes the doctor's professional declaration a sham and a scandal.

Competence now has a far wider definition than in ancient times. Not only must the physician encompass expertly the knowledge pertinent to his own field, but he must be the instrument for bringing all other knowledge to bear on his patient's needs. He now functions as one element in a vast matrix of consultants, technicians, apparatus, and institutions, all of which may contribute to his patient's well-being. He cannot provide all these things himself. To attempt to do so is to pursue the romantic and vanishing illusion of the physician as Renaissance man.

The enormous difficulties of its achievement notwithstanding, competence has become the first ethical precept for the modern physician after integrity. It is also the prime human precept and the one most peculiar to the physician's function in society. Even the current justifiable demands of patients and medical students for greater compassion must not obfuscate the centrality of competence in the physician's existence. The simple intention to help others is commendable but, by itself, not only insufficient but positively dangerous. What is more inhumane or more a violation of trust than incompetence? The consequence of a lack of compassion may be remediable, while a lack of competence may cost the patient his chance for recovery of life, function, and happiness. Clearly, medicine cannot attain the ethical eminence to which it is called without both compassion and competence.

Within this framework, a more rigorous ethic of competence must be elaborated. Continuing education, periodic recertification, and renewal of clinical privileges have become moral mandates, not just hopeful hortatory devices dependent upon individual physician responses. The Hippocratic ethic of the good artisan is now just the point of departure for the wide options technology holds out for individual and social health.

Toward A Corporate Ethic and an Ethical Syncytium

The whole of the Hippocratic corpus, including the ethical treatises, is the work of many authors writing in different historical periods. Thus, the ethical precepts cannot be considered the formal position of a profession in today's sense. There is no evidence of recognition of true corporate responsibility for larger social issues or of sanctions to deter miscreant members.

The Greek physician seems to have regarded himself as the member of an informal aristocratic brotherhood, in which each individual was expected to act ethically and to do so for love of the profession and respect of the patient. His reward was *doxa*, a good reputation, which in turn assured a successful practice. There is notably no sense of the larger responsibilities as a profession for the behavior of each member. Nowhere stated are the potentialities and responsibilities of a group of high-minded individuals to effect reforms and achieve purposes transcending the interests of individual members. In short, the Greek medical profession relied on the sum total of individual ethical behaviors to assure the ethical behavior of the group.

This is still the dominant view of many physicians in the Western world who limit their ethical perspectives to their relationships with their own patients. Medical societies do censure unethical members with varying alacrity for the grosser forms of misconduct or breaches of professional etiquette. But there is as yet insufficient assumption of a corporate and shared responsibility for the actions of each member of the group. The power of physicians as a polity to effect reforms in quality of care, its organization, and its relevance to needs of society is as yet unrealized.

Yet many of the dimensions of medical ethics touched upon in this essay can only be secured by the conscious assumption of a corporate responsibility on the part of all physicians for the final pertinence of their individual acts to promote better life for all. There is the need to develop, as it were, a functioning ethical syncytium in which the actions of each physician would touch upon those of all physicians and in which it is clear that the ethical failings of each member would diminish the stature of every other physician to some degree. This syncytial framework is at variance with the traditional notion that each physician acts as an individual and is primarily responsible only to himself and his patient.

This shift of emphasis is dictated by the metamorphosis of all professions in our complex, highly organized, highly integrated, and egalitarian social order. For most of its history medicine has existed as a select and loosely organized brotherhood. For the past hundred years in our country, it has been more formally organized in the American Medical Association and countless other professional organizations dedicated to a high order of individual ethics. A new stage in the evolution of medicine as a profession is about to begin as a consequence of three clear trends.

First, all professions are increasingly being regarded as services, even as public utilities, dedicated to fulfilling specific social needs not entirely defined by the profession. Professions themselves will acquire dignity and standing in the future, not so much from the tasks they perform, but from the intimacy of the connection between those tasks and the social life of which the profession is a part. Second, the professions are being democratized, and it will be ever more difficult for any group to hold a privileged position. The automatic primacy of medicine is being challenged by the other health professions, whose functions are of increasing importance in patient care. This functionalization of the professions tends to emphasize what is done for a patient and not who does it. Moreover, many tasks formerly performed only by the physicians are being done by other professionals and nonprofessionals. Last, the socialization of all mankind affects the professions as well. Hence, the collectivity will increasingly be expected to take responsibility for how well or poorly the profession carries out the purposes for which it is supported by society.

These changes will threaten medicine only if physicians hold to a simplistic ethic in which the agony of choices among individual and social values is dismissed as spurious or imaginary. The physician is the most highly educated of health professionals. He should be first to take on the burdens of continuing self-reformation in terms of a new ethos—one in which the problematics of priorities and values are openly faced as common responsibilities of the entire profession. We must recognize the continuing validity of traditional ethics for the personal dimensions of patient care and their inadequacy for the newer social dimensions of health in contemporary life. It is the failure to appreciate this distinction that stimulates so much criticism of the profession at the same time that individual physicians are highly respected.

One of the gravest and most easily visible social inequities today is the maldistribution of medical services among portions of our population. This is another sphere in which the profession as a whole must assume responsibility for what individual physicians cannot do alone. The civil rights movement and the revolt of the black minority populations have punctuated the problem. Individual physicians have always tried to redress this evil, some in heroic ways. Now, however, the problem is a major ethical responsibility for the whole profession: we cannot dismiss the issue. We must engender a feeling of ethical diminution of the entire profession whenever there are segments of the population without adequate and accessible medical care. This extends to the provision of primary care for all, insistence on a system of coverage for all communities every hour of the day, proper distribution of the various medical specialties and facilities, and a system of fees no longer based on the usual imponderables, but on more standardized norms.

There are, perforce, reasonable limits to the social ills to which the individual physician and the profession can be expected to attend qua physician. Some have suggested that medicine concern itself with the Vietnam war, the root causes of poverty, environmental pollution, drugs, housing, and racial injustice. It would be difficult to argue that all of these social ills are primary ethical responsibilities of individual physicians or even of the profession. To do so would hopelessly diffuse medical energies and manpower from their proper object—the promotion of health and the cure of illness. The profession can fight poverty, injustice, and war through medicine.

A distinction, therefore, must clearly be made between the physician's primary ethical responsibilities, which derive from the nature of his profession, and those which do not. Each physician must strike for himself an optimal balance between professional and civic responsibilities.

Summary

We have attempted a brief analysis of some of the limitations and omissions in traditional medical ethics as embodied in the Hippocratic corpus and its later exemplifications. These limitations are largely in the realm of social and corporate ethics, realms of increasing significance in an egalitarian, highly structured, and exquisitely interlocked social order.

The individual physician needs more explicit guidelines than traditional codes afford to meet today's new problems. The Hippocratic ethic is one of the most admirable codes in the history of man. But even its ethical sensibilities and high moral tone are insufficient for the complexities of today's problems.

An evolving, constantly refurbished system of medical ethics is requisite in the twentieth century. An axiologic, rather than a deontologic, bias is more in harmony with the questions raised in a world society whose values are in continual flux and reexamination. There is ample opportunity for a critical reappraisal of the Hippocratic ethic and for the elaboration of a fuller and more comprehensive medical ethic suited to our profession as it nears the twenty-first century. This fuller ethic will build upon the noble precepts set forth so long ago in the Hippocratic corpus, It will explicate, complement, and develop those precepts, but it must not be delimited in its evolution by an unwarranted reluctance to question even so ancient and honorable a code as that of the Hippocratic writings.

Notes

1. *American Academy of Arts and Sciences.* "Proceedings" 98:No. 2, 1969.

2. Pellegrino, E. D. The Necessity, Promise, and Dangers of Human Experimentation." *Experiments With Man–World Council Studies, No. 6,* New York: Geneva and Friendship Press, 1969.

3. Annals *of the New York Academy of Arts and Sciences.* "New Dimensions in Legal and Ethical Concepts for Human Research." 169:293–593, 1970.

4. Torrey, E. F. *Ethical Issues in Medicine.* Boston: Little, Brown, 1968.

5. Pellegrino, E. D. "Physicians, Patients, and Society: Some New Tensions in Medical Ethics." In *Human Aspects of Biomedical Innovation,* edited by Everett Mendelsohn, Judith P. Swazey, and Irene Taviss. Cambridge, Mass.: Harvard University Press, 1971, pp. 77–97, 291–220.

6. Sigerest, H. E. *The History of Medicine, vol. 11.* New York: Oxford University Press, 1961, pp. 260, 298.

7. Heidel, W. A. *Hippocratic Medicine: Its Spirit and Method.* New York: Columbia University Press, 1941, p. 149.

8. Jones, W. H. S. Hippocrates, vol. I. Cambridge, Mass.: Harvard University Press, 1923, pp. 299–301, 313–333.

9. Jones, W. H. S. *Hippocrates,* vol. II. Cambridge, Mass.: Harvard University Press, 1923, pp. 263–265, 279–301, 311–313.

10. Leake, C., ed. *Percival's Medical Ethics.* Baltimore: William & Wilkins, 1927, p. 291.

11. Ford, et al. *The Doctor's Perspective.* New York: Year Book, 1967.

12. Eliot, T. S. "The Rock." *The Complete Poems and Plays,* 1909–1950. New York: Harcourt & Brace, 1952, p. 101.

Principles of Medical Ethics (1980)

American Medical Association

──────────────────INTRODUCTION TO READING──────────────────

In 1980 the AMA adopted a completely new set of medical ethical principles. It shows how these concerns with the problems of the original Hippocratic perspective have manifested themselves and gradually emerged to dominate the medical ethics of organized medicine at least in the United States. The committee of the AMA responsible for the writing of the new Principles was chaired by James Todd, who is now AMA Assistant Executive Vice President. The committee reported that medical ethics must be seen increasingly as something to which all members of the society must contribute. It called into question the earlier paternalism of the Hippocratic tradition and emphasized the responsibility of the profession to the society as well as to the individual patient. The new Principles for the first time in any code written by physicians, adopt the language of rights rather than staying exclusively with the more traditional language of benefits and harms. The idea that rights are relevant to morality as well as benefits and harms is alien to professional codes of medical ethics in the Hippocratic tradition. The new Principles show the beginning of the influence of other ethical theories, especially the ethics of modern Western liberalism.

Preamble

The medical profession has long subscribed to a body of ethical statements developed primarily for the benefit of the patient. As a member of this profession, a physician must recognize responsibility not only to patients, but also to society, to other health professionals, and to self. The following Principles adopted by the American Medical Association are not laws, but standards of conduct which define the essentials of honorable behavior for the physician.

I. A physician shall be dedicated to providing competent medical service with compassion and respect for human dignity.

II. A physician shall deal honestly with patients and colleagues, and strive to expose those physicians deficient in character or competence, or who engage in fraud or deception.

III. A physician shall respect the law and also recognize a responsibility to seek changes in those requirements which are contrary to the best interests of the patient.

IV. A physician shall respect the rights of patients, of colleagues, and of other health professionals, and shall safeguard patient confidences within the constraints of the law.

V. A physician shall continue to study, apply and advance scientific knowledge, make relevant information available to patients, colleagues, and the public, obtain consultation, and use the talents of other health professionals when indicated.

VI. A physician shall, in the provision of appropriate patient care, except in emergencies, be free to choose whom to serve, with whom to associate, and the environment in which to provide medical services.

VII. A physician shall recognize a responsibility to participate in activities contributing to an improved community.

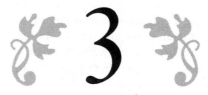

The

Dominant

Western Competitors

Introduction

When the Hippocratic tradition was challenged for its individualism and its lack of commitment to the autonomy of the patient as a decision maker, we began to discover other traditions in Western thought, some of which had well-developed medical ethical traditions of their own. These include the major religious traditions as well as modern secular liberal political philosophy.

Judaism and Catholicism have long held richly nuanced medical ethical systems. They have manifest themselves in hospitals and medical schools within these traditions, but also in the thinking of health-care professionals and lay persons committed to them. As the Hippocratic tradition has become more problematic, we have found it necessary to reexamine the positions and the moral premises of these religious traditions. This is true not only for institutions and individuals who stand within them, but also for health-care providers and public-policy makers who must deal with patients who express judgments about medical care based on these traditions. We are seeing increasingly that they offer coherent, well-considered alternative views about the way health care ought to be provided. In fact, physicians who have long thought of themselves as members simultaneously of the Hippocratic tradition and of some religious tradition are increasingly discovering that on many issues they must choose between the Hippocratic response and the one favored by their religious tradition. At the minimum, the notion of moral epistemology is radically different. While the Hippocratic tradition relies on organized groups of physicians to determine what is morally required for their role, Judaism relies on rabbinical authority and the Talmudic tradition. Catholicism relies on Papal authority as well as scripture, natural law, church councils, and the Catholic tradition. None of these makes much sense to someone committed to the authority of the profession any more than an appeal to the consensus of organized physicians would make sense to those committed to moral authority as understood by these religious traditions.

Although Protestantism would find appeals to the moral authority of organized medicine as strange as would the other major Western religious groups, it, being inherently more pluralistic and more diverse, has not developed as fully articulated a medical ethic as Judaism and Catholicism. Its medical ethical positions, like its theology, are much more diverse. Nevertheless, there are positions that Protestants tend to share. They sometimes stand in contrast to the dominant professional medical ethical positions within the Hippocratic tradition. For example, Protestants tend to emphasize the importance of the lay person as one who is capable of "reading the text," of looking at information and making decisions for himself or herself—radically in contrast to the Hippocratic view that the lay person cannot be trusted with esoteric medical knowledge. Other positions of mainstream Protestantism provide the foundations for a medical ethical system that in turn provides an alternative to the Hippocratic tradition.

JUDAISM

The Oath of Asaph

Asaph Judaeus (ca. 6th Century C.E.)

───────────────INTRODUCTION TO READING───────────────

One of the most ancient and richly developed alternatives to the Hippocratic tradition is the medical ethic of Judaism. Judaism derives its medical ethical positions from its classical sources—the Old Testament (especially the Torah) and the Talmudic sources and their commentaries. Not only are the sources different from Hippocratic professional medical ethics, but the authoritative interpreters are different. Whereas professional medical groups have tended to turn to the profession itself to interpret moral imperatives, Judaism turns to rabbinical authorities and Jewish councils.

The earliest Jewish medical teacher associated with the ethics of medical practice was Asaph Judaeus whose writings included an *Oath,* which is taken as a summary of the ethics of the Jewish physician. The duties of the Jewish physician are not sharply distinguished from the obligations of any Jew. Hence in the Oath of Asaph, which is included in full here, there is relatively less attention to the specific duties of physicians. It dates from the early centuries of the common era, probably the sixth century.

And this is the oath administered by Asaph, the son of Berachyahu, and by Jochanan, the son of Zabda, to their disciples; and they adjured them in these words: Take heed that ye kill not any man with the sap of a root; and ye shall not dispense a potion to a woman with child by adultery to cause her to miscarry; and ye shall not lust after beautiful women to commit adultery with them; and ye shall not disclose secrets confided unto you; and ye shall take no bribes to cause injury and to kill; and ye shall not harden your hearts against the poor and the needy, but heal them; and ye shall not call good evil or evil good; and ye shall not walk in the way of sorcerers to cast spells, to enchant and to bewitch with intent to separate a man from the wife of his bosom or woman from the husband of her youth.

And ye shall not covet wealth or bribes to abet depraved sexual commerce.

And ye shall not make use of any manner of idol-worship to heal thereby, nor trust in the healing powers of any form of their worship. But rather must ye abhor and detest and hate all their worshippers and those that trust in them and cause others to trust in them, for all of them are but vanity and of no avail, for they are naught; and they are demons. Their own carcasses they cannot save; how, then, shall they save the living?

And now, put your trust in the Lord your God, the God of truth, the living God, for He doth kill and make alive, smite and heal. He doth teach man understanding and also to do good. He smiteth in righteousness and justice and healeth in mercy and loving—kindness. No crafty device can be concealed from Him, for naught is hidden from His sight.

He causeth healing plants to grow and doth implant in the hearts of sages skill to heal by His manifold mercies and to declare marvels to the multitude, that all that live may know that He made them, and that beside Him there is none to save. For the peoples trust in their idols to succour them from their afflictions, but they will not save them in their distress, for their hope and their trust are in the Dead. Therefore it is fitting that ye keep apart from them and hold aloof from all the abominations of their idols and cleave unto the name of the Lord God of all flesh. And every living creature is in His hand to kill and to make alive; and there is none to deliver from His hand.

Be ye mindful of Him at all times and seek Him in truth uprightness and rectitude that ye may prosper in all that ye do; then He will cause you to prosper and ye shall be praised by all men. And the peoples will leave their gods and their idols and will yearn to serve the Lord even as ye do, for they will perceive that they have put their trust in a thing of naught and that their labour is in vain; (otherwise) when they cry unto the Lord, He will not save them.

As for you, be strong and let not your hands slacken, for there is a reward for your labours. God is with you when ye are with Him. If ye will keep His covenant and walk in His statutes to cleave unto them, ye shall be as saints in the sight of all men, and they shall say: "Happy is the people that is in such a case; happy is that people whose God is the Lord."

And their disciples answered them and said: All that ye have instructed us and commanded us, that will we do, for it is a commandment of the Torah, and it behooves us to perform it with all our heart and all our soul and all our might: to do and to obey and to turn neither to the right nor to the left. And they blessed them in the name of the Highest God, the Lord of Heaven and earth.

And they admonished them yet again and said unto them: Behold, the Lord God and His saints and His Torah be witness unto you that ye shall fear Him, turning not aside from His commandments, but walking uprightly in His statutes. Incline not to covetousness and aid not the evildoers to shed innocent blood. Neither shall ye mix poisons for a man or a woman to slay his friend therewith; nor shall ye reveal which roots be poisonous or give them into the hand of any man, or be persuaded to do evil. Ye shall not cause the shedding of blood by any manner of medical treatment. Take heed that ye do not cause a malady to any man; and ye shall not cause any man injury by hastening to cut through flesh and blood with an iron instrument or by branding, but shall first observe twice and thrice and only then shall ye give your counsel.

Let not a spirit of haughtiness cause you to lift up your eyes and your hearts in pride. Wreak not the vengeance of hatred on a sick man; and alter not your prescriptions for them that do hate the Lord our God, but keep his ordinances and commandments and walk in all His ways that ye may find favour in His sight. Be ye pure and faithful and upright.

Thus did Asaph and Jochanan instruct and adjure their disciples.

A Comparison of the Oaths of Hippocrates and Asaph

Shimon Glick

───────────INTRODUCTION TO READING───────────

Shimon Glick, a Talmudic scholar and physician who is Professor of Internal Medicine in the Faculty of Health Science, Ben Gurion University of the Negev, Beer-Sheva, Israel, has provided a comparison of the Hippocratic Oath and that of Asaph. He notes not only the change in the reference to the deities, but also a commitment to provide health care for the poor as well as more subtle differences regarding abortion and sexual relations with patients. Also in striking contrast with the Hippocratic Oath is Asaph's acknowledgment of humility, in which God is recognized as the true healer.

The Hippocratic Oath, administered to new physicians the world over for many centuries, has long been considered the hallmark of the ethical Western physician. It is only recently, with the general breakdown of tradition and the questioning of accepted dogmas that the content of the Oath has been questioned, and in many institutions the Oath is being replaced by other expressions of commitment to ethical behaviour on the part of new physicians.

Jews have a long medical tradition replete with outstanding contributions both to the scientific and the ethical aspects of medicine. In view of this long and distinguished association it is worth examining Jewish ethical attitudes. In spite of the many similarities between different deontological bases for medical ethics it is all the more interesting to examine the differences between the Jewish and the classic Hippocratic point of view. By this examination we can perhaps gain better insight into the essence of Judaism and the Jewish physician, and appreciate the unique contributions Jewish values have made to Western medical ethics.

Perhaps the oldest and best known Jewish medical oath is that of Asaph the physician. Since most authorities believe that it was written several centuries after that of Hippocrates and was in large part based on the Hippocratic Oath it is instructive to examine the unique aspects of the Oath of Asaph.

Perhaps first one ought to pose the question as to why the Oath was so late in coming (probably the 6th century of the common era). I would venture the suggestion that the traditional Jewish point of view reflected the Halakha which forbids unnecessary or superfluous oaths. The classical Jewish view is that every Jew, by virtue of his faith, has already sworn allegiance to the Torah at Sinai, rendering superfluous any subsequent oath essentially to uphold his already assumed obligations. The obligations of the physician are, for the most part, not considered unique but are rather a subset of the obligations of any Jew; therefore a separate oath is unnecessary, and if not needed, is actually interdicted. No reasons are given for the subsequent appearance of such an oath, and most suggested reasons are basically merely speculations. Perhaps the inadequacy, in the mind of the Jewish medical educators, of the existing oaths may have been a stimulus. Alternately perhaps it was just a matter of conforming to the accepted non-Jewish practice of oaths at the end of professional training.

The text of the "oath," unlike that of the Hippocratic Oath, which is voiced actively by the students, is rather a covenant made between Asaph and his students in which the teacher outlines the desired particular behaviour patterns and exhorts the students to carry these out. The students respond, accepting his charge, by saying " . . . for it is a commandment of the Torah and we must do it with all our heart, with all our soul and with all our might . . ." In other words, the obligations are merely a reiteration and extension of their already existing obligations as Jews.

In the text of the oaths one of the obvious differences between the oaths of Hippocrates and Asaph is the identity of the divinity invoked. In the Hippocratic Oath a multiplicity of gods and goddesses including Apollo, Askiepios, Hygieia, Panaceia and "all the gods and goddesses" is invoked, although monotheism had been introduced many centuries earlier among the Jewish people. Asaph refers, of course, to the "Lord G-d", a single entity. These differences are not unexpected, given the differing nature of the Greek and the Jewish theologies. But a more substantive, and perhaps more revealing, difference is the vastly different *role* of the divinities in the two oaths. The gods in the Hippocratic Oath are merely witnesses to the taking of the Oath with neither healing powers, nor those of reward or punishment. More strikingly, there is no indication that the gods might be the source of the ethical standard set by the Oath. In contrast in the Oath of Asaph the divinity is invoked as the ultimate source of healing, of reward and punishment, and especially as the prime source of the ethical code. It is the divinity who obliges all mankind to obey him. The text of Asaph is suffused with religious content, almost half of it being devoted to a praise of G-d, his powers and his demands.

In describing rewards for following a proper path of conduct, Hippocrates promises enjoyment of "life and art", and eternal fame among all men, a reasonable array of earthly rewards. The rewards promised to the students of Asaph are largely spiritual, in that, by setting an example of upright behaviour, "the nations will abandon their idols and images and will desire to worship G-d like you". While Asaph also promised success in all the students' endeavors, this promise is clearly secondary in emphasis to the spiritual rewards.

The Hippocratic oath's first subject, occupying almost a third of the text, relates to respect for one's teachers, to the family of one's teachers, and to one's students. The physician promises to teach his teachers' children the art of medicine free of charge, and prescribes that the teaching of medicine be limited to those who have taken the Oath. In spite of much that is laudable in this section it also carries very distinct guild connotations, which indeed characterized Greek medicine. No such references are found in Asaph's Oath, although respect for teachers is a major characteristic of Jewish tradition. But the granting of favoritism in education is antithetical to Judaism, and the subject could receive no priority in the oath of a physician.

The Oath of Asaph expressly emphasizes the obligation to provide health care for the poor: "Do not harden your heart from pitying the poor and healing the needy," a point not mentioned at all in the Hippocratic Oath. This discrepancy is consistent with the marked, socially accepted, stratification of Greek society. Acquiescence to such discrimination could not be countenanced by the Jewish physician.

The students of Asaph are admonished to refrain from drastic therapy unless they "make an examination two or three times—only then you should give your advice". This humility is in the spirit of most of the Oath which clearly designates G-d as the true healer and regards the physician as merely his messenger. The appropriate attitude is further emphasized by the admonition "you shall not be ruled by a haughty spirit". In the Halakha it is expressly forbidden for the physician to care for a patient if there are others in the community more expert than he. While the Hippocratic Oath does indicate "I will not use the knife, not even on sufferers from stone, but will withdraw in favor of such men as are engaged in this work", it is not clear to what extent this attitude reflects humility, an opposition to surgical treatment, or a gentlemen's agreement not to intrude on the surgeons' province.

Both oaths condemn abortion—the Hippocratic Oath "I will not give to a woman an abortion remedy", and Asaph "Do not make a woman (who is) pregnant (as a result) of whoring to take a drink with a view to causing abortion". It would seem that Asaph has a more "liberal" view towards abortion, in contrast with the blanket prohibition by Hippocrates. This permissiveness is consistent with the Halakha which permits abortion under certain circumstances, largely where the life or health of the mother is threatened, in contrast to the prevailing Roman Catholic view and apparently to the Hippocratic approach.

Both oaths warn about illicit sexual encounters, but the differences here are fascinating. Hippocrates renounces "sexual relations with both female and male persons, be they free or slaves" in the course of visits to patients. Asaph warns: "do not covet beauty of form in women with a view to fornicating with them." Thus the latter, while acknowledging the human tendency to succumb, is concerned only about the extraordinary temptation afforded by beautiful women and does not fear "routine" temptation. It does not occur to him to admonish against homosexual relationships, probably in view of the strong Jewish rejection of homosexuality, and the inconceivability that one of Asaph's students might be so tempted.

Overall Asaph's Oath places great emphasis in extent and in tone on general ethical and religious behaviour, above and beyond the specifics of medical practice, while Hippocrates confines himself to the problems unique to medicine. One might say in modern terminology that while Hippocrates viewed the role of the physician in a relatively constricted professional sense, Asaph preached a broader community–oriented approach.

Finally the oath of Asaph provides a striking example of the Jews' precarious position in their countries of residence. In a classic example of how Jews in the Diaspora regarded themselves not merely as individuals, but as representatives of their people, whose actions could reflect badly or well on their compatriots, Asaph admonishes his students "you will be regarded as his saints by all men, and they will say 'Happy the people whose lot is such, happy the people whose G-d is the Lord'". This is a classic example of a call to *Kiddush Hashem*, sanctification of G-d's name, one of the highest goods for the pious Jew.

In summary a simple comparison of two famous physicians' oaths, superficially similar, casts considerable light on the unique nature of the Jewish physician and his ethical standards as compared to the generally accepted world standard.

Acknowledgment

This paper is dedicated to Professor Joshua Leibowitz, a friend and teacher since our first chance meeting in a synagogue in New Haven, Connecticut, almost thirty years ago. I have always cherished his thoughtful advice, his humanity, modesty and learning. His untiring scholarly efforts over hostile circumstances have overcome apathy and ignorance, and have contributed to the field of the history of medicine in general and to the field of Jewish medical history in particular.

I join his many friends and admirers in wishing him continued health and productive years.

An Obligation to Heal in the Judaic Tradition

J. David Bleich

────────────INTRODUCTION TO READING────────────

Rabbi J. David Bleich, a professor at Yeshiva University in New York, is one of the most widely known contemporary scholars of Jewish Medical Ethics. He is also one of the most thorough. As we see in the following essay, the modern understanding of Jewish ethics in the medical sphere is also quite different from traditional, secular, Hippocratic ethics. In particular there is a rigorous commitment to the sacredness of life and the duty to preserve it, a duty that is much more emphatic than in Hippocratic, Christian, or secular traditions. What follows is a shortened form of an essay that originally addressed ethical decision making in the care of defective newborns. The portion reprinted traces the key moral commitments of Jewish ethics applied to medicine.

In recent years medical science and technology have made tremendous strides. Some diseases have been virtually eradicated; for others effective remedies have been virtually eradicated; for others effective remedies have been found. Concomitantly, ways and means have been developed which enable physicians to sustain life even when known cures do not exist. Maladies and deformities often appear in associated syndromes. While heretofore untreatable conditions now respond to medical ministration, such response is often less than total. Particularly in the case of defective newborns, methods now exist which make it possible to correct certain problems only to leave the patient in a deformed or debilitated state. In such cases questions with regard to the value of the life which is preserved become very real.

The physician's practical dilemma can be stated in simple terms: to treat or not to treat. In deciding whether or not to initiate or maintain such treatment the physician is called upon to make not only medical, but also moral, determinations. There are at least two distinguishable components which present themselves in all such quandaries. The first is a value judgment. Is it desirable that the patient be treated? Should value judgments be made with regard to the quality of life to be preserved? The second question pertains to the physician's personal responsibilities. Under what circumstances and to what extent is the physician morally obligated to persist in rendering aggressive professional care?

The value with which human life is regarded in the Jewish tradition is maximized far beyond the value placed upon human life in the Christian tradition or in Anglo-Saxon common law. In Jewish law and moral teaching, the value of human life is supreme and takes precedence over virtually all other considerations. This attitude is most eloquently summed up in a Talmudic passage regarding the creation of Adam:

> Therefore only a single human being was created in the world, to teach that if any person has caused a single soul of Israel to perish, Scripture regards him as if he had caused an entire world to perish; and if any human being saves a single soul of Israel, Scripture regards him as if he had saved an entire world.[1]

Human life is not a good to be preserved as a condition of other values but as an absolute basic and precious good in its own stead. The obligation to preserve life is commensurately all-encompassing.

Life with suffering is regarded as being, in many cases, preferable to cessation of life and with it elimination of suffering. The Talmud, *Sotah 22a*, and Maimonides, *Hilkhot Sotah* 3:20, indicate that the adulterous woman who was made to drink "the bitter waters" (Num. 6:11-31) did not always die immediately. If she possessed other merit, even though guilty of the offense with which she was charged, the waters, rather than causing her to perish immediately, produced a debilitating and degenerative state which led to a protracted termination of life. The added longevity, although accompanied by pain and suffering, is viewed as a privilege bestowed in recognition of meritorious actions. Life accompanied by pain is thus viewed as preferable to death.

Man does not possess absolute title to his life or to his body. He is but the steward of the life which he has been privileged to receive. Man is charged with preserving, dignifying and hallowing that life. He is obliged to seek food and sustenance in order to safeguard the life he has been granted; when falling victim to an illness and disease, he is obliged to seek a cure in order to sustain life. Never is he called upon to determine whether life is worth living—this is a question over which God remains the sole arbiter.

The value placed upon human life is reflected in Halakhah, the corpus of Jewish law, which provides for the suspension of all religious precepts (with the exception of the prohibition against commission of the three cardinal sins: idolatry, murder and certain sexual offenses) when necessary in order to save life.[2] Even the mere possibility of saving human life mandates violation of such laws "however remote the likelihood of saving human life may be."[3] The quality of life which is thus preserved is never a factor to be taken into consideration. Neither is the length of the survivor's life expectancy a controlling factor. Judaism regards not only human life in general as being of infinite and inestimable value, but regards every moment of life as being of infinite value.[4] Obligations with regard to treatment and cure are one and the same whether the person's life is likely to be prolonged for a matter of years or merely for a few seconds. Thus, even on the Sabbath, efforts to free a victim buried under a collapsed building must be maintained even if the victim is found in circumstances such that he cannot survive longer than a brief period of time.[5] Sectarians such as the Sadducees who lived during the period of the Second Commonwealth and the Karaites of the Geonic period who challenged these provisions of Jewish law and, by implication, the value system upon which they are predicated, were branded heretics.[6]

Defective newborns are known and discussed in rabbinic literature. *Sefer Chasidim*, n. 186, a thirteenth-century compendium authored by R. Judah the Pious, describes the case of a child born with severest of physical deformities and mental deficiencies—a monster-like creature which obviously had no human potential whatsoever. A question was raised as to whether or not the monster-birth might be destroyed. The answer was an emphatic negative. The answer is not at all surprising. Noteworthy is the question. The desire to destroy this creature was predicated upon the fact that the monster-like child was born with ferocious-looking teeth and an elongated tail. In light of these characteristics and in view of the general demeanor of the monster-birth, it was felt by some that this creature constituted a life-threatening menace to the community. In circumstances of lesser gravity it would not have occurred to anyone to raise the question. An early nineteenth-century responsum authored by R. Eliezer Fleckeles, *Teshuvah mei-Ahavah*, I, n. 53, makes much the same point in connection with a somewhat less dramatic situation. A child born of a human mother, despite the possession of animal-like organs and features, is a human being whose life must be protected and preserved.[7] Such a creature may not be killed, nor may it, despite its deformity, be permitted to die as a result of benign neglect.

The obligation to save the life of an endangered person is derived by the Talmud from the verse, "Neither shalt thou stand idly by the blood of thy neighbor" (Lev. 19:16).[8] The Talmud and the various codes of Jewish law offer specific examples of situations in which moral obligation exists with regard to rendering aid. These include the rescue of a person drowning in a river, assistance to one being mauled by wild beasts and aid to a person under attack by bandits.

Application of this principle to medical intervention for the purposes of preserving life is not without theological and philosophical difficulties. It is to be anticipated that a theology which ascribes providential concern to the Deity will view sickness as part of the divine scheme. A personal God does not allow his creatures, over whom He exercises providential guardianship, to become ill unless the affliction is divinely ordained as a means of punishment, for purposes of expiation of sin or for some other beneficial purpose entirely comprehensible to the Deity, if not to man. Thus, while the ancient Greeks regarded illness as a curse and the sick as inferior persons because, to them, malady represented the disruption of the harmony of the body which is synonymous with health, in Christianity suffering was deemed to be a manifestation of divine grace because it effected purification of the afflicted and served as an ennobling process. Since illness resulted in a state of enhanced spiritual perfection, the sick man was viewed as marked by divine favor.

Human intervention in causing or speeding the therapeutic process is, then, in a sense, interference with the deliberate design of providence. The patient in seeking medical attention betrays a lack of faith in failing to put his trust in God. This attitude is reflected in the teaching of a number of early and medieval Christian theologians who counseled against seeking medical attention.[9] The Karaites rejected all forms of human healing and relied entirely upon prayer. Consistent with their fundamentalist orientation, they based their position upon a quite liberal reading of Exodus, chapter 16, verse 26. A literal translation of the Hebrew text of the passage reads as follows. "I will put none of the diseases upon thee which I have put upon the Egyptians, for I am the Lord the physician."[10] Hence, the Karaites taught that God alone should be sought as physician.[11]

This view was rejected by rabbinic Judaism, but not without due recognition of the cogency of the theological argument upon which it is based. Rabbinic teaching recognized that intervention for the purposes of thwarting the natural course of the disease could be sanctioned only on the basis of specific divine dispensation. Such license is found, on the basis of Talmudic exegesis, in the scriptural passage dealing with compensation for personal injury:

> And if other men quarrel with one another and one smiteth the other with a stone or with the fist and he die not, but has to keep in bed . . . he must pay the loss entailed by absence from work and cause him to be thoroughly healed (Exod. 21:19–20).

Ostensibly, this passage refers simply to financial liability incurred as the result of an act of assault. However, since specific reference is made to liability for medical expenses, it follows that liability for such expenses implies biblical license to incur those expenses in the course of seeking the ministrations of a practitioner of the healing arts. Thus, the Talmud, Baba Kama 85a, comments "From here [it is derived] that the physician is granted permission to cure." Specific authorization is required, comments Rashi, in order to teach us that ". . . we are not to say, "How is it that God smites and man heals?" In much the same vein, Tosafot and R. Samuel ben Aderet state that without such sanction, "He who heals might appear as if he invalidated a divine decree."[12]

Nontherapeutic lifesaving intervention is Talmudically mandated on independent grounds. The Talmud, Sanhedrin 73a, posits an obligation to rescue a neighbor from danger such as drowning or being mauled by an animal. This obligation is predicated upon spiritual exhortation with regard to the restoration of lost property, "And thou shalt return it to him" (Deut. 22:2). On the basis of a pleanism in the Hebrew text, the Talmud declares that this verse includes an obligation to restore a fellowman's body as well as his property. Hence, there is created an obligation to come to the aid of one's fellowman in a life-threatening situation. Noteworthy is the fact that Maimonides,[13] going beyond the examples supplied by the Talmud, posits this source as the basis of the obligation to render medical care. Maimonides declares that the biblical commandment "And thou shalt return it to him" establishes an obligation requiring the physician to render professional services in the life-threatening situations. Every individual, insofar as he is able, is obligated to restore the health of a fellowman no less than he is obligated to restore his property. Maimonides views this as a binding religious obligation.

Noteworthy is not only Maimonides' expression of this concept to cover medical matters but also his failure to allude at all to the verse "And he shall surely heal." It would appear that Maimonides is of the opinion that without the granting of specific permission, one would not be permitted to tamper with physiological processes; obligations derived from Deuteronomy, chapter 22, verse 2 would be limited to prevention of accident or assault by man or beast. Dispensation to intervene in the natural order is derived from Exodus, chapter 21, verse 20; but once such license is given, medical therapy is not simply elective but acquires the status of a positive obligation.[14] As indicated by Sanhedrin 73a, this obligation mandates not only the rendering of personal assistance as is the case with regard to the restoration of lost property, but, by virtue of the negative commandment, "You shall not stand idly by the blood of your neighbor" (Lev. 19:16), the obligation is expanded to encompass expenditure of financial resources for the sake of preserving the life of one's fellow-man. This seems to have been the interpretation given to Maimonides' comments by Rabbi Joseph Karo who, in his code of Jewish law, combined both concepts in stating:

> The Torah gave permission to the physician to heal; moreover, this is a religious precept and it is included in the category of saving life; and if the physician withholds this services it is considered as shedding blood.[15]

Nachmanides also finds that the obligation of the physician to heal is inherent in the commandment, "And thou shalt love thy neighbor as thyself" (Lev. 19:18).[16] As an instantiation of the general obligation to manifest love and concern for one's neighbor, the obligation to heal encompasses not only situations posing a threat to life or limb or demanding restoration of impaired health but also situations of lesser gravity warranting medical attention for relief of pain and promotion of well-being.[17]

Despite the unequivocal and authoritative rulings of both Maimonides and Rabbi Joseph Karo, there do exist within the rabbinic tradition dissonant views which look somewhat askance at the practice of the healing arts. Abraham Ibn Ezra[18] finds a contradiction between the injunction "And he shall cause to be thoroughly healed" and the account given in II Chronicles, chapter 16, verse 12. Scripture reports that Asa, King of Judah, became severely ill and in his sickness "he sought not to the Lord, but to the physicians." According to Ibn Ezra, Scripture grants license for therapeutic intervention only for treatment of external wounds. Wounds inflicted by man, either by design or by accident, may legitimately be treated by any means known to mankind. That which has been inflicted by man may be cured by man. However, internal wounds or physiological disorders, according to this view, are not encompassed in the injunction "and he shall cause to be thoroughly healed." Such afflictions are presumed to be manifestations of divine rebuke or punishment and only God, Who afflicts, may heal.

Needless to say, Ibn Ezra's position was rejected by normative Judaism as is most eloquently demonstrated by the ruling recorded in *Shulchan Arukh, Orach Chayyim* 328:3. Jewish law not only sanctions but requires suspension of Sabbath restrictions for treatment of a person afflicted by a life-threatening malady. Orach Chayyim 328:3 rules blanketly that all "internal wounds" are to be presumed to be life-threatening for purposes of Halakhah. Quite obviously, Jewish law as coded mandates treatment of even internal disorders by means of all therapeutic techniques. R. Zemach Duran, while acknowledging Ibn Ezra's outstanding competence as a biblical exegete, had little regard for the latter's legal acumen and dismisses him as "not having been proficient in the laws."[19]

Of greater relevance in the formulation of Jewish thought are the comments of Nachmanides in his *Commentary of the Bible*, Leviticus, chapter 26, verse 11.

It is, however, entirely possible that Nachmanides' comments are intended only as a description of conditions prevailing in a spiritual utopia. In developing his theory of providence, Maimonides explains that the quality of providential guardianship extended to man is directly correlative with man's spiritual attainment. To the extent that man is lacking in perfection his condition is regulated by the laws of nature.[20] Thus a pious person privileged to be the recipient of a high degree of providential guardianship would not require medication, but might expect to be healed by God directly. Other individuals, not beneficiaries of this degree of providence, are perforce required to seek a cure by natural means. In doing so they incur no censure whatsoever. Indeed, Nachmanides prefaces his comments with a reference to such times when the people of "Israel are perfect" and specifically states that failure to seek medical attention was normative only "for the righteous" and even for them solely "during the time of prophecy." Lesser individuals living in spiritually imperfect epochs are duty-bound to seek the cures made available by medical science. Understood in this manner, there is no contradiction between Nachmanides and the Talmudic references cited, or, for that manner, between Nachmanides and Maimonides.[21] In terms of normative Jewish law, there is no question that there exists a positive obligation to seek medical care.[22]

However, in the absence of specific spiritual license to practice and to seek the benefits of the healing arts, the Jewish faith community would be a community of faith healers.[23] Thus, despite the serious nature of the halakhic imperative with regard to the preservation of human life, it is not surprising that this imperative is somewhat circumscribed insofar as therapeutic preservation of life is concerned. The limited situation in which treatment may be withheld must be carefully delineated.

There is no basis in Jewish teaching for a distinction between ordinary versus extraordinary forms of therapy per se, and, in fact, no rabbinic authority draws such a distinction which is of great relevance. A patient may be compelled to submit to medically indicated therapy. However, declares R. Jacob Emden, *Mor u-Ketziah Orach Chayyim* 328, a distinction must be made between therapeutic procedures of proven efficacy and those of unproven therapeutic value. Acceptance of a therapeutic procedure of known efficacy, known as *refuah bedukah*, is a moral and halakhic imperative. The patient may not terminate or shorten his life either actively or passively. Since God grants dispensation to seek medical cure, use of medicaments or acceptance of surgical intervention in such situations is mandatory. Man may no more abstain from the use of drugs to cure illness than he may abstain from food and drink. However, if the proposed therapy is of unproven value the patient may legitimately refuse treatment. This is true not only when the treatment itself is potentially hazardous, but even if there is no reason to suspect that the proposed treatment may be harmful in any way. In such instances treatment is discretionary; the patient may licitly decline treatment and rely exclusively upon divine providence. R. Emden declares that one who consistently abstains from such modes of therapy "and does not rely upon a human healer and his cure but leaves the matter in the hands of the trustworthy . . . Healer" is praiseworthy. R. Emden, an eighteenth century authority, himself believed that all medical procedures designed to cure internal afflictions were of the latter category. While R. Emden's position must undoubtedly be modified in the light of present-day medical knowledge, the underlying principle is entirely applicable. The patient is morally bound only with regard to the use of medicaments and procedures of demonstrated efficacy. Applying this principle, the patient may legitimately decline a drug or procedure whose curative powers are questionable. This is not to say that a moral obligation to seek a cure exists only if the physician is in a position to guarantee with certainty that a recovery will ensue. The examples given of demonstrable efficacy, viz., amputation of a limb or applications of salves and bandages, certainly are not of absolute curative power. Despite the most attentive medical ministrations, some patients do not recover. However, the procedures enumerated are of known value in treating certain afflictions and hence must be pursued. Nevertheless, drugs or surgical procedures whose causal efficacy is not known with certitude may be rejected by the patient. Experimental procedures, including those which are non-hazardous in nature, certainly fall within this category.

Although there is clear dispensation to intervene in physiological processes for purposes of effecting a cure, it does not follow that a physician may subject a patient to, or that a patient may voluntarily accept, a mode of therapy which involves an element of risk. The question of the moral propriety of hazardous procedures arises in three different contexts.

1. Situations in which the existing condition is such that if the patient is left untreated he will certainly succumb as a result of his illness.
2. Situations in which the prognosis is uncertain. In such cases, the patient, if not treated, or if treated by non-hazardous procedures may or may not survive, whereas if treated, the hazards of the illness are replaced by the hazards of the treatment.
3. Situations in which the malady is not a life-threatening one, but treatment which is, hazardous in nature is indicated as a means of relieving agony, discomfort or disfigurement.

It is a principle of Jewish law that the obligation to cure and to preserve life is not limited to situations in which it may be anticipated that subsequent to therapy the patient will have a normal life expectancy. As noted, the Talmud, *Yoma* 85a, clearly indicates that a victim trapped under the debris of a fallen wall is to be rescued even if as a result of such efforts his life will be prolonged only a matter of moments. Not only is every human life of infinite value, but every moment of human life is of infinite value. Accordingly, ritual restrictions such as Sabbath laws are suspended even for the most minimal prolongation of life.

However, when minimal duration of life (*chayyei sha'ah*) is weighed against the possibility of cure accompanied by normal life expectancy, Jewish teaching accepts the principle that reasonable risks may be incurred in order to effect a recovery. This is the case even if the proposed therapy is of such a nature that the drug or procedure may prove to be ineffective and the patient's life shortened thereby. Based upon Talmudic discussion, R. Meir Posner, *Bet Meir, Yoreh*

De'ah 339:1 and R. Jacob Reisher, *Shevut Ya'akov*, III, n. 84,[24] specifically permit use of a hazardous drug which might cause death to result "within an hour or two" on behalf of a patient who would otherwise have lived for "a day or two days." Despite the brevity of the period of time which the patient might have been expected to live without therapy, *Shevut Ya'akov* mandated consultation with "proficient medical specialists in the city" and ruled that therapy was to be instituted only if the physicians recommended it by at least a majority of two to one. He further required that the approval of the local rabbinic authority be obtained before such recommendations are acted upon.

An apparent contradiction to this position is found in *Sefer Chasidim*, n. 467. This source describes a folk remedy consisting of "grasses" or herbs administered by "women" in treatment of certain maladies which either cured or killed the person so threatened within a period of days. *Sefer Chasidim* admonishes that they "will certainly be punished for they have killed a person before his time." R. Shlomo Mordechai Shwadron, *Orchot Chayyim*, *Orach Chayyim* 318:10, resolves this contradiction by stating that the instance discussed by *Sefer Chasidim* involved a situation in which there was clearly a possibility for cure without hazardous intervention. According to this analysis *Sefer Chasidim* set forth the commonsense approach that hazardous procedures dare not be instituted unless conventional, non-hazardous approaches have been exhausted.

In none of these sources does one find a discussion or a consideration of the statistical probability of prolonging life versus the mortality rate or the odds of shortening life. Yet certainly, in weighing the advisability of instituting hazardous therapy, the relative possibility of achieving a cure is a factor to be considered. *Bet David* II, n. 340, permits intervention even if there exists but one chance in a thousand that the proposed drug will be efficacious whereas there are nine hundred and ninety-nine chances that it will hasten the death of the patient. A differing view is presented by R. Joseph Hochgelerenter, *Mishnat Chakhamin*, who refuses to sanction hazardous therapy unless there is at least a fifty percent chance of survival.[25] He further requires, as did Shevut Ya'akov, that dispensation be obtained from ecclesiastical authorities on each occasion that such therapy is administered. Rabbi Moses Feinstein, a foremost contemporary authority, however, rules that, where in the absence of intervention death is imminent, a hazardous procedure may be instituted as long as there is a "slim" (*safek rachok*) chance of a cure, even though the chances of survival are "much less than even" and it is in fact almost certain that the patient will die.[26]

A much earlier authority, R. Moses Sofer, refused to sanction a hazardous procedure in which the chances of effecting a cure were "remote"[27] but offers no mathematical criteria with regard to the nature of mortality risks which may be properly assumed.

Tiferet Yisrael raises a quite different question in discussing the permissibility of prophylactic inoculation which are themselves hazardous. In the situation described, the patient, at the time of treatment, is at no risk whatsoever. The fear is that he will contact a potentially fatal disease, apparently smallpox. The inoculation, however, does carry with it a certain degree of immediate risk. *Tiferet Yisrael* justifies acceptance of the risk which he estimates as being "one in a thousand" because the statistical danger of future contagious infection is greater.[28]

At least one contemporary author differentiates between various cases on the basis of the nature of the risk involved, rather than on the basis of anticipated rates of survival. Rabbi Moshe Dov Welner[29] argues that hazardous procedures may be undertaken despite inherent risks only if therapeutic nature of the procedure has been demonstrated. For example, a situation might present itself which calls for administration of a drug with known curative potential but which is also toxic in nature. The efficacy of the drug is known but its toxicity may, under certain conditions, kill the patient. The drug may be administered in anticipation of a cure despite the known statistical risk, argues Rabbi Welner, could not be sanctioned in administering an experimental drug whose curative powers are unknown or have heretofore not been demonstrated.

A related problem is the attitude toward hazardous therapy for alleviation of pain or other symptoms rather than for the cure of a potentially fatal illness. R. Jacob Emden adopts a somewhat ambivalent position with respect to the question.[30] This authority refers specifically to the surgical removal of gall stones, a procedure designed to correct a condition which he viewed as presenting no hazard to life or health but recognized as being excruciatingly painful. He remarks that, in the absence of danger to life, those who submit to surgery "do not act correctly" and that the procedure is not "entirely permissible." R. Emden carefully stops short of branding the procedure sinful.

The permissibility of placing one's life in danger when not afflicted by a life-threatening malady does, however, require justification. The great value placed upon preservation of life augurs against placing oneself in a risk situation. In general, Jewish law teaches that man may not expose himself to danger. An entire section of the Code of Laws (*Yoreh De'ah* II, 116,) is devoted to an enumeration of actions and situations which must be avoided because they present an element of risk. One hypothesis which may be advanced in sanctioning risks undertaken in a medical context is that the verse "and he shall cause to be thoroughly healed" grants blanket dispensation for any sound medical practice. That such dispensation is included within the framework of this mandate may be demonstrated in the following manner: It is beyond dispute that an aggressor is liable for medical expenses even if the wound inflicted is not potentially lethal. It follows that the physician is permitted, and indeed obligated, to treat patients who suffer from afflictions which are not life-threatening. This is certainly the case when the treatment itself poses no danger. The sole question is with regard to justification of hazardous treatment on non-life-threatening afflictions.

Justification for this position may be found in statements of Nachmanides[31] and Rabbenu Nissim Gerondi.[32] These authorities both comment that all modes of therapy are potentially dangerous. In the words of Rabbenu Nissim, "All modes of therapy are a danger for the patient for it is possible that if the physician errs with regard to a specific drug, it will kill the patient." Nachmanides states even more explicitly, "With regard to cures there is naught but danger; what heals one kills another." Nevertheless, healing—even of non-life-threatening afflictions—is sanctioned by Scripture. Apparently then, since even therapy is fraught with danger, the hazards of treatment are specifically sanctioned when incurred in conjunction with a therapeutic protocol. Accordingly, the practice of the healing arts, despite the hazards involved, cannot be branded as sinful even if designed simply for the alleviation of pain.

Utilizations of medical procedures which are ordinary and usual but which carry with them an element of risk may perhaps be justified on other grounds as well. The Talmud in a variety of instances[33] indicates that a person may engage in commonplace activities even though he places himself in a position of danger on doing so. In justifying such conduct the Talmud declares, "Since many have trodden thereon 'the Lord preserveth the simple'" (Ps. 116:6). The principle enunciated in this dictum is that man is justified in placing his trust in God provided that the risk involved is of a type which is commonly accepted as a reasonable one by society at large. It may readily be argued that any accepted therapeutic procedure may be classified in this manner.[34]

The physician may withhold otherwise mandatory treatment only when the patient has reached the state of gesisah, i.e. the patient has become moribund and death is imminent. Jewish laws with regard to care of the dying are spelled out with care and precision. One must not pry his jaws, anoint him, wash him, plug his orifices, remove the pillow from underneath him or place on the ground.[35] It is also forbidden to close his eyes "for whoever closes the eyes with the onset of death is a shedder of blood."[36] Each of these acts is forbidden because the slightest movement of the patient may hasten death. As the Talmud puts it, "The matter may be compared to a flickering flame: as soon as one touches it, the light is extinguished."[37] Accordingly, any movement or manipulation of the dying person is forbidden.

Although euthanasia in any form is forbidden and the hastening of death even by a matter of moment is regarded as tantamount to murder, there is one situation in which treatment may be withheld from the moribund patient in order to provide an unimpeded death. While the death of a goses may not be speeded, there is no obligation to perform any action which will lengthen the life of the patient in this state. The distinction between an active and a passive act applies to a goses and to a goses only. When a patient is, as it were, actually in the clutches of the angel of death and the death process has actually begun, there is no obligation to heal. Therefore, Rema permits the removal of "anything which constitutes a hindrance to the departure of the soul, such as a clattering noise or salt upon his tongue . . . since such acts involve no active hastening of death but only the removal of the impediment."[38] Some authorities not only sanction withholding of treatment but prohibit any action which may prolong the agony of a goses.[39]

It cannot be overemphasized that even acts of omission are permitted only when the patient is in a state of gesisah. At any earlier stage withholding of treatment is tantamount to euthanasia. What are the criteria indicative of the onset of this state? Rema defines this state as being that of the patient who brings up a secretion in his throat on account of the narrowing of his chest."[40] Of course, if the condition is reversible there is an obligation to heal. When the condition of gesisah is irreversible there is no obligation to continue treatment and according to some authorities, even a prohibition against prolonging the life of the moribund patient.

It appears that this state is not determined by a patient's ability to survive solely by natural means for this period unaided by drugs or medication. The implication is that goses is one who cannot, under any circumstances, be maintained alive for a period of seventy-two hours. Testimony with regard to the existence of a state of gesisah as conclusive evidence of impending death implies that the state is not only irreversible but also prolongable even by artificial means. Otherwise there would exist a legal suspicion that life may have been prolonged artificially by means of extraordinary medical treatment. The obvious conclusion to be drawn is that if it is medically feasible to prolong life the patient is indeed not a goses and, therefore, in such instances there is a concomitant obligation to preserve the life of the patient as long as possible.

It follows that a specific physiological condition may or may not correspond to a state of gesisah depending upon the state of medical knowledge of the day. When medicine is of no avail and the patient will expire within seventy-two hours, he is deemed to be in the process of "dying." When, however, medication can prolong life such medicine, in effect, delays the onset of the death process. Accordingly, the patient who receives medical treatment enabling him to survive for a period of three days or more is not yet in the process of "dying." It follows, therefore, that those responsible for his care are not relieved of their duty to minister to his needs and to postpone the onset of death by means of medical treatment.

The aggressiveness with which Judaism teaches that life must be preserved is not at all incompatible with the awareness that the human condition is such that there are circumstances in which man would prefer death to life. The Talmud reports[41] that Rabbi Judah the Prince, redactor of the *Mishnah*, was afflicted by what appears to have been an incurable intestinal disorder and as a result suffered from an apparently debilitating form of dysentery. R. Judah had a female servant who is depicted in rabbinic writings as being a woman of exemplary piety and moral character. This woman is reported to have prayed for the death of R. Judah. On the basis of this narrative, a thirteenth century commentator, Rabbenu Nissim Gerondi[42] states that it is permissible and even praiseworthy to pray for the death of a patient who is gravely ill and in extreme pain. He chides those who are remiss in discharging the obligation of visiting the sick, remarking of such an individual ". . . not only does he not aid [the patient] in living but even when [the patient] would [derive] benefit from death, even that small benefit [prayer for his demise] he does not bestow upon him."

The gift of life, bestowed by God, can be reclaimed only by Him. Man dare not push the divine hand, so to speak, through an overt action but may, through prayer, presume to tell God what to do.

There is one responsum in particular which deals with the question of prayer for termination of suffering through death, but which has important implications for decision making in general. R. Chaim Palaggi, *Chikekei Lev, I, Yoreh De'ah*, n. 50, accepts the view of Rabbenu Nissim but expresses an important *Iaveat*. According to this authority only totally disinterested parties may lead to a premature termination of life. Husband, children, family, and those charged with the care of the patient, according to R. Palaggi, may not pray for death. The considerations underlying this reservation are twofold in nature. (1) Those who are emotionally involved, if they are permitted even such nonphysical methods of intervention as prayer, may be prompted to perform an overt act which would have the effect of shortening life and thus be tantamount to euthanasia; (2) Precisely because of their closeness to the situation they are psychologically incapable of reaching a detached, dispassionate and objective opinion in which considerations of patient benefit are the sole controlling motives. The human psyche is such that the intrusion of emotional involvement and subjective interest preclude a totally objective and disinterested decision.

Decisions that are available therapeutic methods shall not be employed because they are hazardous or of insufficiently demonstrated efficacy or a decision that the patient is already in a state of gesisah are also subject to unconscious bias because of the inability of the family and physician totally to transcend their personal and emotional involvement with the patient. It is entirely in keeping with these considerations that Jewish scholars have insisted that the pertinent facts be placed before a rabbinic decision for adjudication on a case by case basis.

The thrust of the material which has been presented argues in favor of aggressive treatment of defective newborns regardless of the extent of their impairment or the quality of life which may be conserved by such treatment. It is unlikely that its impact upon these physicians who, to a greater or lesser extent, practice selective nontreatment on a routine basis will be sufficiently strong to effect a dramatic volte-face. Nevertheless, this modest effort will have achieved a modicum of success if those engaged in the practice of medicine become sensitized to the issues which have been raised and achieve an awareness of the existence of a rich theological and ethical tradition which cannot acquiesce, much less sanction, the current practice of many physicians.

When analyzing treatment versus nontreatment, informed consent, if it is to be fully informed, should entail an awareness on the part of the person granting consent not only of the medical hazards involved but also of the moral dilemmas present in such a decision. The patient or next of kin should be fully informed with regard to conflicting medical opinion and counsel; He should be equally aware of moral traditions which conflict with a course of action advocated by the medical practitioners. The physician seeking consent is bound in conscience to be absolutely certain that the patient of next of kin is fully informed, both medically and morally.

The rabbinic tradition was fully cognizant of these factors in its insistence upon multiple medical consultation and in its demand that the medical data be placed before a competent rabbinic authority prior to initiation of hazardous therapy or withholding of life-supporting measures. The rabbi served as an ethicist, a qualified expert capable of dispassionate examination of the data and of reaching a determination based upon the ethical principle of his moral tradition.

The rabbi-ethicist presents a role model which might be emulated by society with great moral profit. A qualified and professionally trained ethicist could be an invaluable addition to the hospital staff. In a pluralistic society the ethicist would most emphatically not serve as a decision maker. He would, however, be singularly qualified to analyze and interpret the medical information upon which decision making is based so the patient and his family would be in a position to make an informed medical decision. He would be available to analyze and discuss any moral issues which might be confronted in making such decisions. The ethicist's position would be that of analyst and discussant—not that of advisor. The information transmitted by a trained ethicist in an objective and impartial manner would enable the patient and his family to turn to their own moral and spiritual counselors, if they should desire to do so, for advice consonant with their own religious traditions. The inclusion of an ethicist as a member of the health care team would assure that the decision reached is both a medically and morally informed decision.

Notes

1. Sanhedrin 37a.

2. Yoreh De'ah 157:1.

3. Orach Chayyim 329:3.

4. See R. Yechiel Michal Tucatzinsky, *The Death Penalty According to the Torah in the Past and the Present*, Ha-Torah ve-ha-Medinah 2 IV, 34 (1952) and V–VI 331–334 (1953–1954).

5. Orach Chayyim 329:4.

6. See Hamburger, Real-Encyclopaedie fur Bibel und Talmud, Supplement II 37 (1901); Zimmels, Magicians, Theologians and Doctors 172 n. 72 (1952).

7. It is of interest to compare this view with that of Martin Luther who refused to baptize deformed children and who declared that they ought to be drowned because they have no soul. See McKenzie, *The Infancy of Medicine: An Enquiry into the Influence of Folklore Upon the Evolution of Scientific Medicine 313* (1927).

8. Sanhedrin 73a.

9. See Allbutt, Greek Medicine in Rome 402 (1921).

10. See Abraham Ibn Ezra, Commentary on the Bible, ad locum.

11. See A. Harkavy, Likutei Kadmoniyot II, 148 (1903); Harry Friedenwald, The Jews and Medicine 9 (1944).

12. See commentaries of Tosafot and Rashba, ad locum.

13. Commentary on the Mishnah, Nedarim 4:4; cf. Maimonides, Mishneh Torah, Hilkhot Nedarim 6:8.

14. Cf. R. Barukh Ha-Levi Epstein, Torah Temimah, Exodus 21:19 and Deuteronomy 22:2. This explanation of Maimonides' apparent contradiction of the Talmudic text as well as the comments of Torah Temimah contradict Jakobovits' statement to the effect that Maimonides' system does not require biblical sanction for the practice of medicine. See Immanuel Jakobovits, *Jewish Medical Ethics* 260 n. 8 (1959). See infra note 83.

15. Yoreh De'ah 336:1. See Eliezer Waldenberg, *Ramat Rachel* no. 21 and id. *Tritz Eliezer X*, n. 25, chap. 7.

16. Nachmanides, Torah Ha-Adam, Kitvei Ramban II, 43 (B. Cheval ed. 5724).

17. Waldenberg, Ramat Rachel n. 21.

18. Ibn Ezra, *supra note* 67, Exodus 21:19.

19. R. Zemach Duran, Teshuvot Tashbatz I, n. 51. Nevertheless Ibn Ezra's interpretation of Exodus 21:19 is followed by the fourteenth-century biblical exegete, Rabbenu Bachya, in his commentary on that passage and R. Johnathan Eybeschutz, Kereiti U-Peleiti, Tiferet Yisra'El, Yoreh De'Ah 188:5.

20. Maimonides, Guide of the Perplexed III, chaps. 17–18.

21. This appears to be the manner in which Nachmanides was interpreted by R. David Ben Shmuel Ha-Levi, Taz, Yoreh De'Ah 336:1; see also R. Eliyahu Dessler, Mikhtav MeiEliyahu III, 170–175 (5725) and Waldenberg, supra note 74, n. 20, 3.

22. See Bachya Ibn Pakuda, Chovat Ha-Levavot, Sha'Ar Ha-Bitachon chap. 4; R. Simon Ben Zemach Duran, Teshuvot Tashbatz III, n. 82; R. Joel Serkes, Bayit Chadash, Yoreh De'Ah 336:2 R. Abraham Gumbiner, Magen Avraham, Orach Chayyim 328:6; R. Moses Sofer, Teshuvot Chatam Sofer, Orach Chayyim n. 176; Besamim Rosh n. 386; R. Ya'akov Ettlinger, Binyan Zion n. 111; R. Nissim Abraham Ashkenazi, Ma'Aseh Avraham, Yoreh De'Ah n. 55; R. Nathan Nate Landau, Kenaf Renanah, Orach Chayyim n. 60; R. Ovadiah Yosef, Yabi'a Omer, IV, Choshen Mishpat n. 6, 4; R. Moses Ben Abraham Mat, Matteh Mosheh IV, chap. 3; R. Samson Morpug, Shemesh Tzdakah, Yoreh De'Ah n. 29; R. Chaim Yosef David Azulai, Birkei Yosef, Yoreh De'Ah 336:2; R. Yehudah Eyash, Shivtei Yehudah n. 336; Waldenberg supra note 74 n. 20; id. tzitz Eli'ezer IX, n. 17, chap.6, 17; X, n. 25, chap. 19; XI, n. 41, chap. 20; R. Ya'Akov Prager, Sheilat Ya-Akov n. 5.

23. See R. Abraham Danzig, Chokhmat Adam 141:25.

24. See also Ettlinger, supra note 82; Waldenberg, supra note 82, IV, n. 13; R. Israel Lipshitz, Tiferet Yisrael, YOMA, 8:41; R. Shlomo Eger, Gilyon Maharsha, Yoreh De'Ah 155:1.

25. This is also the position of Waldenberg, supra note 82, X, n. 25, chap. 5, 5. Cf. R. Chaim Ozer Grodzinski, Teshuvot Achi'Ezer, Yoreh De'Ah n. 16, 8.

26. Igrot Moshe, Yoreh De'Ah II, n. 58.

27. Teshuvot Chatam Sofer, Yoreh De'Ah n. 76.

28. Bo'Az, Yoma 8:3.

29. Ha-Torah Ve-Ha-Medinah VII-VIII, 314 (1956–1957).

30. R. Jacob Embden, Mor U-Ketziah, Orach Chayyim 338.

31. Nachmanides, supra note 73.

32. Rabbenu Nissim Gerondi, Commentary to Sanhedrin 84b.
33. Shabbat 128b; Avodah Zarah 30b; Niddah 31a; & Yevamot 72a.
34. Cf. R. Ya'Akov Breish, Chelkat Ya'Akov III, n. 11.
35. Yoreh De'Ah 339:1.
36. Id.
37. Shabbat 151b: & Semachot 1:4.
38. Yoreh De'Ah 339:1.
39. Teshuvot Bet Ya'Akov n. 59; Moshe, supra note 86, II, n. 174; cf also R. Moses Isserles, Darkei Mosheh, Yoreh De'Ah 339; however, Shevut Ya'Akov I, n. 13, Bi'Ur Halakhah, Orach Chayyim 329:2; and Waldenberg, supra note 74, n. 28, see no prohibition against prolonging the life of a goses; the latter two authorities view prolongation by means of accepted medical treatment as obligatory.
40. Even Ha'Ezer 121:7 and Choshen Mishpat 221:2.
41. Ketubot 104a.
42. Rabbenu Nissim Gerondi, Commentary to Nedarim 40a.

ROMAN CATHOLOCISM

Ethical and Religious Directives for Catholic Health Care Services

National Conference of Catholic Bishops

———————————— INTRODUCTION TO READING ————————————

Roman Catholic moral theology also has a long history of interest in medical ethics. Like Judaism its medical ethic is derived from its systematic theological commitments. As such, it may not always be compatible with the Hippocratic tradition. Moreover, its source of authority is more appropriately church authority rather than medical authority. Centuries of writings articulate positions within Catholicism on classical moral dilemmas including not only abortion and contraception, but also the care of the terminally ill and all other categories of medical problems. In the selection that follows, a code of ethics adopted by the National Conference of Catholic Bishops demonstrates many of the classical Catholic positions including the doctrine of double effect, the distinction between ordinary and extraordinary means, and the criterion of proportionality.

Preamble

Health care in the United States is marked by extraordinary chance. Not only is there continuing change in clinical practice due to technological advances, but the health care system in the United States is being challenged by both institutional and social factors as well. At the same time, there are a number of developments within the Catholic Church affecting the ecclesial mission of health care. Among these are significant changes in religious orders and congregations, the increased involvement of lay men and women, a heightened awareness of the church's social role in the world and developments in moral theology since the Second Vatican Council. A contemporary understanding of the Catholic health care ministry must take into account the new challenges presented by transitions both in the church and in American society.

Throughout the centuries, with the aid of other sciences a body of moral principles has emerged that expresses the church's teaching on medical and moral matters and has proven to be pertinent and applicable to the ever-changing circumstances of health care and its delivery. In response to today's challenges, these same moral principles of Catholic teaching provide the rationale and direction for this revision of the "Ethical and Religious Directives for Catholic Health Care Services."

These directives presuppose our statement "Health and Health Care," published in 1981.[1] There we presented the theological principles that guide the church's vision of health care, called for all Catholics to share in the healing mission of the church, expressed our full commitment to the health care ministry and offered encouragement to all those who are involved in it. Now, with American health care facing even more dramatic changes, we reaffirm the church's commitment to health care ministry and the distinctive Catholic identity of the church's institutional health care services.[2] The purpose of these ethical and religious directives then is twofold: first, to reaffirm the ethical standards of behavior in health care which flow from the church's teaching, about the dignity of the human person; second, to provide authoritative guidance on certain moral issues which face Catholic health care today.

The ethical and religious directives are concerned primarily with institutionally based Catholic health care services. They address the sponsors, trustees, administrators, chaplains, physicians, health care personnel and patients or residents of these institutions and services. Since they express the church's moral teaching, these directives also will be helpful to Catholic professionals engaged in health care services in other settings. The moral teachings that we profess here flow principally from the natural law, understood in the light of the revelation Christ has entrusted to his church. From this source the church has derived its understanding of the nature of the human person, of human acts and of the goals that shape human activity.

The directives have been refined through an extensive process of consultation with bishops, theologians, sponsors, administrators, physicians and other health care providers. While providing standards and guidance, the directives do not cover in detail all of the complex issues that confront Catholic health care today. Moreover, the directives will be reviewed periodically by the National Conference of Catholic Bishops, in the light of authoritative church teaching, in order to address new insights from theological and medical research or new requirements of public policy.

The directives begin with a general introduction that presents a theological basis for the Catholic health care ministry. Each of the six parts that follows is divided into two sections. The first section is in expository form; it serves as an introduction and provides the context in which concrete issues can be discussed from the perspective of the Catholic faith. The second section is in prescriptive form; the directives promote and protect the truths of the Catholic faith as those truths are brought to bear on concrete issues in health care.

General Introduction

The church has always sought to employ our Savior's concern for the sick. The Gospel accounts of Jesus' ministry draw special attention to his acts of healing: He cleansed a man with leprosy (Mt. 8:1–4; Mk. 1:40-42); he gave sight to two people who were blind (Mt. 20:29–34; Mk. 10:46–52); he enabled one who was mute to speak (Lk. 11:14); he cured a woman who was hemorrhaging (Mt. 9:20–22; Mk. 5:25–34); and he brought a young girl back to life (Mt. 9:18, 23–25; Mk. 5:35–42). Indeed, the Gospels are replete with examples of how the Lord cured every kind of ailment and disease (Mt. 9:35). In the account of Matthew, Jesus' mission fulfilled the prophecy of Isaiah: "He took away our infirmities and bore our diseases". (Mt. 8:17; cf. Is. 53:4). Jesus' healing mission went further than caring only for physical affliction. He touched people at the deepest level of their existence; he sought their physical, mental and spiritual healing (Jn. 6:35; 11:25–27). He "came so that they might have life and have it more abundantly" (Jn. 10: 10).

The mystery of Christ casts light on every facet of Catholic health care: to see Christian love as the animating principle of health care; to see healing and compassion as a continuation of Christ's mission; to see suffering as a participation in the redemptive power of Christ's passion, death and resurrection; and to see death, transformed by the resurrection, as an opportunity for a final act of communion with Christ.

For the Christian, our encounter with suffering and death can take on a positive and distinctive meaning through the redemptive power of Jesus' suffering and death. As St. Paul says, we are "always carrying about in the body the dying of Jesus, so that the life of Jesus may also be manifested in our body" (2 Cor. 4:10). This truth does not lessen the pain and fear, but gives confidence and grace for bearing suffering rather than being overwhelmed by it. Catholic health care ministry bears witness to the truth that, for those who are in Christ, suffering and death are the birth pangs of the new creation. "God himself will always be with them. He will wipe every tear from their eyes and there shall be no more death or mourning, wailing or pain, for the old order has passed away" (Rv. 21:3–4).

In faithful imitation of Christ, the church has served the sick, suffering and dying in various ways throughout history. The zealous service of individuals and communities has provided shelter for the traveler, infirmaries for the sick and homes for children, adults and the elderly.[3] In the United States, the many religious communities as well as dioceses that sponsor and staff this country's Catholic health care institutions and services have established an effective Catholic presence in health care. Modeling their efforts on the Gospel parable of the good Samaritan, these communities of women and men have exemplified authentic neighborliness to those in need (Lk 10:25–37). The church seeks to ensure that the service offered in the past will be continued into the future.

While many religious communities continue their commitment to the health care ministry, lay Catholics increasingly have stepped forward to collaborate in this ministry. Inspired by the example of Christ and mandated by the Second Vatican Council, lay faithful are invited to a broader and more intense field of ministries than in the past.[4] By virtue of their baptism, lay faithful are called to participate actively in the church's life and mission.[5] Their participation and leadership in the health care ministry, through new forms of sponsorship and governance of institutional Catholic health care, are essential for the church to continue her ministry of healing and compassion. They are joined in the church's health care mission by many men and women who are not Catholic.

Catholic health care expresses the healing ministry of Christ in a specific way within the local church. Here the diocesan bishop exercises responsibilities that are rooted in his office as pastor, teacher and priest. As the center of unity in the diocese and coordinator of ministries in the local church, the diocesan bishop fosters the mission of Catholic health care in a way that promotes collaboration among health care leaders, providers, medical professionals, theologians and other specialists. As pastor, the diocesan bishop is in a unique position to encourage the faithful to greater responsibility in the healing ministry of the church. As teacher, the diocesan bishop ensures the moral and religious identity of the health care ministry in whatever setting it is carried out in the diocese. As priest, the diocesan bishop oversees the sacramental care of the sick. These responsibilities will require that Catholic health care providers and diocesan bishops engage in ongoing communication on ethical and pastoral matters that require his attention.

In a time of new medical discoveries, rapid technological developments and social change, what is new can either be an opportunity for genuine advance in human culture or it can lead to policies and actions that are contrary to the true dignity and vocation of the human person. In consultation with medical professionals, church leaders review these developments, judge them according to the principles of right reason and the ultimate standard of revealed truth, and offer authoritative teaching and guidance about the moral and pastoral responsibilities entailed by the Christian faith.[6] While the church cannot furnish a ready answer to every moral dilemma, there are many questions about which she provides normative guidance and direction. In the absence of a determination by the magisterium, but never contrary to church teaching, the guidance of approved authors can offer appropriate guidance for ethical decision making.

Created in God's image and likeness, the human family shares in the dominion which Christ manifested in his healing ministry. This sharing involves a stewardship over all material creation (Gn. 1:26) that should neither abuse nor squander nature's resources. Through science the human race comes to understand God's wonderful work; and through technology it must conserve, protect and perfect nature in harmony with God's purposes. Health care professionals pursue a special vocation to share in carrying forth God's life-giving and healing work.

The dialogue between medical science and Christian faith has for its primary purpose the

common good of all human persons. It presupposes that science and faith do not contradict each other. Both are grounded in respect for truth and freedom. As new knowledge and new technologies expand, each person must form a correct conscience based on the moral norms for proper health care.

Part 1
The Social Responsibility of Catholic Health Care Services

Introduction

Their embrace of Christ's healing mission has led institutionally based Catholic health care services in the United States to become an integral part of the nation's health care system. Today this complex health care system confronts a range of economic, technological, social and moral challenges. The response of Catholic health care institutions and services to these challenges is guided by normative principles that inform the church's healing ministry.

First, Catholic health care ministry is rooted in a commitment to promote and defend human dignity; this is the foundation of its concern to respect the sacredness of every human life from the moment of conception until death. The first right of the human person, the right to life entails a right to the means for the proper development of life such as adequate health care.[7]

Second, the biblical mandate to care for the poor requires us to express this in concrete action at all levels of Catholic health care. This mandate prompts us to work to ensure that our country's health care delivery system provides adequate health care for the poor. In Catholic institutions, particular attention should be given to the health care needs of the poor, the uninsured and the underinsured.[8]

Third, Catholic health care ministry seeks to contribute to the common good. The common good is realized when economic, political and social conditions ensure protection for the fundamental rights of all individuals, and enable all to fulfill their common purpose and reach their common goals.[9]

Fourth, Catholic health care ministry exercises responsible stewardship of available health care resources. A just health care system will be concerned both with promoting equity of care—to assure that the right of each person to basic health care is respected—and with promoting the good health of all in the community. The responsible stewardship of health care resources can be accomplished best in dialogue with people from all levels of society, in accordance with the principle of subsidiarity and with respect for the moral principles which guide institutions and persons.

Fifth, within a pluralistic society Catholic health care services will encounter requests for medical procedures contrary to the moral teachings of the church. Catholic health care does not offend the rights of individual conscience by refusing to provide or permit medical procedures that are judged morally wrong by the teaching authority of the church.

Directives

1.   A Catholic institutional health care service is a community which provides health care to those in need of it. This service must be animated by the Gospel of Jesus Christ and guided by the normal tradition of the church.

2.   Catholic health care should be marked by a spirit of mutual respect among caregivers which disposes them to deal with those it serves and their families with the compassion of Christ, sensitive to their vulnerability at a time of special need.

3.   In accord with its mission, Catholic health care should distinguish itself by service to and advocacy for those people whose social condition puts them at the margins of our society and makes them particularly vulnerable to discrimination: the poor, the uninsured and the underinsured; children, the unborn, single parents and the elderly; those with incurable diseases and chemical dependencies; and racial minorities, immigrants and refugees. In particular, the person with mental or physical disabilities, regardless of the cause or severity, must be treated as a unique person of incomparable worth, with the same right to life and to adequate health care as all other persons.

4.   A Catholic health care institution, especially a teaching hospital, will promote medical research consistent with its mission of providing health care and with concern for the responsible stewardship of health care resources. Such medical research must adhere to Catholic moral principles.

5.   Catholic health care services must adopt these directives as policy, require adherence to them within the institution as a condition for medical privileges and employment, and provide appropriate instruction regarding the directives for administration, medical and nursing staff and other personnel.

6.   A Catholic health care organization should be a responsible steward of the health care resources available to it. Collaboration with other health care providers in ways that do not compromise Catholic social moral teaching can be an effective means of such stewardship.[10]

7.   A Catholic health care institution must treat its employees respectfully and justly. This responsibility includes: equal employment opportunities for anyone qualified for the task, irrespective of a person's race, sex, age, national origin or disability; a workplace that promotes employee participation; a work environment that ensures employee safety and well-being; just compensation and benefits; and recognition of the rights of employees to organize and bargain collectively without prejudice to the common good.

8.   Catholic health care institutions have a unique relationship to both the church and the wider community they serve. Because of the ecclesial nature of this relationship, the relevant requirements of canon law will be observed with regard to the foundation of a new Catholic health care institution, the substantial revision of the mission of an institution and the sale, sponsorship transfer or the closure of an existing institution.

9.   Employees of a Catholic health care institution must respect and uphold the religious mission of the institution and adhere to these directives. They should maintain professional standards and promote the institution's commitment to human dignity and the common good.

Part 2
Pastoral and Spiritual Responsibility of Catholic Health Care

Introduction

The dignity of human life flows from creation in the image of God (Gn. 1:26), from redemption by Jesus Christ (Eph. 1:10; 1 Tm.. 2:4–6) and from our common destiny to share a life with God beyond all corruption (1 Cor. 15:42–57). Catholic health care has the responsibility to treat those in need in a way that respects the human dignity and eternal destiny of all. The words of Christ have provided inspiration for Catholic health care: "I was ill and you cared for me" (Mt. 25:36). The care provided assists those in need to experience their own dignity and value, especially when these are obscured by the burdens of illness or the anxiety of imminent death.

Since a Catholic health care institution is a community of healing and compassion, the care offered is not limited to the treatment of a disease or bodily ailment but embraces the physical, psychological, social and spiritual dimensions of the human person. The medical expertise offered through Catholic health care is combined with other forms of care to promote health and relieve human suffering. For this reason, Catholic health care extends to the spiritual nature of the person.

"Without health of the spirit, high technology focused strictly on the body offers limited hope for healing the whole person."[11] Directed to spiritual needs that are often appreciated more deeply during times of illness, pastoral care is an integral part of Catholic health care. Pastoral care encompasses the full range of spiritual services, including a listening presence, help in dealing with powerlessness, pain and alienation, and assistance in recognizing and responding to God's will with greater joy and peace. It should be acknowledged, of course, that technological advances in medicine have reduced the length of hospital stays dramatically. It follows, therefore, that the pastoral care of patients, especially administration of the sacraments, will be provided more often than not at the parish level, both before and after one's hospitalization. For this reason, it is essential that there be very cordial and cooperative relationships between the personnel of pastoral care departments and the local clergy and ministers of care.

Priests, deacons, religious and laity exercise diverse but complementary roles in this pastoral care. Since many areas of pastoral care call upon the creative response of these pastoral caregivers to the particular needs of patients or residents, the following directives address only a limited number of specific pastoral activities.

Directives

10. A Catholic health care organization should provide pastoral care to minister to the religious and spiritual needs of all those it serves. Pastoral care personnel, clergy, religious and lay alike, should have appropriate professional preparation, including an understanding of these directives.

11. Pastoral care personnel should work in close collaboration with local parishes and community clergy. Appropriate pastoral services and/or referrals should be available to all in keeping with their religious beliefs or affiliation.

12. For Catholic patients or residents provision for the sacraments is an especially important part of Catholic health care ministry. Every effort should be made to have priests assigned to hospitals and health care institutions to celebrate the eucharist and provide the sacraments to patients and staff.

13. Particular care should be taken to provide and to publicize opportunities for patients or residents to receive the sacrament of penance.

14 Properly prepared lay Catholics can be appointed to serve as extraordinary ministers of holy communion, in accordance with canon law and the policies of the local diocese. They should assist pastoral care personnel—clergy, religious and laity—by providing supportive visits, advising patients regarding the availability of priests for the sacrament of penance and distributing holy communion to the faithful who request it.

15. Responsive to a patient's desires and condition, all involved in pastoral care should facilitate the availability of priests to provide the sacrament of anointing of the sick, recognizing that through this sacrament Christ provides

grace and support to those who are seriously ill or weakened by advanced age. Normally, the sacrament is celebrated when the sick person is fully conscious. It may be conferred upon the sick who have lost consciousness or the use of reason if there is reason to believe that they would have asked for the sacrament while in control of their faculties.

16. All Catholics who are capable of receiving communion should receive viaticum when they are in danger of death, while still in full possession of their faculties.[12]

17. Except in cases of emergency (i.e., danger of death), any request for baptism made by adults or for infants should be referred to the chaplain of the institution. Newly born infants in danger of death, including those miscarried, should be baptized if this is possible.[13] In case of emergency, if a priest or deacon is not available, anyone can validly baptize.[14] In the case of emergency baptism, the chaplain or the director of pastoral care is to be notified.

18. When a Catholic who has been baptized but not yet confirmed is in danger of death, any priest may confirm the person.[15]

19. A record of the conferral of baptism or confirmation should be sent to the parish in which the institution is located and posted in its baptism and confirmation registers.

20. Catholic discipline generally reserves the reception of the sacraments to Catholics. In accord with Canon 844.3, Catholic ministers may administer the sacraments of Eucharist, penance and anointing of the sick to members of the Oriental churches which do not have full communion with the Catholic Church or of other churches in the judgment of the Holy See are in the same condition as the Oriental churches, if such persons ask for the sacraments on their own and are properly disposed.

With regard to other Christians not in full communion with the Catholic Church, when the danger of death or other grave necessity is present, the four conditions of Canon 844.4 also must be present, namely, they cannot approach a minister of their own community, they ask for the sacraments on their own, they manifest Catholic faith in these sacraments and they are properly disposed. The diocesan bishop has the responsibility to oversee this pastoral practice.

21. The appointment of priests and deacons to the pastoral care staff of a Catholic institution must have the explicit approval or confirmation of the local bishop in collaboration with the administration of the institution. The appointment of the director of the pastoral care staff should be made in consultation with the diocesan bishop.

22. For the sake of appropriate ecumenical and interfaith relations, a diocesan policy should be developed with regard to the appointment of non-Catholic members to the pastoral care staff of a Catholic health care institution. The director of pastoral care at a Catholic institution should be a Catholic; any exception to this norm should be approved by the diocesan bishop.

Part 3
The Professional-Patient Relationship

Introduction

A person in need of health care and the professional health care provider who accepts that person as a patient enter into a relationship that requires, among other things, mutual respect, trust, honesty and appropriate confidentiality. The resulting free exchange of information must avoid manipulation, intimidation or condescension. Such a relationship enables the patient to disclose personal information needed for effective care and permits the health care provider to use his or her professional competence most effectively to maintain or restore the patient's health. Neither the health care professional nor the patient acts independently of the other; both participate in the healing process.

Today, a patient often receives health care from a team of providers, especially in the setting of the modern acute-care hospital. But the resulting multiplication of relationships does not alter the personal character of the interaction between health care providers and the patient. The relationship of the persons seeking health care and the professionals providing that care is an important part of the foundation on which diagnosis and care are provided. Diagnosis and care therefore entail a series of decisions with ethical as well as medical dimensions. The health care professional has the knowledge and experience to pursue the goals of healing, the maintenance of health and the compassionate care of the dying, taking into account the patient's convictions and spiritual needs, and the moral responsibilities of all concerned. The person in need of health care depends on the skill of the health care provider to assist in preserving life and promoting health of body, mind and spirit. The patient, in turn, has responsibility to use these physical and mental resources in the service of moral and spiritual goals to the best of his or her ability.

When the health care professional and the patient use institutional Catholic health care, they also accept its public commitment to the church's understanding of and witness to the dignity of the human person. The church's moral teaching on health care nurtures a truly interpersonal professional-patient relationship. This professional-patient relationship is never separated, then, from the Catholic identity of the health care institution. The faith that inspires Catholic health care guides medical decisions in ways that fully respect the dignity of the person and the relationship with the health care professional.

Directives

23. The inherent dignity of the human person must be respected regardless of the nature of the person's health problem or social status. The respect for human dignity extends to all persons who are served by Catholic health care.

24. In compliance with federal law, a Catholic health care institution will make available to patients information about their rights, under the laws of their state, to make an advance directive for their medical treatment. The institution, however, will not honor an advance directive that is contrary to

Catholic teaching. If the advance directive conflicts with Catholic teaching, an explanation should be provided as to why the directive cannot be honored.

25. Each person may identify in advance a representative to make health care decisions as his or her surrogate in the event that the person loses the capacity to make health care decisions. Decisions by the designated surrogate should be faithful to Catholic moral principles and to the person's intentions and values or, if the person's intentions are unknown, to the person's best interests. In the event that an advance directive is not executed, those who are in a position to know best the patient's wishes—usually family members and loved ones—should participate in the treatment decisions for the person who has lost the capacity to make health care decisions.

26. The free and informed consent of the person or the person's surrogate is required for medical treatments and procedures, except in an emergency situation when consent cannot be obtained and there is no indication that the patient would refuse consent to the treatment.

27. Free and informed consent requires that the person or the person's surrogate receive all reasonable information about the essential nature of the proposed treatment and its benefits; its risks, side effects, consequences and cost; and any reasonable and morally legitimate alternatives, including no treatment at all.

28. Each person or the person's surrogate should have access to medical and moral information and counseling so as to be able to form his or her conscience. The free and informed health care decision of the person or the person's surrogate is to be followed so long as it does not contradict Catholic principles.

29. All persons served by Catholic health care have the right and duty to protect and preserve their bodily and functional integrity.[16] The functional integrity of the person may be sacrificed to maintain the health or life of the person when no other morally permissible means is available.[17]

30. The transplantation of organs from living donors is morally permissible when such a donation will not sacrifice or seriously impair any essential bodily function and the anticipated benefit to the recipient is proportionate to the harm done to the donor. Furthermore, the freedom of the prospective donor must be respected, and economic advantages should not accrue to the donor.

31. No one should be the subject of medical or genetic experimentation, even if it is therapeutic, unless the person or surrogate first has given free and informed consent. In instances of nontherapeutic experimentation, the surrogate can give this consent only if the experiment entails no significant risk to the person's well-being. Moreover, the greater the person's incompetency and vulnerability, the greater the reasons must be to perform any medical experimentation, especially nontherapeutic.

32. While every person is obliged to use ordinary means to preserve his or her health, no person should be obliged to submit to a health care procedure that the person has judged, with a free and informed conscience, not to provide a reasonable hope of benefit without imposing excessive risks and burdens on the patient, or excessive expense to family or community.[18]

33. The well-being of the whole person must be taken into account in deciding about any therapeutic intervention or use of technology. Therapeutic procedures that are likely to cause harm or undesirable side effects can be justified only by a proportionate benefit to the patient.

34. Health care' providers are to respect each person's privacy and confidentiality regarding information related to the person's diagnosis, treatment and care.

35. Health care professionals should be educated to recognize the symptoms of abuse and violence, and are obliged to report cases of abuse to the proper authorities in accordance with local statutes.

36. Compassionate and understanding care should be given to a person who is the victim of sexual assault. Health care providers should cooperate with law enforcement officials, offer the person psychological and spiritual support, and accurate medical information. A female who has been raped should be able to defend herself against a potential conception from the sexual assault. If, after appropriate testing, there is no evidence that conception has occurred already, she may be treated with medications that would prevent ovulation, sperm capacitation or fertilization. It is not permissible, however, to initiate or to recommend treatments that have as their purpose or direct effect the removal, destruction or interference with the implantation of a fertilized ovum.[19]

37. An ethics committee or some alternate form of ethical consultation should be available to assist by advising on particular ethical situations, by offering educational opportunities, and by reviewing and recommending policies. To these ends there should be appropriate standards for medical ethical consultation within a particular diocese that will respect the diocesan bishop's pastoral responsibility as well as assist members of ethics committees to be familiar with Catholic medical ethics and, in particular, these directives.

Part 4
Issues in Care for the Beginning of Life

Introduction

The church's commitment to human dignity inspires an abiding concern for the sanctity of human life from its very beginning, and with the dignity of marriage and of the marriage act by which human life is transmitted. The church cannot approve medical practices that undermine the biological, psychological and moral bonds on which the strength of marriage and the family depends.

Catholic health care ministry witnesses to the sanctity of life "from the moment of conception until death."[20] The church's defense of life encompasses the unborn, and the care of women and their children during and after pregnancy. The church's commitment to life is seen in its willingness to collaborate with others to alleviate the causes of the high infant mortality rate and to provide adequate health care to mothers and their children before and after birth.

The church has the deepest respect for the family, for the marriage covenant and for the love that binds a married couple together. This includes respect for the marriage act by which husband and wife express their love and cooperate with God in the creation of a new human being. The Second Vatican Council affirms: "This love is an eminently human one. . . . It involves the good of the whole person. . . . The actions within marriage by which the couple are united intimately and chastely are noble and worthy ones. Expressed in a manner which is truly human, these actions signify and promote that mutual self-giving by which spouses enrich each other with a joyful and thankful will."[21] Marriage and conjugal love are by their nature ordained toward the begetting and educating of children. Children are really the supreme gift of marriage and contribute very substantially to the welfare of their parents. . . . Parents should regard as their proper mission the task of transmitting human life and educating those to whom it has been transmitted. . . . They are thereby cooperators with the love of God the Creator, and are, so to speak, the interpreters of that love."[22]

For legitimate reasons of responsible parenthood, married couples may limit the number of their children by natural means. The church cannot approve contraceptive interventions which "either in anticipation of the marital act, or in its accomplishment or in the development of its natural consequences have the purpose, whether as an end or a means, to render procreation impossible."[23] Such interventions violate "the inseparable connection, willed by between the two meanings of the conjugal act: the unitive and procreative meaning."[24]

With the advance of the biological and medical sciences, society has at its disposal new technologies for responding to the problem of infertility. While we rejoice in the potential for good inherent in many of these technologies, we cannot assume that what is technically possible is always morally right. Reproductive technologies that substitute for the marriage act are not consistent with human dignity. Just as the marriage act is joined naturally to procreation, so procreation is joined naturally to the marriage act. As Pope John XXIII observed: "The transmission of human life is entrusted by nature to a personal and conscious act and as such is subject to all the holy laws of God: the immutable and inviolable laws which must be recognized and observed. For this reason, one cannot use means and follow methods which could be licit in the transmission of the life of plants and animals."[25] Because the moral law is rooted in the whole of human nature, human persons, through intelligent reflection on their own spiritual destiny, can discover and cooperate in the plan of the Creator.[26]

Directives

38. When the marital act of sexual intercourse is not able to attain its procreative purpose, assistance that does not separate the unitive and procreative ends of the act, and does not substitute for the marital act itself, may be used to help married couples conceive.[27]

39. Those techniques of assisted conception that respect the unitive and procreative meanings of sexual intercourse and do not involve the destruction of human embryos or their deliberate generation in such numbers that it is clearly envisaged that all cannot implant and some are simply being used to maximize the chances of others implanting, may be used for infertility.

40. Heterologous fertilization (that is, any technique used to achieve conception by the use of gametes coming from at least one donor other than the spouses) is prohibited because it is contrary to the covenant of marriage, the unity of the spouses and the dignity proper to parents and the child.[28]

41. Homologous artificial fertilization (that is, any technique used to achieve conception using the gametes of the two spouses joined in marriage) is prohibited when it separates procreation from the marital act in its unitive significance, e.g., any technique used to achieve extracorporal conception.[29]

42. Because of the dignity of the child and of marriage, and because of the uniqueness of the mother-child relationship, participation in contracts or arrangements for surrogate motherhood is not permitted. Moreover, the commercialization of such surrogacy denigrates the dignity of women, especially the poor.[30]

43. A Catholic health care institution that provides treatment for infertility should offer not only technical assistance to infertile couples but also should help couples pursue other solutions, e.g. counseling, adoption.

44. Catholic health care institutions should provide prenatal, obstetric and postnatal services for mothers and their children in a manner consonant with its mission.

45. Abortion, that is, the directly intended termination of pregnancy before viability or the directly intended destruction of a viable fetus, is never permitted. Every procedure whose sole immediate effect is the termination of pregnancy before viability is an abortion, which, in its moral context includes the interval between conception and implantation of the embryo. Catholic health care institutions are not to provide abortion service even based upon the principle of material cooperation. In this context, Catholic health care institutions need to be concerned about the danger of scandal in any association with abortion providers.

46. Catholic health care providers should be ready to offer compassionate physical, psychological, moral and spiritual care to those persons who have suffered from the trauma of abortion.

47. Operations, treatments and medications that have as their direct purpose the cure of a proportionately serious pathological condition of a pregnant woman are permitted when they cannot be safely postponed until the unborn child is viable, even if they will result in the death of the unborn child.

48. In case of extrauterine pregnancy, no intervention is morally licit which constitutes a direct abortion.[31]

49. For a proportionate reason, labor may be induced after the fetus is viable.[32]

50. Prenatal diagnosis is permitted when the procedure does not threaten the life or physical integrity of the unborn child or the mother and does not

subject them to disproportionate risks, when the diagnosis can provide information to guide preventative care for the mother or pre- or postnatal care for the child and when the parents, or at least the mother, give free and informed consent. Prenatal diagnosis is not permitted when undertaken with the intention of aborting an unborn child with a serious defect.

51. Nontherapeutic experiments on a living embryo or fetus are not permitted, even with the consent of the parents. Therapeutic experiments are permitted for a proportionate reason with the free and informed consent of the parents or, if the father cannot be contacted, at least of the mother. Medical research that will not harm the life or physical integrity of an unborn child is permitted with parental consent.[33]

52. Catholic health institutions may not promote or condone contraceptive practices, but should provide, for married couples and the medical staff who counsel them, instruction both about the church's teaching on responsible parenthood and in methods of natural family planning.

53. Direct sterilization of either men or women, whether permanent or temporary, is not permitted in a Catholic health care institution when its sole immediate effect is to prevent conception. Procedures that induce sterility are permitted when their direct effect is the cure or alleviation of a present pathology and a simpler treatment is not available.[34]

54. Genetic counseling may be provided in order to promote responsible parenthood and to prepare for the proper treatment and care of children with genetic defects, in accordance with Catholic moral teaching and the intrinsic rights and obligations of married couples regarding the transmission of life.

Part 5
Issues in Care for the Dying

Introduction

Christ's redemption and saving grace embrace the whole person, especially in his or her illness, suffering and death.[35] The Catholic health care ministry faces the reality of death with the confidence of faith. In the face of death—for many, a time when hope seems lost—the church witnesses to her belief that God has created each person for eternal life.[36]

Above all, as a witness to its faith, a Catholic health care institution will be a community of respect, love and support to patients or residents and their families as they face the reality of death, that is hardest to face is the process of dying itself, especially the dependency, helplessness and the pain that so often accompany terminal illness. One of the primary purposes of medicine in caring for the dying is the relief of pain and the suffering caused by it. Effective management of pain in all its forms is critical in the appropriate care of the dying.

The truth that life is a precious gift from God has profound implications for the question of stewardship over human life. We are not the owners of our lives and hence do not have absolute power over life. We have a duty to preserve our life and to use it for the glory of God; but the duty to preserve life is not absolute, for reject life-prolonging procedures that are insufficiently beneficial or excessively burdensome. Suicide and euthanasia are never morally acceptable options.

The task of medicine is to care even when it cannot cure. Physicians and their patients must evaluate the use of the technology at their disposal. Reflection on the innate dignity of human life in all its dimensions and on the purpose of medical care is indispensable for formulating a true moral judgment about the use of technology to maintain life. The use of life-sustaining technology is judged in light of the Christian meaning of life, suffering and death. Only in this way are two extremes avoided: on the one hand, an insistence on useless or burdensome technology even when a patient may legitimately wish to forgo it and, on the other hand, the withdrawal of technology with the intention of causing death.[37]

Some state Catholic conferences, individual bishops and the NCCB Committee on Pro-Life Activities have addressed the moral issues concerning medically assisted hydration and nutrition. The bishops are guided by the church's teaching forbidding euthanasia, which is "an action or an omission which of itself or by intention causes death, in order that all suffering may in this way be eliminated."[38] These statements agree that hydration and nutrition are not morally obligatory either when they brings no comfort to a person who is imminently dying or when they cannot be assimilated by a person's body. The NCCB Committee on Pro-Life Activities report, in addition, points out the necessary distinctions between questions already resolved by the magisterium and those requiring further reflection, as, for example, the morality of withdrawing medically assisted hydration and nutrition from a person who is in the condition which is recognized by physicians as the "persistent vegetative state."[39]

Directives

55. Catholic health care institutions offering care to persons in danger of death from illness, accident, advanced age or similar condition should provide them with appropriate opportunities to prepare for death. Persons in danger of death should be provided with whatever information is necessary to help them understand their condition, and have the opportunity to discuss their condition with their family members and care providers. They should also be offered the appropriate medical information which would make it possible to address the morally legitimate choices available to them. They should be provided the spiritual support as well as the opportunity to receive the sacraments in order to prepare well for death.

56. A person has a moral obligation to use ordinary or proportionate means of preserving his or her life. Proportionate means are those that in the judgment of the patient offer a reasonable hope of benefit and do not entail an excessive burden or impose excessive expense on the family or the community.[40]

57. A person may forgo extraordinary or disproportionate means of preserving life. Disproportionate means are those that in the patient's judgment do not offer a reasonable hope of benefit or entail an excessive burden or impose excessive expense on the family or the community.[41]

58. There should be a presumption in favor of providing nutrition and hydration to all patients, including patients who require medically assisted nutrition and hydration, as long as this is of sufficient benefit to outweigh the burdens involved to the patient.

59. The free and informed judgment made by a competent adult patient concerning the use or withdrawal of life-sustaining procedures should always be respected and normally complied with, unless contrary to Catholic moral teaching.

60. Euthanasia is an action or omission which of itself or by intention causes death, in order to alleviate suffering. Catholic health care institutions may never condone or participate in euthanasia or assisted suicide in any way. Dying patients who request euthanasia should receive loving care, psychological and spiritual support, and appropriate remedies for pain and other symptoms so that they can live with dignity until the time of natural death.[42]

61. Patients should be kept as free of pain as possible so that they may die comfortably and with dignity, and in the place where they wish to die. Since a person has the right to prepare for his or her death while fully conscious, he or she should not be deprived of consciousness without a compelling reason. Medicines capable of alleviating or suppressing pain may be given to a dying person even if this therapy may indirectly shorten the person's life, so long as the intent is not to hasten death. Patients experiencing suffering that cannot be alleviated should be helped to appreciate the Christian understanding of redemptive suffering.

62. The determination of death should be made by the physician or competent medical authority in accordance with responsible and commonly accepted scientific criteria.

63. Catholic health care institutions should encourage and provide the means whereby those who wish to do so may arrange for the donation of their organs and bodily tissue for ethically legitimate purposes, so that they may be used for donation and research after death.

64. Such organs should not be removed until it has been medically determined that the patient has died. In order to prevent any conflict of interest, the physician who determines death should not be a member of the transplant team.

65. The use of tissue or organs from an infant may be permitted after death has been determined and with the informed consent of the parents or guardians.

66. Catholic health care institutions should not make use of human tissue obtained by direct abortions, even for research and therapeutic purposes.[43]

Part 6
Forming Partnerships with
Health Care Organizations and Providers

Introduction

Until recently, most health care providers enjoyed a degree of independence from one another. In ever-increasing ways, Catholic health care providers have become involved with other health care organizations and providers. For instance, many Catholic health care systems and institutions share in the joint purchase of technology and services with other local facilities or physicians' groups. Another phenomenon is the growing number of Catholic health care systems and institutions joining co-sponsoring integrated delivery networks or managed-care organizations in order to contract with insurers or other health care payers. In some instances, Catholic health care systems sponsor a health care plan or health maintenance organization. In many dioceses new partnerships will result in a decrease in the number of health care providers at times leaving the Catholic institution as the sole provider of health care services. At whatever level, new partnerships forge a variety of inter-woven relationships: between the various institutional partners, between health care providers and the community, between physicians and health care services, and between health care services and payers.

On the one hand, new partnerships can be viewed as opportunities for Catholic health care institutions and services to witness to their religious and ethical commitments and so influence the healing profession. For example, new partnerships can help to implement the church's social teaching. New partnerships can be opportunities to realign the local delivery system in order to provide a continuum of health care to the community; they can witness to a responsible stewardship of limited health care resources; and they can be opportunities to provide to poor and vulnerable persons a more equitable access to basic care.

On the other hand, new partnerships can pose serious challenges to the viability of the identity of Catholic health care institutions and services, and their ability to implement these directives in a consistent way, especially when partnerships are formed with those who do not share Catholic moral principles. The risk of scandal cannot be underestimated when partnerships are not built upon common values and moral principles. Partnership opportunities for some Catholic health care providers may even threaten the continued existence of other Catholic institutions and services, particularly when partnerships are driven by financial considerations alone. Because of the potential dangers involved in the new partnerships that are emerging, an increased collaboration among Catholic-sponsored health care institutions is essential and should be sought before other forms of partnerships.

The significant challenges that new partnerships may pose, however, do not necessarily preclude their possibility on moral grounds. The potential dangers require that new partnerships undergo systematic and objective moral analysis which takes into account the various factors that often pressure institutions and services into new partnerships that can diminish the autonomy and ministry of the Catholic partner. The following directives are offered to assist institutionally based Catholic health care services in this process of analysis. To this end the National Conference of Catholic Bishops has established the Ad Hoc Committee on Health Care Issues and the Church as a resource for bishops and health care leaders. An appendix at the end offers a clarification of the terms relative to the principles governing cooperation and their application to concrete situations.

Directives

67. Decisions that may lead to serious consequences for the identity or reputation of Catholic health care services or entail the high risk of scandal should be made in consultation with the diocesan bishop or his health care liaison.

68. Any partnership that will affect the mission or religious and ethical identity of Catholic health care institutional services must respect church teaching and discipline. Diocesan bishops and other church authorities should be involved as such partnerships are developed, and the diocesan bishop should give the appropriate authorization before they are completed. The diocesan bishop's approval is required for partnerships sponsored by institutions subject to his governing authority; for partnerships sponsored by religious institutes of pontifical right, his *nihil obstat* should be obtained.

69. When a Catholic health care institution is participating in a partnership which may be involved in activities judged morally wrong by the church, the Catholic institution should limit its involvement in accord with the moral principles governing cooperation.

70. The possibility of scandal, e.g. generating a confusion about Catholic moral teaching, is an important factor that should be considered when applying the principles governing cooperation. Cooperation, which in all other respects is morally appropriate, may be refused because of the scandal that would be caused in the circumstances.

Conclusion

Sickness speaks to us of our limitations and human frailty. It can take the form of infirmity resulting from the simple passing of years or injury from the exuberance of youthful energy. It can be temporary or chronic, debilitating and even terminal. Yet, the follower of Jesus faces illness and the consequences of the human condition aware that our Lord always shows compassion toward the infirm.

Jesus not only taught his disciples to be compassionate, but he also told them who should be the special object of their compassion. The parable of the feast with its humble guests was preceded by the instruction: "When you hold a banquet, invite the poor, the crippled, the lame, the blind"(Lk. 14:13). These were people whom Jesus healed and loved.

Catholic health care is a response to the challenge of Jesus to go and do likewise. Catholic health care services rejoice in the challenge to be Christ's healing compassion in the world and see their ministry not only as an effort to restore and preserve health, but also as a spiritual service and a sign of that final healing which will one day bring about the new creation that is the ultimate fruit of Jesus' ministry and God's love for us.

Appendix
The Principles Governing Cooperation

The principles governing cooperation differentiate the action of the wrong-doer from the action of the cooperator through two major distinctions. The first is between formal and material cooperation. If the cooperator intends the object of the wrongdoer's activity, then the cooperation is formal and, there-fore, morally wrong. Since intention is not simply an explicit act of the will, formal cooperation can also be implicit. Implicit formal cooperation is attrib-uted when, even though the cooperator denies intending the wrongdoer's object, no other explanation can distinguish the cooperator's object from the wrongdoer's object. If the cooperator does not intend the object of the wrong-doer's activity, the cooperation is material and can be morally licit.

The second distinction deals with the object of the action and is expressed by immediate and mediate material cooperation. Material cooperation is immediate when the object of the cooperator is the same as the object of the wrongdoer. Immediate material cooperation is wrong, except in some instances of duress. The matter of duress distinguishes immediate material cooperation from implicit formal cooperation. But immediate material cooper-ation—without duress—is equivalent to implicit formal cooperation and, therefore, is morally wrong. When the object of the cooperator's action remains distinguishable from that of the wrongdoer's, material cooperation is mediate and can be morally licit.

Moral theologians recommend two other considerations for the proper evaluation of material cooperation. First, the object of material cooperation should be as distant as possible from the wrongdoer's act. Second, any act of material cooperation requires a proportionately grave reason.

Prudence guides those involved in cooperation to estimate questions of intention, duress, distance, necessity and gravity. In making a judgment about cooperation, it is essential that the possibility of scandal should be eliminated. Appropriate consideration should also be given to the church's prophetic responsibility.

Notes

1. National Conference of Catholic Bishops. "Health and Health Care" (Washington, U.S. Catholic Conference. 1981). Also in Origins II (1981): 396–402.

2. Health care services under Catholic auspices are carried out in a variety of institutional settings, e.g. hospitals, clinics, outpatient facilities, urgent care centers, hospices, nursing homes and parishes. Depending on the context, these directives will employ the term *institution and/or services* in order to encompass the variety of settings in which Catholic health care is provided.

3. "Health and Health Care," p. 5.

4. Second Vatican Council, Decree on the Apostolate of the Laity, *Apostolicam Actuositatem*, No. 1.

5. Pope John Paul II, apostolic exhortation *Christifideles Laici* (1988), No. 29.

6. As examples see Congregation for the Doctrine of the Faith, Declaration on Procured Abortion (1974); Congregation for the Doctrine of the Faith, Declaration on Euthanasia (1980); Instruction on Respect for Human Life in Its Origin and on the Dignity of Procreation, Donum Vitae (1987).

7. Pope John XXIII, encyclical *Pacem in Terris* (1963), No. 11; "Health and Health Care," pp. 5, 17–18; Catechism of the Catholic Church, No. 2211.

8. Pope John Paul II, encyclical *Sollicitudo Rei Socialis* (1988). No, 43.

9. National Conference of Catholic Bishops, "Economic Justice for All: Pastoral Letter on Catholic Social Teaching and the U.S. Economy (Washington: U.S. Catholic Conference, 1986), no. 80.

10. The duty of responsible stewardship demands responsible collaboration. But in collaborative efforts, Catholic institutionally based health care services must be attentive to occasions when the policies and practices of other institutions are not compatible with the church's authoritative moral teaching. At such times, Catholic health care institutions should determine whether or to what degree collaboration would be morally permissible. To make that judgment, the governing boards of Catholic institutions should adhere to the moral principles on cooperation. See Part 6.

11. "Health and Health Care," p. 12.

12. Cf. Canons 921-923.

13. Cf. Canon 867.2 and Canon 871.

14. To confer baptism in an emergency, one must have the proper intention (to do what the church intends by baptism) and pour water on the head of the person to be baptized, meanwhile pronouncing the words: "I baptize you in the name of the Father, and of the Son, and of the Holy Spirit."

15. Cf. Canon 883. 3.

16. For example, while the donation of a kidney represents loss of biological integrity, such a donation does not compromise functional integrity since human beings are capable of functioning with only one kidney.

17. Cf. Directive 53.

18. Declaration on Euthanasia, Part IV. Cf. also Directives 56–57.

19. It is recommended that a sexually assaulted woman be advised of the ethical restrictions which prevent Catholic hospitals from using abortifacient procedures; cf. Pennsylvania Catholic Conference, "Guidelines for Catholic Hospitals Treating Victims of Sexual Assault," Origins 22 (1993): 810.

20. Pope John Paul II, address of Oct. 29. 1983, to the 35th general assembly of the World Medical Association, Acta Apostolicae Sedis 76 (1984): 390.

21. Second Vatican Council, Pastoral Constitution on the Church in the Modern World., *Gaudium et Spes* (1965). No. 49.

22. Ibid., No. 50.

23. Pope Paul VI, encyclical *Humane Vitae* (1968), No. 14.

24. Ibid., No. 12.

25. Pope John XXIII, encyclical *Mater et Magistra* (1961), No. 193. quoted in *Donum Vitae*, No. 4.

26. Pope John Paul II, encyclical *Veritatis Splendor* (1993), No. 50.

27. "Homologous artificial insemination within marriage cannot be admitted except for those cases in which the technical means is not a substitute for the conjugal act but serves to facilitate and to help so that the act attains its natural purpose," *Donum Vitae*. Part II, B, No. 6; cf. also Part 1, No. 1, and Part 1, No. 6.

28 Ibid., Part II. A. No. 2.

29. Artificial insemination as a substitute for the conjugal act is prohibited by reason of the voluntarily achieved dissociation of the two meanings of the conjugal act. Masturbation, through which the sperm is normally obtained, is another sign of this dissociation: Even when it is done for the purpose of procreation, the act remains deprived of its unitive meaning: 'It lacks the sexual relationship called for by the moral order, namely the relationship which realizes "the full sense of mutual self-giving and human procreation in the context of true love."'" Donum Vitae, Part II, B, No. 6.

30. Ibid., Part II, A, No. 3.

31. Cf. Directive 45.

32. *Donum Vitae*, Part 1. No. 2.

33. Cf. ibid., Part I, No. 4.

34. Cf. Congregation for the Doctrine of the Faith, "Responses on Uterine Isolation and Related Matters," July 31, 1993, Origins 24 (1994): 211–212.

35. Pope John Paul II, Apostolic Letter, "Suffering Mankind," Origins 14 (1985): 762; apostolic letter *Salvifici Doloris*, (1984), Nos. 25–27.

36. National Conference of Catholic Bishops, "Order of Christian Funerals" (Collegeville, Minn.: The Liturgical Press, 1989), No. 1.

37. Declaration on Euthanasia.

38. Ibid., Part II, p.4.

39. U.S. Bishops' Pro-Life Committee, "Nutrition and Hydration: Moral and Pastoral Reflections," Origins 21 (1992), 705–712. On the importance of consulting authoritative teaching in the formation of conscience and in taking moral decisions, see *Veritatis Splendor*, Nos. 63–64.

40. Declaration on Euthanasia, Part IV.

41. Ibid.

42. Cf. ibid.

43. *Donum Vitae*, Part I, No. 4.

PROTESTANTISM

The Patient as Person

Paul Ramsey

──────────────INTRODUCTION TO READING──────────────

Protestants reflect very great diversity in their ethical and religious positions. As such it is difficult to identify any one representative Protestant
medical ethic. Part of the core commitment of Protestantism is a respect
for the lay person's capacity to develop and articulate his or her own moral
and religious positions. On any given issue there can be a wide range of
often conflicting views.

　　While positions vary tremendously, there is a common orientation and
method shared by many working explicitly within the Protestant context.
The following essay by Paul Ramsey, a former professor of religion at
Princeton and Protestant scholar, is taken from the preface to his pioneer-
ing book, *The Patient as Person*. It traces key Protestant themes—covenant
fidelity, faithfulness defined by covenant, the role of all, including lay
persons, in decisions, and the uniqueness of the religious perspective.

The problems of medical ethics that are especially urgent in the present day . . .
are by no means technical problems on which only the expert (in this case the
physician) can have an opinion. They are rather the problems of human beings
in situations in which medical care is needed. Birth and death, illness and injury
are not simply events the doctor attends. They are moments in every human
life. The doctor makes decisions as an expert but also as a man among men; and
his patient is a human being coming to his birth or to his death, or being
rescued from illness or injury in between.

　　Therefore, the doctor who attends *the case* has reason to be attentive to the
patient as person. Resonating throughout his professional actions, and crucial
in some of them, will be a view of man, an understanding of the meaning of the
life at whose first or second exodus he is present, a care for the life he attends in
its afflictions. In this respect the doctor is quite like the rest of us, who must yet
depend wholly on him to diagnose the options, perhaps the narrow range of
options, and to conduct us through the one that is taken.

　　To take up for scrutiny some of the problems of medical ethics is, therefore, to bring under examination at once a number of crucial human moral
problems. These are not narrowly defined issues of medical ethics alone. Thus

this volume has—if, I may say so—the widest possible audience. It is addressed to patients as persons, to physicians of patients who are persons—in short, to everyone who has had or will have to do with disease or death. The question, What ought the doctor to do? is only a particular form of the question, What should be done?

This, then, is a book *about ethics*, written by a Christian ethicist. I hold that medical ethics is consonant with the ethics of a wider human community. The former is (however special) only a particular case of the latter. The moral requirements governing the relations of physician to patients and researcher to subjects are only a special case of the moral requirements governing any relations between man and man. Canons of loyalty to patients or to joint adventurers in medical research are simply particular manifestations of canons of loyalty of person to person generally. Therefore, in the following chapters I undertake to explore a number of medical covenants among men. These are the covenant between physician and patient, the covenant between researcher and "subject" in experiments with human beings, the covenant between men and a child in need of care, the covenant between the living and the dying, the covenant between the well and the ill or with those in need of some extraordinary therapy.

We are born within covenants of life with life. By nature, choice, or need we live with our fellowmen in roles or relations. Therefore we must ask, What is the meaning of the *faithfulness* of one human being to another in every one of these relations? This is the ethical question.

At crucial points in the analysis of medical ethics, I shall not be embarrassed to use as an interpretative principle the Biblical norm of *fidelity to covenant*, with the meaning it gives to *righteousness* between man and man. This is not a very prominent feature in the pages that follow since it is also necessary for an ethicist to go as far as possible into the technical and other particular aspects of the problems he ventures to take up. Also, in the midst of any of these urgent human problems, an ethicist finds that he has been joined— whether in agreement or with some disagreement—by men of various persuasions, often quite different ones. There is in actuality a community of moral discourse concerning the claims of persons. This is the main appeal in the pages that follow.

Still we should be clear about the moral and religious premises here at the outset. I hold with Karl Barth that covenant-fidelity is the inner meaning and purpose of our creation as human beings, while the whole of creation is the external basis and condition of the possibility of covenant. This means that the conscious acceptance of covenant responsibilities is the inner meaning of even the "natural" or systemic relations or roles we enter by choice, while this fabric provides the external framework for human fulfillment in explicit covenants among men. The practice of medicine is one such covenant. *Justice, fairness, righteousness, faithfulness, cannons of loyalty, the sanctity of life, hesed, agape* or *charity* are some of the names given to the moral quality of attitude and of action owed to all men by any man who steps into a covenant with another man—by any man who, so far as he is a religious man, explicitly acknowledges that we are a covenant people on a common pilgrimage.

The chief aim of the chapters to follow is, then, simply to explore the meaning of *care*, to find the actions and abstentions that come from adherence to *covenant*, to ask the meaning of the *sanctity* of life, to articulate the requirements of steadfast *faithfulness* to a fellow man. We shall ask, What are the moral claims upon us in crucial medical situations and human relations in which some decision must be made about how to show respect for, protect, preserve, and honor the life of fellow man?

Just as man is a *sacredness in the social and political order,* so he is a *sacredness in the natural, biological order.* He is a sacredness in bodily life. He is a person who within the ambience of the flesh claims our care. He is an embodied soul or ensouled body. He is therefore a sacredness in illness and in his dying. He is a sacredness in the fruits of the generative processes. (From some point he is this if he has any sanctity, since it is undeniably the case that men are never more than, from generation to generation, the products of human generation.) The sanctity of human life prevents ultimate trespass upon him even for the sake of treating his bodily life, or for the sake of others who are also only a sacredness in their bodily lives. Only a being who is a sacredness in the social order can withstand complete dominion by "society" for the sake of engineering civilizational goals—withstand, in the sense that the engineering of civilizational goals cannot be accomplished without denying the sacredness of the human being. So also in the use of medical or scientific techniques.

It is of first importance that this be understood, since we live in an age in which *hesed* (steadfast love) has become *maybe* and the "sanctity" of human life has been reduced to the ever more reducible motion of the "dignity" of human life. The latter is a sliver of a shield in comparison with the awesome respect required of men in all their dealings with men if man has a touch of sanctity in this his fetal, mortal, bodily, living and dying life.

Today someone is likely to say: "Another 'semanticism' which is somewhat of an argument-stopper has to do with the sacredness of inviolability of the individual."[1] If such a principle is asserted in gatherings of physicians, it is likely to be met with another argument-stopper: It is immoral not to do research (or this experiment must be done despite its necessary deception of human beings). This is then a standoff of contrary moral judgments or intuitions or commitments.

The next step may be for someone to say that medical advancement is hampered because our "society" makes an absolute of the inviolability of the individual. This raises the spectre of a medical and scientific community freed from the shackles of that cultural norm, and proceeding upon the basis of an ethos all its own. Alternatively, the next move may be for someone to say: Our major task is to reconcile the welfare of the individual with the welfare of mankind; both must be served. This, indeed, is the principal task of medical ethics. However, there is no "unseen hand" guaranteeing that, for example, *good* experimental designs will always be morally *justifiable*. It is better not to begin with the laissez-faire assumption that the rights of men and the needs of future progress are always reconcilable. Indeed, the contrary assumption may be more salutary.

Several statements of this viewpoint may well stand as mottos over all that follows in this volume. "In the end we may have to accept the fact that some limits do exist to the search for knowledge."[2] "The end does not always justify the means, and the good things a man does can be made complete only by the things he refuses to do."[3] "There may be valuable scientific knowledge which it is morally impossible to obtain. There may be truths which would be of great and lasting benefit to mankind if they could be discovered, but which cannot be discovered without systematic and sustained violation of legitimate moral imperatives. It may be necessary to choose between knowledge and morality, in opposition to our long-standing prejudice that the two must go together."[4] "To justify whatever practice we think is technically demanded by showing that we are doing it for a good end . . . is both the best defense and the last refuge of a scoundrel."[5] "A[n experimental] study is ethical or not in its inception; it does not become ethical or not because it turned up valuable data."[6] These are salutary warnings precisely because by them we are driven to make the most searching inquiry concerning more basic ethical principles governing medical practice.

Because physicians deal with life and death, health and maiming, they cannot avoid being conscious or deliberate in their ethics to some degree. However, it is important to call attention to the fact that medical ethics cannot remain at the level of surface intuitions or in an impasse of conversation-stoppers. At this point there can be no other resort than to ethical theory—as that elder statesman of medical ethics, Dr. Chauncey D. Leake, Professor of Pharmacology at the University of California Medical Center, San Francisco, so often reminds us. At this point physicians must in greater measure become moral philosophers, asking themselves some quite profound questions about the nature of proper moral reasoning, and how moral dilemmas are rightly to be resolved. If they do not, the existing medical ethics will be eroded more and more by what it is alleged must be done and technically can be done.

In the medical literature there are many articles on ethics which are greatly to be admired. Yet I know that these are not part of the daily fare of medical students, or of members of the profession when they gather together as professionals or even for purposes of conviviality. I do not believe that either the codes of medical ethics or the physicians who have undertaken to comment on them and to give fresh analysis of the physician's moral decisions will suffice to withstand the omnivorous appetite of scientific research or of a therapeutic technology that has a momentum and a life of its own.

The Nuremberg Code, The Declaration of Helsinki, various "guidelines" of the American Medical Association, and other "codes" governing medical practice constitute a sort of "catechism" in the ethics of the medical profession. These codes exhibit a professional ethics which ministers and theologians and members of other professions can only profoundly respect and admire. Still, a catechism never sufficed. Unless these principles are constantly pondered and enlivened in their application they become dead letters. There is also need that these principles be deepened and sensitized and opened to further humane revision in face of all the ordinary and the newly emerging situations which a doctor confronts—as do we all—in the present day. In this task none of the sources of moral insight, no understanding of the humanity of man or for answering questions of life and death, can rightfully be neglected.

There is, in any case, no way to avoid the moral pluralism of our society. There is no avoiding the fact that today no one can do medical ethics until someone first does so. Due to the uncertainties in Roman Catholic moral theology since Vatican II, even the traditional medical ethics courses in schools under Catholic auspices are undergoing vast changes, abandonment, or severe crisis. The medical profession now finds itself without one of the ancient land-marks—or without one opponent. Research and therapies and actionable schemes for the self-creation of our species mount exponentially, while Nuremberg recedes.

The last state of the patient (medical ethics) may be worse than the first. Still there is evidence that this can be a moment of great opportunity. An increasing number of moralists—Catholic, Protestant, Jewish and unlabeled men—are manifesting interest, devoting their trained powers of ethical reasoning to questions of medical practice and technology. This same gallop-ing technology gives all mankind reason to ask how much longer we can go on assuming that what can be done or should be, without uncovering the ethical principles we mean to abide by. These questions are now completely in the public forum, no longer the province of scientific experts alone.

The day is past when one could write a manual on medical ethics. Such books by Roman Catholic moralists are not to be criticized for being deduc-tive. They were not; rather they were commendable attempts to deal with concrete cases. These manuals were written with the conviction that moral reasoning can encompass hard cases, that ethical deliberation need not remain highfalutin but can "subsume" concrete situations under the illuminating power of human moral reason. However, the manuals can be criticized for seeding finally to "resolve" innumerable cases and to give the once and for all "solution" to them. This attempt left the impression that a rule book could be written for medical practice. In a sense, this impression was the consequence of a chief virtue of the authors, i.e., that they were resolved to think through a problem, if possible, *to the end* and precisely with relevance and applicability in concrete cases. Past medical moralists can still be profitably read by anyone who wishes to face the challenge of how he would go about prolonging ethical reflection into action.

Medical ethics today must, indeed, be "casuistry"; it must deal as compe-tently and exhaustively as possible with the concrete features of actual moral decisions of life and death and medical care. But we can no longer be so confi-dent that "resolution" or "solution" will be forthcoming.

To take up the questions of medical ethics for probing, to try to enter into the heart of these problems with reasonable and compassionate moral reflec-tion, is to engage in the greatest of joint ventures: the moral becoming of man.

This is to see in the prism of medical cases the claims of any man to be honored and respected. So might we enter thoughtfully and actively into the moral history of mankind's fidelity to covenants. In this everyone is engaged.

Notes

1. Wolf Wolfensberger, "Ethical Issues in Research with Human Subjects" *Science* 155:48, January 6, l967.

2. Paul A. Freund, *Is the Law Ready for Human Experimentation?* Trial 2 (October-November 1966):49; "Ethical Problems in Human Experimentation." *New England Journal of Medicine* 273 (No. 10):692, 10 September 1965.

3. Dunlop (1965), quoted in Douglass Hubble, "Medical Science, Society and Human Values." *British Medical Journal* 5485:476, 19 February 1966.

4. James P. Scanlan, "The Morality of Deception in Experiments." *Bucknell Review* 13 (No.1):26, March 1965.

5. John E. Smith, "Panel Discussion: Moral Issues in Clinical Research." *Yale Journal of Biology and Medicine* 36:463, June 1964.

6. Henry K. Beecher, *Research and the Individual: Human Studies.* Boston: Little, Brown, 1970, p. 25.

Within Shouting Distance: Paul Ramsey and Richard McCormick on Method

Lisa Sowle Cahill

──────────────INTRODUCTION TO READING──────────────

The differences on certain issues between Catholic and Protestant medical ethics are well known. The methods and concepts used in the two traditions are less thoroughly analyzed. In the following essay Lisa Sowle Cahill, a scholar familiar with both traditions, compares the work of Paul Ramsey with that of Richard McCormick, one of the leading Catholic scholars working in medical ethics today. She shows how Ramsey insists on working within explicitly Christian sources like the Bible while McCormick, taking a more traditional Catholic position, makes use of rational ethics as well as Christian sources. McCormick's Catholic ethics is teleological; the focus is on the end, the highest good. Ramsey, by contrast, is more deontological; he focuses on moral obligation and obedience to covenant, rather than good ends. Cahill traces other contrasts in their ethics including the relative priority of the individual and the common good and the role of moral rules. She concludes that they are "within shouting distance."

Those reflecting on medical ethics from the perspective of religious commitment and its theological elucidation are confronted with the peculiar problem of reconciling the language of a community of faith and obligation with a perceived responsibility to and for the larger human community and with a concomitant need for public discourse. In their medical-ethical arguments, two prominent Christian ethicists, Paul Ramsey and Richard McCormick, develop working paradigm for successful public conversation. Ramsey is not only a representative of themes which often characterize Protestant ethics, but also has contributed a quantity of recent and detailed analysis of the crises of values in research and health care. McCormick affirms the major historical and systematic influences within Roman Catholicism. Moreover, he develops, from within natural law moral theology itself, revisions not only of past moral judgments but of formal principles and metaphysical foundations of the former. Ramsey's vision remains distinctively Christian, even when this weakens his case for a universal ethical appeal; McCormick forcefully correlates religious and secular values, but does not so clearly demonstrate the functional significance for ethics of his theology, precisely as Christian. The purpose of the present analysis is to determine to what extent the ethics of each author is informed by his theological commitments, and how the differences between the two illustrate underlying theological disputes.

The Sources and Scope of Christian Ethics

Ramsey is committed to develop for Christian decision making the biblical norm of agape, or self-sacrificial neighbor love. He disclaims interest in discovering secular translations of it, but does expect a "convergence" of religion and humanism at the level of concrete judgments. Thus Ramsey makes the peculiar claim that, while his reasoning has a unique and nonreducible source, his conclusions may well convince those who reject his presuppositions (Ramsey 1970b, p. xi; 1977b, p. 59; 1978a, p. xiii). So does Ramsey modify his "confessional" Christian position as he engages in the task of effective proclamation in a pluralistic setting.

McCormick, on the other hand, defines his position within a theological ethics which systematically has anticipated a coincidence between natural or rational ethics and Christian ethics. The premise of the "law of nature" is, as he states it, an objective moral order discernible both prediscursively and reflectively (McCormick 1978a, pp. 250–253). Human consciousness grasps in actual experience "the goods or values man can seek, the values that define his human opportunity, his flourishing" (1978b, p. 217). The revelation in Jesus Christ discloses the coherence of these values in God, friendship with whom is the destiny to which persons are invited. This revelation does not, however, generate distinct moral norm which supersede those discernible by reason (McCormick 1977, p. 69; 1978c, p. 100; 1979, pp. 98–99). Rational discourse about obligation in medical practice, as in other personal and social relationships, is in principle an adequate basis of ethics for both Christian and secular humanist.

If a move toward at least a practical universalism is needed to avoid the "separatism" of theological ethics in relation to public ethics, Ramsey must find an alternative to McCormick's reasonable order of values which will compromise his own presuppositions and concerns. He therefore buttresses his expectation of confluence between religious and humanistic ethics by several innovative qualifications of his original particularistic position. On this issue, Ramsey's perspective develops chronologically and in relation to specific problems which have absorbed his attention.

In his first major and only foundational work, *Basic Christian Ethics*, Ramsey envisions Christian ethics as witness to Christ in its practical dimensions. The righteousness and faithfulness of God establish the covenant to which the human response is "obedient love" (1951, pp. xi, 13). Ramsey's more topical writings manifest three modifications of, albeit not departures from, his original insistence that the Christian moral ought is not evident to reason (1951, p. 14; see also 1967a, pp. 108–109; 1977b, p. 59,). These are: (1) the derivation of moral norms from natural "covenants" distinct from but congruent with revealed ones; (2) the affirmation of Christian values in Western culture; and (3) the suggestion that God's redemptive covenant itself is all-inclusive.

In *Deeds and Rules in Christian Ethics*, Ramsey explains his own ethics as "mixed agapism" relying on reason as well as revelation, not because these are independent sources, but because God's covenant is established with all persons in Christ (Ramsey 1967, pp. 29, 122). Therefore "traces of agapistic attitudes and actions" characterize "our common humanity" (1967, p. 43). Appeals to a universal covenant abound, but are introduced briefly and rhetorically, rather than systematically.[1]

Recent writings also presuppose a comprehensive moral community, suggested in conjunction with Ramsey's appropriation of "performative language analysis" (see esp. Evans 1963; cf Ramsey 1968a, pp. 121–125; 1977b, pp. 60–66; see also a section of an unpublished manuscript entitled "Religious Faith a Performative Morality," available from author) to interpret God's covenantal initiative and humankind's obedient response. Ramsey's premise of a covenant revealed to a particular community but effectively established for "all" persons backs up an inclusive understanding of obligation without abandoning his biblical base. A similar inclusiveness can be defended by the "natural law" affirmation of God as the end toward which all persons implicitly are oriented in their actualization of ordered finite values.

Deontology "versus" Teleology

Ramsey's and McCormick's latest controversies have focused at the formal level on an issue which has long been fundamental for both, that is, a paradigm to interpret human moral agency and derive concrete norms. In terms also appropriate to the parallel Anglo-American philosophical debate, the choice lies between a teleological model and a deontological one (see Broad 1944, esp. pp. 206–207). This controversy is relevant to theological ethics, insofar as deontology historically has been associated with scriptural confessionalism, and teleology with the Aristotelian-Thomistic ethics of natural virtue. The discussion rapidly proceeds to whether and when teleologists can be characterized as utilitarians, the latter having become a distinctly pejorative epithet in Christian ethics. In teleology, as concerned with some *goal*, it is precisely consequences which determine normative moral evaluation, although not necessarily measurable consequences for specific historical communities, as is assumed by those who would paint all teleologists with a utilitarian brush. Deontologists frequently insist that considerations of justice, equality, or fairness are essential in the fulfillment of moral *duty*. Thus those actions which treat persons as means to desirable social states ought to be prohibited absolutely. However, not every *telos* excludes some persons from participation for the benefit of others, or justifies any conceivable act given the right configuration of social-benefits-producing circumstances. For example, Aristotle's "happiness" or Aquinas's "friendship with God" are not quantifiable, nor limited in their possible range of distribution, and not reserved for some at the expense of others.

Ramsey has been committed consistently to a deontological model of ethics, as alone expressing the character of Christian moral obligation as obedient response in covenant. Consideration of consequences remains secondary to the determination of the unconditional demands of agape or covenant fidelity (Ramsey 1951, pp. 107, 115–116, 124, 130; 1961c, p. 3, 8; 1967, pp. 108, 109; 1970a, pp. 29–31; 1970b, pp. 2, 25, 58, 256; 1971, pp. 700–706; 1975, pp. xv–xvi, 13; 1979, pp. 8–10). The "ethics of agent agape" and of "agent care" in *Ethics at the Edges of Life* reaffirms obligation as the starting point for medical ethics, not any calculation of the good or harmful consequences of affording treatment to any individual, especially on the basis of social usefulness or merit (Ramsey 1978a, p. 218).

McCormick, by contrast, models moral agency teleologically, God is loved and pursued through the free realization of values which participate in the absolute good, God (*summum bonum*). Moral choice is the preference of some values over others and may be evaluated by an intelligent perception of their objective hierarchical relations (*ordo bonorum*). Those acts are good acts which realize the highest available good in a given situation. McCormick has been accused of utilitarianism (e.g., Carney 1978), because it appears occasionally that his criterion for concrete value preference is an empirical and relatively immediate social good rather that the comprehensive transcendent good, God. (I shall return to the merits of this accusation and to the general characterization of McCormick as a teleologist in a later portion of this essay.)

The debate over teleology "versus" deontology will be pursued here through the issues remaining, namely, the function of moral rules, the relative priority of the individual and the common good, and the ethics of causing death in a medical setting. These are specifics about which Ramsey and McCormick claim that certain conclusions are coherent with, or even entailed by, the teleological and deontological perspectives. My own perception is that the usefulness of the distinction is largely limited to descriptions of the basic character of moral agency (e.g., as responsive obedience to divine mandates or as purposive striving toward union with God).

Individual and Society

McCormick's teleology of common moral experience and Ramsey's theological deontology become differentiated more precisely when focused on a problem endemic to social ethics: the relative priority of individual and community. Disagreements between these colleagues have been pronounced regarding proxy consent to nontherapeutic research on children and fetuses.[2] Themes coalesce there which are also represented in other analyses by both. Ramsey essentially asserts that both natural and Christian covenant-fidelity yield "informed consent" as an inviolable requirement of medical practice. The sacredness of the individual must not be compromised for the sake of benefits to others. Since agapic concern directs itself above all to the weak and vulnerable, children ought most to be protected against consequentialist incursions. Although self-sacrifice is mandatory for the Christian, it has moral significance and justifiability only when its subject is a volunteer, a status impossible of attainment by the fetus, child, or mentally incompetent person.

McCormick attempts to highlight the essential and natural sociality of persons in-community while not denigrating their dignity. Rather than stressing the inviolability of noncompetent research subjects, McCormick locates them within the fabric of the "common good," in whose benefits they share. One ought reasonably to consent in social justice to contribute to the good of others, if at little or no risk to oneself. In such circumstances, consent of noncompetents may be presumed and their participation enlisted as obligatory, not supererogatory.

Though Ramsey has been branded an individualist and McCormick caricatured as a utilitarian, more profit might be gained by appreciation of the theological commitments conserved in the conclusions of each. Backing Ramsey's insistence on respect for the individual is his affirmation of steadfast concern for the "neighbor." By framing this concern deontologically, he ensures its vitality and imperviousness to the imperatives of long-range social ideals in whose light is contemplated the exclusion of those deemed less useful or less able to protect their interests. He does not leave communal needs (those of "all God's other children" [Ramsey 1968b, p. 151]) completely out of account, but here responds to a perceived immediate threat to one pole of the individual-community dialectic. McCormick's perceptions of imminent danger may lie in the opposite direction; in addition, his theological tradition makes available a relatively coherent method for balancing both individual rights and the welfare of the whole community (e.g., social encyclicals of nineteenth- and twentieth-century popes). The method's controlling concept is that of the "common good," a notion inclusive of persons, of their association in community, and of the totality itself, as more than a simple aggregate of individuals. This notion is distinctive in its comprehension of all persons equally and by its ordering to a transcendent communion, that of persons in God. McCormick defines justifiable experimentation on the premise that communal interaction is an essential component of the realization of values, and proposes it with the conviction that those values persons "tend toward" or seek are common ones.

From this exchange, it becomes evident that the links McCormick and Ramsey build between Christian presuppositions and moral conclusions are determined largely by the authors' particular ethical concerns, and that while these concerns and conclusions are defended within a teleological or deontological vision of moral agency, neither vision is entailed by Christian faith or necessarily conducive to some moral judgments rather than others. While on the problem at hand and generally, Ramsey defends the inviolability of individual freedom as a requirement of agape, he has sometimes (on justifiable warfare, on conscientious objection to civil law) defended strictures of social existence. While McCormick presently and characteristically endorses the reasonableness of exacting from all individuals their minimal social obligations, his natural law framework allows an occasional shift to the interests of individuals (e.g., on neonatal care, on contraception). For both of these ethicists, theology provides a court within which to hear a moral case but the outcome is decided only with the assistance of *amici curiae* (e.g., philosophy, the social and empirical sciences).

Moral Norms and Exceptions

The justification of moral norms is a burden which theologians of the past two decades have shared with philosophers, and which has been borne in rather different directions by Paul Ramsey and Richard McCormick. Their recent joint effort to light the path, *Doing Evil to Achieve Good* (McCormick and Ramsey 1978), discloses tenacious differences. The effort of each to account for rules and delimit their function within his respective theological tradition evinces distinct historical concerns. Ramsey decried a Protestant "relativism" in ethics as long ago as *Christian Ethics* (1951, p. 77) and devoted *Deeds and Rules in Christian Ethics* to a cure for the "professional allergy" to rules which he diagnosed among contemporary theologians (1967, p. 3). Ramsey pursues a definition of rules consistent with biblical agape. An unmistakable evolution occurs from *Basic Christian Ethics* (1951) through *Deeds and Rules* (1967) and an important article, "The Case of the Curious Exception" (1968a), to the *Ethics at the Edges of Lif* (1978a); however, tracing the genealogy of the latest offspring is no easy matter.

The neo-Thomism of the moral manuals spawned a notorious Catholic legalism which it has been incumbent upon ethicists critically loyal to that tradition to reduce if not dismember. In the 1960s and 1970s, continental theologians challenged the notions of "intrinsic evil" and absolute norms; McCormick's "Ambiguity in Moral Choice" (1978b) both summarized the state of the question and broke new ground through a deepened understanding of the relation of norms to values. That attempt precipitated *Doing Evil to Achieve Good* (McCormick and Ramsey 1978), a collection of exchanges on norms which prohibit or permit acts having both a positive and negative relation to values (via "the principle of double effect"). The Catholic effort, however, is not simply to overturn the dictates of an absolutist morality; more broadly, it is an attempt to come to terms both with the real insights of the tradition and with an element that tradition neglected, that is, the centrality of Scripture and its normative imperative for any "Christian" ethics.

For Ramsey, rules indicate the continuity of covenant obligation. However, the primary meaning of covenant fidelity has shifted from a Christian love freely transforming every situation, even beyond prior rules (1961c, pp. 179, 190: "in the instant agape controls"), to the enactment of stable social institutions which protect the individual, albeit also as a requirement of agape (1978a, p. 217: "What rule of practice best expresses covenant fidelity?"). Early on, Ramsey developed the phrases "love-transformed-justice" and "in-principled-love" (1961a, 1961b) to signify that norms are consonant with Christian love itself, whether responsive to the one or many neighbors. The first indicates love building on the orders of natural justice, the second the intrinsic specification of love within covenant. Recently, for example, on medical ethics, Ramsey concentrates on the derivation of rules from love itself, though both themes continue.

His formal definition of rule Ramsey draws from John Rawls's "classic article," "Two Concepts of Rules" (Rawls 1955; cf Ramsey 1967, chap. 4). Rawls's own intention is to outline a more defensible utilitarian theory by pointing out the distinction between justifying a "practice" and justifying an action falling under it. A practice as an institutionalized structure of activity is justified by utilitarian (or, for Ramsey, agapic) considerations. Once the practice is established, each act included under it is not reconsidered independently. Ramsey assimilates Rawls's terms to the language of theological ethics, though he is more interested in their function in his own system than in consistency with their original meaning. He proposes exceptionless general rules in Christian ethics, and derives their content from three sources. The first is Christian discernment of the individual and of what love requires toward the individual, for example, nontherapeutic research on children is prohibited generally and unexceptionably. The second source is discernment of the most loving social practice, or the practice that most adequately and generally embodies agape (Ramsey adverts to Robert Veatch's "red light rule" [Veatch and Branson 1976]; see Ramsey 1978a, p. 217). For example, the rule which prohibits inducing death delimits the most generally loving acts, and to admit exceptions would weaken it. Third, "a natural sense of justice and injustice" penetrates to the good for persons and formulates it in binding principles

(Ramsey 1967, p. 127; see also Ramsey 1977b, p. 59). The first two sources represent Christian love's intrinsic requirements, captured in its perception of essential humanity and of the best possible social existence (Ramsey 1967, p. 143). The third is an independent source, presumed to be congenial with the first two, for any or all of the three reasons mentioned earlier in this essay.

Nevertheless, Ramsey formulates Christian rules of practice with a view to individual rights within a larger society conducive to encroachments. His denunciations of "atomistic individualism," which echo through *Ethics at the Edges*, therefore are surprising until one realizes that what Ramsey condemns is the refusal of individuals to make or keep covenant with others and to acknowledge that some requirements of covenant bind all and always (e.g., Ramsey 1967, p. 44; 1978a, p. 13). Far from sacrificing individual interests to social goods, those who enjoin compelling rules "would build a floor under the individual fellowman by minimum faithfulness-rules or canons of loyalty to him that are unexceptionable" (Ramsey 1968a, p. 133). A pressing question is whether the universalization of requirements for moral relations among individuals is adequate as "social" ethics, or whether it is finally a more equalitarian individualism. In attending to "rules of practice" as instruments of individual rights, Ramsey leaves aside the question of community as more than a mechanism for reconciling claims of individuals, and of the role and responsibility of persons within and to it.

Although whether rules can be absolute is not an issue for theological ethics alone, McCormick and Ramsey handle it with theological concerns in mind. McCormick undertakes a "reasonable" analysis of human moral agency as value actualization. While Ramsey is interested in the logical character of exceptions, he asks primarily if they are consistent with covenant fidelity, especially for the Christian. "The Case of the Curious Exception" (Ramsey 1968a), an article to which Ramsey continues to refer the reader (see Ramsey 1978a, p. 212, n. 37), explains the logical relation of the "exception" to the "exceptionless rule. " The distinctive insight is that "exceptions" to norms veritably disappear when properly considered. If an exception has specifiable features, then it must be repeatable; and if repeatable, it is no exception at all, but an act falling under a different principle. In this case, some "exempting-condition" is present which destroys the exception's "singular" character. In other cases, what seems to be an exception to a rule is really another qualification of the rule-generating principle, based on a deepened understanding of it. If so, "qualifying conditions" are present which turn violation into fulfillment. For example, telling a falsehood to save a life might be construed as form of serving truth, rather than as "lying." In such instances, exceptions are not created by consequence features of acts, but by a deeper understanding of the covenant faithfulness expressed in those acts. Ramsey thereby provides some flexibility to moral rules without resorting to consequentialism. Ultimately, these two types of exceptions converge (see Ramsey 1976a). The more precisely defined and universalizable "exception" to a prior rule is justified in relation to the same principle that generated the original rule. For example, just as proxy consent to hazardous research is ruled out by the standard of care, so such research becomes "exceptionally" justified if it is a last resort for therapy.

Sometimes, though, Ramsey seems to disallow even duty-generated exceptions. In one of his responses to McCormick on pediatric experimentation (Ramsey 1976b), he advises that when neglect of research is as immoral as the infringement of rights it requires, the Christian, at least, might better "sin bravely." This phrase captures nicely a Protestant acknowledgment of moral gray areas and even paradox, to be contrasted with the Catholic drive to reconcile values in rationally perspicacious choices.

Exceptionable Norms in an Ethics of Reasonable Values

Doing Evil to Achieve Good is an enormously complex discussion of an equally complex principle, that of "double effect." I will confine my remarks to the collection's central subject, Richard McCormick's revisionist justification of norms.[3] The Catholic tradition of ethics, appealing for a reasoned consideration of moral agency, has generated rule absolutely prohibiting some acts as "intrinsically evil." By this principle it has permitted others, despite morally objectionable aspects. In the justifiable act, the associated evil is described as "tolerated" or "indirectly intended," not desired in itself or even the means of producing the good effect. Thus destruction of a fetus in utero to save the mother was not permitted, though removal of a cancerous and pregnant uterus for the same purpose was.

Originally written in 1973, "Ambiguity in Moral Choice" (in McCormick and Ramsey 1978) was McCormick's first extended attempt to reinterpret this principle by focusing on "proportionate reason," rather than "directness" of action and intention. McCormick showed that there can be teleologically justified exceptions to moral norms forbidding "physical," "premoral," "nonmoral" or "ontic"evils (synonymous terms for disvalues such as error, pain, death) and that, in fact, the norms themselves are justified on the same grounds. A "premoral" value is precisely one which is not absolute. Premoral values and disvalues are relevant to moral judgments insofar as they are in general either to be sought (life) or avoided (death); however the obligation to actualize them concretely depends upon the weight of other values simultaneously at stake. *Moral* values, on the other hand, ought never to be violated since they do not in principle conflict. Moral norms specify the relation of acts to values in the *ordo bonorum*; acts can be enjoined or prohibited generally, because and to the extent that they affirm or deny values. Exceptions occur because goods per se to be realized conflict concretely with equal or higher goods. In conflict situations, the commendable act is the act which realizes the highest value then possible. The only "absolute" norms enjoin moral values (fidelity, truthfulness, justice); norms cannot specify material acts which always or never embody these values. Killing might be "unjust" in most circumstances, but "just" in exceptional ones, while "Never act unjustly" is an unconditional prohibition. It is *proportionate reason*, observes McCormick, that justifies killing at all. One may kill to preserve one's life but not one's purse. *Moral* evil is precisely to do avoidable (disproportionate) concrete harm, that is, to do premoral evil deliberately, and without adequate cause (see McCormick 1978a, pp. 255–260). A premoral evil may be directly done if the value promoted outweighs the disvalue caused, if no less harmful alternative is available, and if the greater value will not "in the long run" be undermined by the manner of its protection now (McCormick 1978b, p. 45). only moral evil ought never be intended directly. Direct intention of a moral evil would entail approval, since moral values are not mutually exclusive (honesty and fidelity); the difficulty is rather to determine which acts best concretize them by appropriately reconciling premoral values (telling a lie to save a friend).

Ramsey's chapter does not alter considerably his own position on rules or that of his adversary. It is largely an attack upon consequentialism and a defense of the requirement of "indirectness" as part of the principle under discussion. If values in conflict, either moral or nonmoral, are incommensurable, he insists, one may not justifiably be sacrificed for the other except indirectly. McCormick's reply is that indirectness does not resolve incommensurability (1978a, p. 227) and, further, that even "incommensurables" must be commensurated approximately and the due trepidation—as is often done in moral choices (1978a, pp. 229–230, 251–253). This assessment, of course, relies on a confidence not shared by Ramsey, namely, trust in a providentially ordered moral universe, where conflicts are permeable and resolvable by reason, however falteringly (McCormick 1978a, pp. 217, 222).

A more substantial objection may be Ramsey's resistance to the inclusion of charity within the domain of proportionate reason (Ramsey 1978b, pp. 131–137). Given his starting point, McCormick is pressed to incorporate a distinctively Christian self-understanding, and a Christian norm, charity, as more than superfluous appendages to ethics. Some lack of success in doing so to the satisfaction of his non-Catholic peers is a liability shared with the rest of natural law moral theology. In "Ambiguity in Moral Choice," McCormick remarks that "self-sacrifice to save the neighbor can truly be proportionate" (1978b, p. 48), a statement open to the inference that which is obligatory precisely at cost to oneself McCormick has proposed also that organ donation or participation in therapeutic experimentation may be "personally good for" the subject and that this good is "the good of expressed charity" (1974, p. 220). Yet McCormick himself undoubtedly agrees that "charity" in the New Testament sense is not commended because of "sticky benefits." Although the virtue of the agent justifies an act of sacrifice in a general sense, the dominant and immediate motivation is the neighbor's good (McCormick 1975b, p. 508). Nevertheless, there apparently remains here, as in Ramsey's covenant ethics, an impermeable tension between rational discourse and the biblical norm of sacrifice.

By this revised theory of proportionate reason, McCormick claims to repudiate crude consequentialism. He names himself a "moderate teleologist"

(McCormick 1978a, pp. 239–255) because, besides consequences, "proportionate reason" refers to an intrinsic relationship of acts to goods sought. Or, citing Louis Janssens, "the principle which has been affirmed in the end must not be negated by the means" (McCormick 1978a, p. 202; cf Janssens 1972, p. 142).

Having defined teleology to include consideration both of consequences and of "feature-dependent" norms, McCormick enfolds the goats with the sheep by insisting that "all of the contributors to this volume are teleologists in the sense just explained." Some, indeed, are "crypto-teleologists (e.g., Ramsey) who remain in the closet" (McCormick 1978a, p. 200). Ramsey as well as McCormick generally maintains the separation between teleology and deontology, asserting that only one is an adequate model for Christian ethics; at the same time, both struggle to define the chosen model inclusively. In Ramsey's frequent deontological apologiae, teleology consistently is reduced to utilitarianism ("producing *teloi*") and rejected (e.g., Ramsey 1967, p. 108). Yet, in the same paragraph in which he brands McCormick a consequentialist, Ramsey affirms, "Traditional Christian ethics assumed that the greatest good for persons is friendship with God and that this is not measurable at all" (1978b, p. 70). McCormick's arguments are approved to the extent that they incorporate nonteleological elements (Ramsey 1978b, p. 117); however, when Ramsey issues his own imperatives, "duty" can demand efforts to "stem the tide" toward harmful effects of present legislative or to other social decisions (1978a, p. 329). Ramsey makes the effort to demonstrate that both "consequential" and "intrinsic" moral considerations are required in a deontological model ("mixed agapism"); McCormick's effort is to demonstrate that the same is true in a teleological one ("moderate teleology").

It might be concluded from this that the controversy over these models is to a large degree unnecessary.[4] The issue is not whether either model inadequately accounts for moral experience by minimizing or excluding one of these factors. The issues are rather (1) which model more appropriately portrays the fundamental quality of that experience, given the shape of one's "metaethical" (e.g., religious and theological) convictions, symbols, and communal self-understanding; and (2) how the diverse more specific elements of moral theory and decision can be defined coherently within that model (e.g., a fulfillment of duties, accountability for consequences, a sense of moral purposiveness, justification of rules and exceptions, etc.).

Notes

1. Variations of the phrase "love for every man for whom Christ died" are numerous (see esp. Ramsey 1961c, pp. xvi, xviii, xx, 54, 114, 305; 1968b, pp. 150–151). All indicate that any individual must be regarded as redeemed by the grace of Christ. Ramsey also cites Karl Barth's affirmation that covenant is "the inner meaning and purpose" of creation, inferring that natural and Christian morality are complementary (see Ramsey 1961a, p. 28; 1967, p. 67; 1970b, p. 2xii).

2. The controversy has been prolonged and sometimes acerbic; see, e.g., Ramsey (1968a, 1970b, 1975, 1976b, 1977a); McCormick (1973b, 1975a, 1976); McCormick and Walters (1975).

3. Helpful analyses of this work, especially the exchanges of McCormick and Ramsey, are provided by Allen (1979) and Langan (1979).

4. Other authors agree, albeit for varied reasons, e.g., Maguire (1978). See also Broad (1944, p. 207); Ramsey (1967, p. 108); and McCormick (1978a, pp. 197-200).

References

Allen, Joseph L. "Paul Ramsey and His Respondents Since The Patient as Person." *Religious Studies Review* 5:89–95, 1979.

Broad, C. D. Five *Types of Ethical Theory*. New York: Harcourt, Brace & Co., 1944.

Carney, Frederick S. "On McCormick and Teleological Morality." *Journal of Religious Ethics* 6:81–107,1978.

Evans, Donald. *The Language of Self-Involvement*. London: SCM Press, 1963.

Janssens, Louis. "Ontic Evil and Moral Evil." *Louvain Studies* 4:115–156, 1972.

Langan, John. "Direct and Indirect—Some Recent Exchanges Between Paul Ramsey and Richard McCormick." *Religious Studies Review* 5:95–101, 1979.

McCormick, Richard A. "Proxy Consent in the Experimentation Situation." In *Love and Society*, edited by James Johnson and David Smith. Missoula, Mont.: Scholars Press, 1973(b).

McCormick, Richard A. "To Save or Let Die." *America* 30:6–10, 1974.

McCormick, Richard A. "Fetal Research, Morality, and Public Policy." *Hastings Center Report* 5 (No. 3):41–46, 1975(a).

McCormick, Richard A. "Transplantation of Organs: A Commentary on Paul Ramsey." *Theological Studies* 36:503–509, 1975(b).

McCormick, Richard A. "Experimentation in Children: Sharing in Sociality." *Hastings Center Report* 6, (No. 6):41–46, 1976.

McCormick, Richard A. "Notes on Moral Theology: 1976." *Theological Studies* 38:57–114, 1977.

McCormick, Richard A. "A Commentary on the Commentaries." In McCormick and Ramsey; 1978(a).

McCormick, Richard A. "Ambiguity in Moral Choice." In McCormick and Ramsey; 1978(b).

McCormick, Richard A. "Notes on Moral Theology, 1977: The Church in Dispute." *Theological Studies* 39:76–138, 1978(c).

McCormick, Richard A. "Notes on Moral Theology, 1978." *Theological Studies* :59–112, 1979.

McCormick, Richard A., and Ramsey, Paul, eds. *Doing Evil to Achieve Good*. Chicago: Loyola University Press, 1978.

McCormick, Richard A., and Walters, LeRoy. "Fetal Research and Public Policy." *America* 132:473–476, 1975.

Maguire, Daniel. *The Moral Choice*. New York: Prentice-Hall, 1978.

Ramsey, Paul. *Basic Christian Ethics*. New York: Scribner's, 1951.

Ramsey, Paul. *Christian Ethics and the Sit-In*. New York: Association Press, 1961(a).

Ramsey, Paul. "Faith Effective Through In-Principled Love." *Christianity and Crisis* 20:76–78, 1961 (b).

Ramsey, Paul. *War and the Christian Conscience: How Shall Modern War Be Conducted Justly?* Durham, N.C.: Duke University Press, 1961(c).

Ramsey, Paul. *Deeds and Rules in Christian Ethics*. New York: Scribner's, 1967.

Ramsey, Paul. "The Case of the Curious Exception." In *Norm and Context in Christian Ethics*, edited by Gene Outka and Paul Ramsey. New York: Scribner's, 1968(a).

Ramsey, Paul. *The Just War: Force and Political Responsibility*. New York: Scribner's, 1968(b).

Ramsey, Paul. *Fabricated Man*. New Haven, Conn.: Yale University Press, 1970(a).

Ramsey, Paul. *The Patient as Person*. New Haven, Conn: Yale University Press, 1970(b).

Ramsey, Paul. "The Ethics of a Cottage Industry in an Age of Community and Research Medicine." *New England Journal of Medicine* 284:700–706, 1971.

Ramsey, Paul. *The Ethics of Fetal Research*. New Haven, Conn.: Yale University Press, 1975.
Ramsey, Paul. "Conceptual Foundations for an Ethics of Medical Care: A Response."
In Veatch and Branson 1976(a).
Ramsey, Paul. "The Enforcement of Morals: Nontherapeutic Research on Children."
Hastings Center Report 6 (No. 4):21–30, 1976(b).
Ramsey, Paul. "Children as Research Subjects: A Reply." *Hastings Center Report* 7 (No.
2):40–41, 1977(a).
Ramsey, Paul. "Kant's Moral Philosophy or a Religious Ethics?" In *Knowledge, Value and
Belief*, edited by H. Tristram Engelhardt, Jr., and Daniel Callahan. Hastings-on-
Hudson, N.Y.: Hastings Center, 1977(b).
Ramsey, Paul. *Ethics at the Edges of Life*. New Haven, Conn.: Yale University Press, 1978(a).
Ramsey, Paul. "Incommensurability and Indeterminacy in Moral Choice." In McCormick
and Ramsey 1978(b).
Ramsey, Paul. "On In Vitro Fertilization." Testimony before the Ethics Advisory Board,
Department of Health, Education and Welfare. Chicago: Americans United for
Life,1979.
Rawls, John. "Two Concepts of Rules." *Philosophical Review* 64:3–32, 1955.
Veatch, Robert M., and Branson, Roy, eds. *Ethics and Health Policy*. Cambridge, Mass.:
Ballinger Publishing Co., 1976.

Code, Covenant, Contract, or Philanthropy

William F. May

──────────────── INTRODUCTION TO READING ────────────────

One of the more serious differences between medical ethics articulated by
medical professional groups and that articulated by religious groups is the
grounding of the ethics. Professional organizations see themselves as
generating for themselves a set of moral norms which gives rise to a code
of ethics coming from only one side of the lay-professional relationship. It
overlooks the possibility that some people on the other side of the relationship may have different conceptions of what is expected morally in the
relation. When the profession and the lay population differ on questions of
what the moral duties of health professionals and lay people are, the traditional medical professional response was to claim that the profession had
the authority to determine what these duties were.

There are other approaches to establishing what the norms are. In
Catholic thought the church is considered authoritative rather than the
profession. Working from Scripture and church tradition as well as reason,
the Pope, church councils, priests, and theologians are the ones who articulate the moral norms for both lay people and physicians as well as other
health professionals.

An alternative way of determining the norms involves a more inclusive
approach. Some would favor bringing lay people and professionals
together to see if they can jointly agree on some compromise set of

principles, rules or standards. While in secular circles the metaphor of forming a *social contract* is sometimes used, religious thinkers, especially Protestant religious thinkers, often prefer to speak of forming a *covenant*. The term covenant implies to some a less legalistic or business-like kind of agreement. In the essay that follows William May challenges the ethics of professional codes, supporting in their place an ethic of covenant between lay and professional. While May goes to some lengths to distinguish a covenant from a contract, he seems to have in mind contracts of the legal-istic, business variety rather than the more philosophical notion used in secular political philosophy of a "social contract," which is seen by many Western philosophers as the way of articulating the foundations of the moral norms of a society.

Questions in medical ethics cannot be resolved apart from the professional matrix in which most decisions are made. What is the nature of the relation-ship between physicians and their patients? How best can we conceptualize professional ethics and understand its binding power? The times press these questions, while tradition offers us several starting points, alternative ways of interpreting professional obligations: the concepts of code and covenant, and the allied notions of philanthropy and contract.

The Hippocratic Oath, as Ludwig Edelstein notes in his unsurpassed study of that document,[1] contains two distinct sets of obligations—those that pertain to the doctor's treatment of his patients and those that are owed his teacher and his teacher's progeny. Edelstein characterizes the first set of oblig-ations, those owed patients, as an ethical code and the second set, those toward the professional guild, as a covenant.

This distinction between code and covenant is extremely revealing and useful. Code itself, furthermore, may be divided into the unwritten codes of practical behavior, transmitted chiefly in a clinical setting from generation to generation of physicians, and into the written codes, beginning with the Hippocratic Oath and concluding with the various revisions of the AMA codes that have had wide currency in this country. Technical proficiency is the prized ideal in the unwritten and informal codes of behavior passed on from doctor to doctor; the ideal of philanthropy (that is, the notion of gratuitous service to humankind) looms large in the more official engraved tablets of the profession. Then, the notion of covenant stands in contrast not only with the ideals of technical proficiency and philanthropy but also with the legal instrument of a contract to which, at first glance, a covenant seems so similar. With these distinctions, then, let us begin.

The Hippocratic Oath

As elaborated in the Hippocratic Oath, the duties of a physician toward his patients include a series of absolute prohibitions: against performing surgery, against assisting patients in attempts at suicide or abortion, breaches in confidentiality, and against acts of injustice or mischief toward the patient and his household, including sexual misconduct. More positively, the physician must act always for the benefit of the sick—the chief illustration of which is to apply dietetic measures according to the physician's best judgment and ability—and, more generally, to keep them from harm and injustice. These various professional obligations to the patient have a religious reference, as the physician declares, "In purity and holiness I will guard my life and art," and petitions, "If I fulfill this oath and do not violate it, may it be granted to me to enjoy life and art . . .; if I transgress it and swear falsely, may the opposite of all this be my lot."

The second set of obligations, directed to the physician's teacher, his teacher's children and his own, require him to accept full filial responsibilities for his adopted father's personal and financial welfare, and to transmit without fee his art and knowledge of the teacher's progeny, to his own, and to other pupils, but only those others who take the oath according to medical law.

It will be the contention of this essay that the development of the practice of modern medicine, for understandable reasons, has tended to reinforce the ancient distinction between these two obligations, that is, between code and covenant; and that it has opted for code as the ruling ideal in relations to patients. The choice has not had altogether favorable consequences for the moral health of the profession.

The Characteristics of a Code

For the purposes of this essay, it can be said, a code shapes human behavior in a fashion somewhat similar to habits and rules. A habit, as Peter Winch has pointed out[2] is a matter of doing the same thing on the same kind of occasion in the same way. A moral rule is distinct from a habit in that the agent in this instance *understands what is meant* by doing the same thing on the same kind of occasion in the same way. Both habits and rules are categorical, universal, and to this degree ahistorical: they do not receive their authority from particular events by which they are authorized or legitimated. They remain operative categorically on all similar occasions: Never assist patients in attempts at suicide or abortion; never break a confidence except under certain specified circumstances.

A code is usually categorical and universal in the aforementioned senses, but not in the sense that it is binding on any and all groups. Hammurabi's code is obligatory only for particular peoples. Moreover, inner circles within certain societies—whether professional or social groups—develop their special codes of behavior. We think of code words or special behaviors among friends, workers in the same company, or professionals within a guild. These codes offer directives not only for the content of action, but also for its form. In its concern with appropriate form, a code moves in the direction of the aesthetic. It is concerned not only with what is done but with how it is done; it touches on matters of style and decorum. Thus medical codes include directives not only on the content of therapeutic action, but also on the fitting style for professional behavior including such matters as suitable dress, discretion in the household, appropriate behavior in the hospital, and prohibitions on self-advertisement.

This tendency to move ethics in the direction of aesthetics is best illustrated in the work of the modern novelist most associated with the ideal of a code. The ritual killing of a bull in the short stories and novels of Hemingway symbolizes an ethic in which stylish performance is everything.

> . . . the bull charged and Villalta charges and just for a moment they became one. Villalta became one with the bull and then it was over.
>
> —Hemingway, *In Our Time*

For the Hemingway hero, there is no question of permanent commitments to particular persons, causes, or places. Robert Jordan of *For Whom the Bell Tolls* does not even remember the "cause" for which he came to Spain to fight. Once he is absorbed in the ordeal of war, the test of a man is not a cause to which he is committed but his conduct from moment to moment. Life is a matter of eating, drinking, loving, hunting, and dying well. Hemingway writes about lovers, but rarely about marriage or the family. Catherine in *Farewell to Arms* and Robert Jordan in *For Whom the Bell Tolls* inevitably must die. Just for a moment, lovers become one and then it is over.

The bullfighter, the wartime lover, the doctor—all alike—must live by a code that eschews involvement; for each there comes a time when the thing is over; matters are terminated by death. But this does not mean that men cannot live beautifully, stylishly, fittingly. Discipline is all. There is a right and a wrong way to do things. And the wrong way usually results from a deficiency in technique or from an excessive preoccupation with one's ego. The bad bullfighter either lacks technique or he lets his ego—through fear or vanity—get in the way of his performance. The conditions of beauty are technical proficiency and a style wholly purified of disruptive preoccupation with oneself. Literally, however, when the critical moment is consummated, it is over; it cannot shape the future. Partners must fall away; only the code remains.

For several reasons, the medical profession has been attracted to the ideal of code for its interpretation of its ethics. First, a code requires one to subordinate the ego to the more technical question of how a thing is done and done well. At its best, the discipline of a code has an aesthetic value. It encourages a proficiency that is quietly eloquent. It conjoins the good with the beautiful. Since the technical demands of medicine have become so great, the standards of the guild are transmitted largely by apprenticeship to those who preeminent skills define the real meaning of the profession without significant remainder. All the rest is a question of disciplining the ego to the point that nervousness, fatigue, faintheartedness, and temptations to self-display (including gross efforts at self-advertisement) have been smoothed away.

A code is additionally attractive in that it does not, in and of itself, encourage personal involvement with the patient; and it helps free the physician of the destructive consequences of that personal involvement. Compassion, in the strictest sense of the term—"suffering with"—has its disadvantages in the professional relationship. It will not do to pretend that one is the second person of the Trinity, prepared to make with every patient the sympathetic descent into his suffering, pain, particular form of crucifixion, and hell. It is enough to offer whatever help one can through finely honed services. It is important to remain emotionally free so as to be able to withdraw the self when those services are no longer pertinent, when as Hemingway says, "it is over."

Finally, a code provides the modern doctor with a basic style of operation that shapes not only his professional but his free time, not only his vocation but his avocations. The self-same pleasure he derives from proficiency in his professional life, he transposes now to his recreational life—flying, skiing, traveling, daily in the precincts of suffering and death he learns that life is available only from moment to moment. As a hard-pressed professional, he knows that both his life and free time are limited—like the soldier's furlough. It makes sense to live by a code that operates from moment to moment, savoring pleasure in stylish action. Thus his code not only frees him from some of the awkwardness and distress that sentient beings are prey to in the midst of agony; but, when he is momentarily free of the battle, it provides him with a style and allows him to live, like most warriors who have tasted death, by the canons of hedonism, which money places specially within his reach.

The Ideal of a Covenant

A covenant, as opposed to a code, has its roots in specific historical events. Like a code, it may give inclusive shape to subsequent behavior, but it always has reference to specific historical exchange between partners leading to a promissory event. Edelstein is quite right in distinguishing code from covenant in the Hippocratic Oath. Rules governing behavior toward patients have a different ring to them from that fealty which a physician owes to his teacher. Loyalty to one's instructor is founded in a specific historical event—that original transaction in which the student received his knowledge and art. He accepts, in effect, a specific gift from his teacher which deserves his lifelong loyalty, a gift that he perpetuates in his own right and turn as he offers his art without fee to his teacher's children and to his own progeny. Covenant ethics is responsive in character.

In its ancient and most influential form, a covenant usually included the following elements: (1) an original experience of gift between the soon-to-be covenanted partners; (2) a covenant promise based on this original or anticipated exchange of gifts, labors, or services; and (3) the shaping of subsequent life for each partner by the promissory event. God "marks the forehead" of the Jews forever, as they respond by accepting an inclusive set of ritual and moral commandments by which they will live. These commands are both specific enough (e.g., the dietary laws) to make the future duties of Israel concrete, yet summary enough (e.g., love the Lord; thy God with all thy heart. . . .) to require a fidelity that exceeds any specification.

The most striking contemporary restatement of an ethic based on covenant is offered by Hemingway's great competitor and contemporary as a novelist—William Faulkner. While the Hemingway hero lives from moment to moment, Faulkner's characters take their bearings from a covenant event. Like Hemingway, Faulkner also writes about a ritual slaying, but with a difference. In "Delta Autumn," a young boy, Isaac McCaslin, "comes of age" in the course of a hunt:

> And the gun levelled rapidly without haste and crashed and he walked to the buck still intact and still in the shape of that magnificent speed and bled it with Sam Father's knife and Sam dipped his hands in the hot blood and marked his face forever . . . Faulkner, "Delta Autumn"

The Hemingway hero slays his bull and then it is over; but young Isaac McCaslin binds the whole of his future in the instant.

> I slew you; my bearing must not shame your quitting of life. My conduct forever onward must become your death.

From then on, just as the marked Jew, the errant, harassed, and estranged Jew, recovers the covenant of Mt. Sinai through ritual renewal, Isaac returns to the delta every autumn to renew the hunt and to suffer his own renewal despite the alienation and pain and defeat which he has subsequently known across a lifetime. This covenant moreover looms over all else—his relationship to the land, to women, to blacks, to all of which and whom he is bound.

For some of the reasons already mentioned, the bond of covenant, in the classical period, tended to define and bind together medical colleagues to one another, but it did not figure large in interpreting the relations between the doctor and his patients. This gift establishes a bond between them and prompts him to assume certain lifetime duties not only toward the teacher (and his financial welfare), but toward his children. This symbolic bond with one's teacher acknowledged in the Hippocratic Oath is strengthened in modern professional life by all those exchanges between colleagues—referrals, favors, personal confidences, and collaborative work on cases. Thus loyalty to colleagues is a responsive act for gifts already, and to be received.

Duties to patients are not similarly interpreted in the medical codes as a responsive act of gifts or services received. This is the essential feature of covenant which is conspicuously missing in the interpretation of professional duties from the Hippocratic Oath to the modern codes of the AMA.

The Code Ideal of Philanthropy vs. Covenantal Indebtedness

The medical profession includes in its written codes an ideal that seldom looms large in the ethic of any self-selected inner group—the ideal of philanthropy. The medical profession proclaims its dedication to the service of mankind.

This ideal is implicitly at work in the Hippocratic Oath and the culture out of which it emerged;[3] It continues in the Code of Medical Ethics originally adopted by the American Medical Association at its national convention in 1847, and it is elaborated in contemporary statements of that code.

This ideal of service, in my judgment, succumbs to what might be called the conceit of philanthropy when it is assumed that the professional's commitment to his fellowman is a gratuitous, rather than responsive or reciprocal, act. Statements of medical ethics that obscure the doctor's prior indebtedness to the community are tainted with the odor of condescension. The point is obvious if one contrasts the way in which the code of 1847 interprets the obligations of patients and the public. On this particular question, I see no fundamental change from 1847 to 1957.

Clearly the duties of the patient are founded on what he has received from. the doctor:

> The members of the medical profession, upon whom is enjoined the performance of so many important and arduous duties toward the community, and who are required to make so many sacrifices of comfort, ease, and health, for the welfare of those who avail themselves of their services, certainly have a right to expect a just sense of the duties which they owe to their medical attendants.[4]

In like manner, the section on the Obligations of the Public to Physicians emphasizes those many gifts and services which the public has received from the medical profession and which are basis for its indebtedness to the profession.

> The benefits accruing to the public, directly and indirectly, from the active and unwearied beneficence of the profession, are so numerous and important, that physicians are unjustly entitled to the utmost consideration and respect from the community.[5]

But turning to the preamble for the physician's duties to the patient and the public, we find no corresponding section in the code of 1847 (or 1957) which founds the doctor's obligation on those gifts and services which he has received from the community. Thus we are presented with the picture of a relatively self-sufficient monad, who, out of the nobility and generosity of his disposition and the gratuitously accepted conscience of his profession, has taken upon himself the noble life of service. The false posture in all this cries out in one of the opening sections of the 1847 code. Physicians "should study, also, in their deportment so as to unite tenderness with firmness, and condescension with authority, so as to inspire the minds of their patients with gratitude, respect and confidence."

I do not intend to demean the specific content of those duties which the codes set forth in their statement of the duties of physicians to their patients, but I am critical of the setting or context in which they are placed. Significantly the code refers to the Duties of physicians to their patients but to the Obligations of patients to their physicians. The shift from "Duties" to "obligations" may seem slight, but in fact, I believe it is a revealing adjustment in language. The AMA thought of the patient and public as indebted to the profession for its services but the profession has accepted its duties to the patients and public out of noble conscience rather than a reciprocal sense of indebtedness.

Put another way, the medical profession imitates God not so much because it exercises power of life and death over others, but because it does not really think itself beholden, even partially, to anyone for those duties to patients which it lays upon itself. Like God, the profession draws its life from itself alone. Its action is wholly gratuitous.

Now, in fact, the physician is in very considerable debt to the community. The first of these debts is already adumbrated in the original Hippocratic Oath. He is obliged to someone or some group for his education. In ancient times, this led to a special sense of covenant obligation to one's teacher. Under the conditions of modern medical education, this indebtedness is both substantial (far exceeding the social investment in the training of any other professional) and widely distributed (including not only one's teachers but those public monies on the basis of which the medical school, the teaching hospital, and research into disease are funded).

In view of the fact that many more qualified candidates apply for medical school than can be admitted and many more doctors are needed than the schools can train, the doctor-to-be has a second order of indebtedness for privileges that have almost arbitrarily fallen his way. While the 1847 codes refers to the "privileges" of being a doctor it does not specify the social origins of those privileges. Third, and not surprisingly, the codes do not make reference to that extraordinary social largesse that befalls the physician, in payment for services, in a society where need abounds and available personnel is limited. Further, the codes do not concede the indebtedness of the physician to those patients who have offered themselves as subjects for experimentation or as teaching material (either in teaching hospitals or in early years of practice). Early practice includes, after all, the element of increased risk for patients who lay their bodies on the line as the doctor "practices" on them. The pun in the word but reflects the inevitable social price of training. This indebtedness to the patient was most recently and eloquently acknowledged by Judah Folkman, M.D., of Harvard Medical School in a Class Day Address.

> In the long run, it is better if we come to terms with the uncertainty of medical practice. Once we recognize that all our efforts to relieve suffering might on occasion cause suffering, we are in a position to learn from our mistakes and appreciate the debt we owe our patients for our education. It is a debt which we must repay—it is like tithing.

> I doubt that the debt we accumulate can be repaid our patients by trying to reduce the practice of medicine to a forty-hour week or by dissolving the quality of our residency programs just because certain groups of residents in that country have refused, through legal tactics, to be on duty more than every fourth or fifth night or any nights at all.

And it can't be repaid by refusing to see Medicaid patients when the state can't afford to pay for them temporarily.

But we can repay the debt in many ways. We can attend postgraduate courses and seminars, be available to patients at all hours, teach, take recertifications examinations; maybe in the future even volunteer for national service; or, most difficult of all, carry out investigation or research.[6]

The physician, finally, is indebted to his patients not only for a start in his career. He remains unceasingly in their debt in its full course. This continuing reciprocity of need is somewhat obscured for we think of the mature professional as powerful and authoritative rather than needy. He seems to be a self-sufficient virtuoso whose life is derived from his competence while others appear before him in their neediness, exposing their illness, their crimes, or their ignorance, for which the professional—doctor, lawyer, or teacher—offers remedy.

In fact, however, a reciprocity of giving and receiving is at work in the professional relationship that needs to be acknowledged. In the profession of teaching, for example, the student needs the teacher to assist him in learning, but so also the professor needs his students. They provide him with regular occasion and forum in which to work out what he has to say and to rediscover his subject afresh through the discipline of sharing it with others. Likewise, the doctor needs his patients. No one can watch a physician nervously approach retirement without realizing how much he needed his patients to be himself.

A convenantal ethics helps acknowledge this full context of need and indebtedness in which professional duties are undertaken and discharged. It also relieves the professional of the temptation and pressure to pretend that he is a demigod exempt from human exigency.

Contract or Covenant

While criticizing the ideal of philanthropy, I have emphasized the elements of exchange, agreement, and reciprocity that mark the professional relationship. This leaves us with the question as to whether the element of gratuitous should be suppressed altogether in professional ethics. Does the physician merely respond to the social investment in his training, the fees paid for his services, and the terms of an agreement drawn up between himself and his patients, or does some element of gratuitous remain?

To put this question another way: is covenant simply another name for a contract in which two parties calculate their own best interests and agree upon some joint project in which both derive roughly equivalent benefits for goods contributed to each? If so, this essay would appear to move in the direction of those who interpret the doctor-patient relationship as a legal agreement and who want, on the whole, to see medical ethics draw closer to medical law.

The notion of the physician as contractor has certain obvious attractions. First, it represents a deliberate break with more authoritarian models (such as priest or parent) for interpreting the role. At the heart of a contract is informed consent rather than blind trust; a contractual understanding of the therapeutic relationship encourages full respect for the dignity of the patient, who has not, through illness, forfeited his sovereignty as a human being. The notion of a contract includes an exchange of information on the basis of which an agreement is reached and a subsequent exchange of goods (money or services); it also allows for a specification of rights, duties, conditions, and qualifications limiting the agreement. The net effect is to establish some symmetry and mutuality in the relationship between the doctor and patient.

Second, a contract provides for the legal enforcement of its items—on both parties—and thus offers both parties some protection and recourse under the law for making the other accountable for the agreement.

Finally, a contract does not rely on the pose of philanthropy, the condescension of charity. It presupposes that people are primarily governed by self-interest. When two people enter into a contract, they do so because each sees it to his own advantage. This is true not only of private contracts but also of that primordial social contract in and through which the state came into being. So argued the theorists of the 18th century. The state was not established by some heroic act of sacrifice on the part of the gods or men. Rather men entered in the social contract because each found it to his individual advantage. It is better to surrender some liberty and property to the state than to suffer the evils that would beset men except for its protection. Subsequent enthusiasts about the social instrument of contracts[7] have tended to measure human progress by the degree to which a society is based on contract rather than status. In ancient world, the Romans made the most striking advances in extending the areas in which contract rather than custom determined commerce between people. In the modern world, the bourgeoisie extended the instrumentality of contracts farthest into the sphere of economics; the free churches, into the arena of religion. Some educationists today have extended the device into the classroom (as students are encouraged to contract units of work for levels of grade); more recently some women's liberationists would extend it into marriage; and still others would prefer to see it define the professional relationship. The movement, on the whole, has the intention of laicizing authority, legalizing relationships, activating self-interests, and encouraging collaboration.

In my judgement, some of these aims of the contractualists are desirable, but it would be unfortunate if professional ethics were reduced to a commercial contract without significant remainder. First, the notion of contract suppresses the element of gift in human relationships. Earlier I verged on denying the importance of this ingredient in professional relations, when I criticized the medical profession for its conceit of philanthropy, for its self-interpretation as the great giver. In fact, this earlier objection should be limited to the failure of the medical profession to acknowledge those gifts and goods it has itself received. It is unbecoming to adopt the pose of spontaneous generosity when the profession has received so much from the community and from patients, past and present.

But the contractualist approach to professional behavior falls into the opposite error of minimalism. It reduces everything to tit-for-tat: do no more for your patients than what the contract calls for; perform specified services for certain fees and no more. The commercial contract is a fitting instrument in the purchase of an appliance, a house, or certain services that can be specified fully in advance of delivery. The existence of a legally enforceable agreement in professional transactions may also be useful to protect the patient or client against the physician or lawyer whose services fall below a minimal standard. But it would be wrong to reduce professional obligation to the specifics of a contract alone.

Professional services in the so-called helping professions are directed to subjects who are in the nature of the case rather unpredictable. One deals with the sickness, ills, crimes, needs, and tragedies of humankind. These needs cannot be exhaustively specified in advance for each patient or client. The professions must be ready to cope with the contingent, the unexpected. Calls upon services may be required that exceed those anticipated in a contract or for which compensation may be available in a given case. These services, moreover, are more likely to be effective in achieving the desired therapeutic result if they are delivered in the context of a fiduciary relationship that the patient or client can really trust.

The Limitations of Contract

Contract and covenant, materially considered, seem like first cousins; they both include an exchange and an agreement between parties. But, in spirit, contract and covenant are quite different. Contracts are external; covenants are internal to the parties involved. Contracts are signed to be expediently discharged. Covenants have a gratuitous, growing edge to them that nourishes rather than limits relationships. To the best of my knowledge, no one has put quite so effectively the difference between the two as the novelist already cited in the earlier discussion of covenant.

At the outset of Faulkner's *Intruder in the Dust,* a white boy, hunting with young blacks, falls into a creek on a cold winter's day. After the boy clambers out of the river, Lucas Beauchamp, a proud, commanding black man, brings him, shivering, to his house where Mrs. Beauchamp takes care of him. She takes off his wet clothes and wraps him in Negro blanket, feeds him Negro food, and warms him by the fire.

When his clothes dry off, the boy dresses to go, but, uneasy about his debt to the other, he reaches into his pocket for some coins and offers seventy cents compensation for Beauchamp's help. Lucas rejects the money firmly and commands the two black boys to pick up the coins from the floor where they have fallen and return them to the white boy.

Shortly thereafter, still uneasy about the episode at the river and his frustrated effort to pay off Lucas for his help, the boy buys some imitation silk for Lucas's wife and gets his Negro friend to deliver it. But a few days later, the white boy goes to his own backdoor stoop to find a jug of molasses left there for him by Lucas. So he is back to where he started, beholden to the black man again.

Several months later, the boy passes Lucas on the street and scans his face closely, wondering if the black man remembers the incident between them. He can't be sure. Four years pass, and Lucas is accused of murdering a white man. He is scheduled to be taken to jail. The boy goes early before the crowd gathers and ponders whether the old man remembers their past encounter. Just as Lucas is about to enter the jailhouse, he wheels and points his long arm in the direction of the boy and says, "Boy, I want to see you." The boy obeys and visits Lucas in the jailhouse, and eventually he and his aunt are instrumental in proving Lucas's innocence.

Faulkner's story is a parable for the relationship of the white man to the black man in the South. The black man has labored in the white man's fields, built and cared for his house, fed, clothed, and nurtured his children. In accepting these labors, the white man has received his life and substance from the black man over and over again. But he resists this involvement and tries to pay off the black man with a few coins. He pretends that their relationship is transient and external, to be managed at arm's length.

For better or for worse, blacks and whites in this country are bound up in a common life and destiny together. The problem between them will not be resolved until they accept the covenant between them which is entailed in the original acceptance of labor.

There is a donative element in the nourishing of covenant—whether it is the covenant of marriage, friendship, or professional relationship. Tit-for-tat characterizes a commercial transaction, but it does not exhaustively define the vitality of that relationship in which one must serve and draw upon the deeper reserves of another.

This donative element is important not only in the doctor's care of the patient but in other aspects of health care. In a fascinating study of *The Gift Relationship*, the late Richard M. Titmuss compares the British system of obtaining blood by donations with the American partial reliance on the commercial purchase and sale of blood.[8] The British system obtains more and better blood, without the exploitation of the indigent, which the American system has condoned and which our courts have encouraged when they refused to exempt non-profit blood banks from the anti-trust laws. By court definition, blood exchange becomes a commercial transaction in the United States. Titmuss expanded his theme from human blood to social policy by offering sober criticism of the increased commercialism of American medicine and society at large. Recent court decisions have tended to shift more and more of what had previously been considered as services into the category of commodity transactions, with negative consequences he believes for the health of health delivery systems.[9] Hans Jonas has had to reckon with the importance of voluntary sacrifice to the social order in a somewhat comparable essay on "Human Experimentation." Others have done so on the subject of organ transplants.

The kind of minimalism encouraged by a contractualist understanding of the professional relationship produces a professional too grudging, too calculating, too lacking in spontaneity, too quickly exhausted to go the second mile with his patients along the road of their distress.

Contract medicine not only encourages minimalism, it also provokes a peculiar kind of maximalism, the name for which is "defensive medicine." Especially under the pressure of malpractice suits, doctors are tempted to order too many examinations and procedures for self- protection. Paradoxically, contractualism simultaneously tempts the doctor to do too little and too much for the patient: too little in that one extends oneself only to the limits of what is specified in the contract; yet, at the same time, too much in that one orders procedures useful in protecting oneself as the contractor even though they are not fully indicated by the condition of the patient. The link between these apparently contradictory strategies of too little and too much is the emphasis in contractual decisions grounded in self-interest.

Three concluding objections to contractualism can be stated summarily. Parties to a contract are better able to protect their self-interest insofar as they are informed about the goods bought and sold. Insofar as contract medicine encourages increased knowledge on the part of the patient, well and good. Nevertheless the physician's knowledge so exceeds that of his patient that the patient's knowledgeability alone is not a satisfactory constraint on the physician's behavior. One must, at least in part, depend upon some internal fiduciary checks which the professional and his guild take on.

Another self-regulating mechanism in the traditional contractual relationship is the consumer's freedom to shop and choose among various vendors of services. Certainly this freedom of choice needs to be expanded for the patient by an increase in the number of physicians and paramedical personnel. However, the crisis circumstances under which medical services are often needed and delivered does not always provide the consumer with the kind of leisure or calm required for discretionary judgement. Thus normal marketplace controls cannot be fully relied upon to protect the consumer in dealings with the physician.

For a final reason, medical ethics should not be reduced to the contractual relationship alone. Normally conceived, ethics establishes certain rights and duties that transcend the particulars of a given agreement. The justice of any specific contract may then be measured by these standards. If, however, such rights and duties adhere only to the contract, then a patient may legitimately be persuaded to waive his rights. The contract would solely determine what is required and permissible. An ethical principle should not be waivable (except to give way to a higher ethical principle). Professional ethics should not be so defined as to permit a physician to persuade a patient to waive rights that transcend the particulars of their agreement.

Transcendence and Covenant

This essay has developed two characteristics of conventional ethics in the course of contrasting it with the ideal of philanthropy and the legal instrument of contracts. As opposed to the ideal of philanthropy that pretends to wholly gratuitous altruism, covenantal ethics places the service of the professional within the full context of goods, gifts, and services received; thus covenantal ethics is responsive. As opposed to the instrument of contract that presupposes agreement reached on the basis of self-interest, covenantal ethics may require one to be available to the covenant partner above and beyond the measure of self-interest; thus covenantal ethics has an element of the gratuitous in it.

We have to reckon now with the potential conflict between these characteristics. Have we developed our notion of covenant too reactively to alternatives without paying attention to the inner consistency of the concept itself? On the one hand, we had cause for suspicion of those idealists who founded professional duties on a philanthropic impulse, without so much as acknowledging the sacrifice of others by which their own lives have been nourished. Then we had reasons for drawing back from those legal realists and positivists who would circumscribe professional life entirely within the calculus of commodities bought and sold. But now, brought face to face, these characteristics conflict. Response to debt and gratuitous service seem opposed principles of action.

Perhaps our difficulty results from the fact that we have abstracted the concept of covenant from its original context within the transcendent. The indebtedness of a human being that makes his life—however sacrificial—inescapably responsive cannot be fully appreciated by totaling up the varying sacrifices and investments made by others in his favor. Such sacrifices are there; and it is lacking in honesty not to acknowledge them. But the sense that one is exhaustibly the object of gift presupposes a more transcendent source of donative activity than the sum of gifts received from others. For the Biblical tradition this transcendent was the secret root of every gift between human beings, of which the human order of giving and receiving could only be a sign. Thus the Jewish scriptures enjoin: when you harvest your crops, do not pick your fields too clean. Leave something for the sojourner for you were once sojourners in Egypt. Farmers obedient to this injunction were responsive, but not simply mathematically responsive to gifts received from the Egyptians or from strangers now drifting through their own land. At the same time, their actions could not be constructed as wholly gratuitous. Their ethic of service to the needy flowed from Israel's original and continuing state of neediness and indebtedness before God. Thus action which at a human level appears gratu-itous, in that it is not provoked by a specific gratuity from another human being, is at its deepest level but gift answering gift. This responsivity is theo-logically expressed in the New Testament as follows: "In this is love, not that we loved God, but that he loved us . . . if God so loved us, we also ought to love one another" (1 John 4:10–11). In some such way, covenant ethics shies back from the idealist assumption that professional action is and ought to be wholly gratuitous, and from the contractualist assumption that it be carefully governed by quotidian self-interest in every exchange.

A transcendent reference may also be important not only in setting forth the proper context in which human service takes place but also in laying out the specific standards by which it is measured. Earlier we noted some dangers in reducing rights and duties to the terms of a particular contract. We observed the need for a transcendent norm by which contracts are measured (and limited). By the same token, rights and duties cannot be wholly derived from the particulars of a given covenant. What limits ought to be placed on demands of an excessively dependent patient? At what point does the keeping of one's covenant do an injustice to obligations entailed in others? These are questions that warn against a covenantal ethics that sentimentalizes any and all involve-ments, without reference to a transcendent by which they are both justified and measured.

Further Reflections on Covenant

So far we have discussed those features of a covenant that affect the doctor's conduct toward his patient. The concept of covenant has further consequences for the patient's self-interpretation, for the accountability of health institu-tions, for the placement of institutional priorities within other national commitments, and, finally, for such collateral problems as truth-telling.

Every model for the doctor/patient relationship establishes not only a certain image of the doctor, but also a specific concept of the self. The image of the doctor as priest or parent encourages dependency in the patient. The image of doctor as skillful technician prompts the patient to think less in terms of his personal dependence, but still it encourages a somewhat impersonal passivity, with the doctor and his technical procedures the only serious agent in the relationship. The image of doctor as covenanter or contracter bids the patient to become a more active participant both in the prevention and the healing of the disease. He must bring to the partnership a will to life and a will to health.

Differing views of disease are involved in these differing patterns of rela-tionship to the doctor. Disease today is usually interpreted by the layman as an extraordinary state, discrete and episodic, disjunct from the ordinary condi-tion of health. Illness is a special time when the doctor is in charge and the layman renounces authority over his life. This view, while psychologically understandable, ignores the growth during apparent periods of health of those pathological conditions that invite the dramatic breakdown when the doctor "takes over."

The cardio-vascular accident is a case in point. Horacio Fabrega[10] has urged an interpretation of disease and health that respects more fully the processive rather than the episodic character of both disease and health. This interpretation, I assume, would encourage the doctor to monitor more continuously health/disease than ordinarily occurs today, to share with the patient more fully the information so obtained, and to engage the layperson in health maintenance.

The concept of covenant has two further advantages for defining the professional relationship, not enjoyed by models such as parent, friend, or technician. First, covenant is not so restrictively personal a term as parent or friend. It reminds the professional community that it is not good enough for the individual doctor to be a good friend or parent to the patient; that it is important also for whole institutions—the hospital, the clinic, the professional group—to keep covenant with those who seek their assistance and sanctuary. Thus the concept permits a certain broadening of accountability beyond personal agency.

At the same time, however, the notion of covenant also permits one to set professional responsibility for this one human good (health) within social limits. The professional covenant concerning health should be situated within a larger set of covenant obligations that both the doctor and patient have toward other institutions and priorities within the society at large. The traditional models for the doctor/patient relationship (parent, friend) tend to establish an exclusivity of relationship that obscures those larger responsibilities. At a time when health needs command 120 billion dollars out of the national budget, one must think about the place held by the obligation to the limited human good of health among a whole range of social and personal goods for which men are compacted together as a society.

A covenantal ethic has implications for other collateral problems in biomedical ethics, some of which have been explored in the searching work of Paul Ramsey, *The Patient as Person*. I will restrict myself simply to one issue that has not been viewed from the perspective of covenant: the question of truth-telling.

Key ingredients in the notion of covenant are promise and fidelity to promise. The philosopher J.I. Austin drew the distinction, now famous, between two kinds of speech: descriptive and performative utterances. In ordinary declarative or descriptive sentences, one describes a given term within the world. (It is raining. The tumor is malignant. The crisis is past.) In performative utterances, one does not merely describe a world, in effect, one alters the world by introducing an ingredient that would not be there apart from the utterance. Promises are such performative utterances. (I, John, take thee, Mary. We will defend your country in case of attack. I will not abandon you.) To make or to go back on a promise is a very solemn matter precisely because a promise is world-altering.

In the field of medical ethics, the question of truth-telling has tended to be discussed entirely as a question of descriptive speech. Should the doctor, as technician, tell the patient he has a malignancy or not? If not, may he lie or must he merely withhold the truth?

The distinction between descriptive and performative speech expands the question of the truth in professional life. The doctor, after all, not only tells descriptive truths, he also makes or implies promises. (I will see you next Tuesday; or, Despite the fact that I cannot cure you, I will not abandon you.) In brief, the moral question for the doctor is not simply a question of telling truths, but of being true to his promises. Conversely, the total situation for the patient includes not only the disease he's got, but also whether others ditch him or stand by him in his extremity. The fidelity of others will not eliminate the disease, but it affects mightily the human context in which the disease runs its course. What the doctor has to offer his patient is not simply proficiency but fidelity.

Perhaps more patients could accept the descriptive truth if they experienced the performative truth. Perhaps also they would be more inclined to believe in the doctor's performative utterances if they were not handed false diagnoses of false promises. That is why a cautiously wise medieval physician once advised his colleagues: "Promise only fidelity!"

The Problem of Discipline

The conclusion of this essay is not that covenantal ethics should be preferred to the exclusion of some of those values best symbolized by code and contract. If we turn now to the problem of professional discipline, we can see that both alternatives have resources for self-criticism.

Those who live by a code of technical proficiency have a standard on the basis of which to discipline their peers. The Hemingway novel, especially, *The Sun Also Rises*, is quite clear about this. Those who live by a code know how to ostracize deficient peers. Indeed, any "in-group," professional or otherwise, can be quite ruthless about sorting out those who are "quality" and those who do not have the "goods." Medicine is no exception. Ostracism, in the form of discreetly refusing to refer patients to a doctor whose competence is suspected, is probably the commonest and most effective form of discipline in the profession today.

Defenders of an ethic based on code might argue further that deficiencies in enforcement today result largely from too strongly developed a sense of covenantal obligations to colleagues and too weakly developed a sense of code. From this perspective, then, covenant is the source of the problem in the profession rather than the basis for its amendment. Covenantal obligation to colleagues inhibits the enforcement of code.

A code alone, however, will not in and of itself solve the problem of professional discipline. It provides a basis for excluding from one's own inner circle an incompetent physician. But, as Eliot Freidson has pointed out in *Professional*

Dominance, under the present system the incompetent professional, when he is excluded from a given hospital, group practice, or informal circle of referrals, simply moves his practice and finds another circle of people of equal incompetence in which he can function. It will take a much stronger, more active and internal sense of covenant obligation to patients on the part of the profession to enforce standards within the guild beyond local informal patterns of ostracism. In a mobile society with a scarcity of doctors, local ostracism simply hands on problem-physicians to other patients elsewhere. It does not address them.

Code patterns of discipline not only fall short of adequate protection for the patient; they may also fail in collegial responsibility to the troubled physician. To ostracize may be the lazy way of handling a colleague when it fails altogether to make a first attempt at remedy and to address the physician himself in his difficulty.

At the same time, it would be unfortunate if the indispensable interest and pride of the medical profession in technical proficiency were allowed to lapse out of an expressed preference for a professional ethic based on covenant. Covenant fidelity to the patient remains unrealized if it does not include proficiency. A rather sentimental existentialism unfortunately assumes that it is enough for human beings to be "present" to one another. But in crisis, the ill person needs not simply presence but skill, not just personal concern but highly disciplined services targeted on specific needs. Code behavior, handed down from doctor to doctor, is largely concerned with the transmission of technical skills. Covenant ethics, then must include rather than exclude the interests of the codes.

Neither does this essay conclude with a preference for covenant to the total exclusion of the interests of enforceable contract. While the reduction of medical ethics to contract alone incurs the danger of minimalism, patients ought to have recourse against those physicians who fail to meet minimal standards. One ought not to be dependent entirely upon disciplinary measures undertaken within the profession. There ought to be appeal to the law in cases of malpractice and for breach of contract explicit or implied.

On the other hand, in the case of injustice a legal appeal cannot be sustained without assistance and testimony from physicians who take their obligations to patients seriously. If, in such cases, fellow physicians simply herd around and protect their colleagues like a wounded elephant, the patient with just cause is not likely to get far. Thus the instrumentation of contract and other avenues of legal redress can be sustained only by a professional sense of obligation to the patient. Needless to say, it would be better for all concerned if professional discipline and continuing education were so vigorously pursued within the profession as to cut down drastically on the number of cases that needed to reach the courts.

The author inclines to accept covenant as the most inclusive and satisfying model for framing questions of professional obligation. Covenant fidelity includes the code obligation to become technically proficient; it reenforces the legal duty to meet minimal terms of contract; but it also requires much more. This surplus of obligation moreover may be redound not only to the benefit of patients but also to the advantage of troubled colleagues and their welfare.

Notes

1. Edelstein, Ludwig. *Ancient Medicine.* Baltimore: Johns Hopkins Press, 1967.

2. Winch, Peter. *The Idea of a Social Science and Its Relation to Philosophy.* New York: Humanities Press, 1958.

3. See P. Lain Entralgo, *Doctor and Patient* (New York: McGraw-Hill, 1969), for his analysis of the classic fusion of *techne* with *philanthropia;* skill in the art of healing combined with a love of mankind defines the good physician.

4. Chapter I, Article II, "Obligation of Patients to Their Physicians," *Code of Medical Ethics,* American Medical Association, May 1847. Chicago: AMA Press, 1987.

5. *Ibid.*, Chapter III, Article II.

6. New York Times, editorial and comment, 6 June 1975.

7. Sir Henry Summer Maine, *Ancient Law.* London: Oxford University Press, 1931.

8. Titmuss, Richard M. *The Gift Relationship:* From *Human Blood to Social Polity.* New York: Pantheon, 1971.

9. Titmuss does not observe that physicians in the United States had already prepared for this commercialization of medicine by their substantial fees for services (as opposed to salaried professors in the teaching field or salaried health professionals in other countries).

10. Fabrega, Horacio. Jr., "Concepts of Disease: Logical Features and Social Implications." *Perspectives in Biology and Medicine* 15: University of Chicago Press, Summer 1972.

4

Medical Ethics in Liberal Political Philosophy

Introduction

In addition to the religious traditions, secular thought also has the potential of providing an alternative to Hippocratic medical ethics. The most important secular philosophical system is that of liberal political philosophy. In the United States it manifests itself in such crucial political documents as the Declaration of Independence and the Bill of Rights of the Constitution. Internationally, it is reflected in the United National Universal Declaration of Human Rights, various documents of the World Health Organization, and the recent agreed-upon Convention on Human Rights and Biomedicine of the Council of Europe.

Political liberalism provides the philosophical underpinnings of the hundreds of court decisions, both domestically and internationally, that have essentially overturned the core ethical positions of the Hippocratic tradition. It underlies the Karen Ann Quinlan decision, the evolution of the doctrine of informed consent, the movement for the right of access to health care, and the Nuremberg trials together with the evolution of the affirmation of the rights of subjects of biomedical and behavioral research. It stands behind the moral notions of the rights of patients to consent to treatment, to have information

135

about themselves held in privacy regardless of professional judgments about the benefit of such privacy, and the right to refuse treatment.

Liberalism is traced to the political philosophy of Locke, Hobbes, Rousseau, Kant, and the thought of the enlightenment of the eighteenth century. It is grounded in religious and philosophical developments of earlier centuries. Some would associate it with the trends in Judeo-Christian theology that affirm the dignity of the individual and the importance of the individual as one who makes choices and interprets moral norms independent of political or religious authority. Thus the Protestant reformation is, in some sense, a precursor to liberalism, especially in its more left-wing and sectarian forms.

Its chief characteristics include the affirmation of the freedom or liberty of the individual. Political liberalism takes various forms. Some liberals stress the priority of the individual as one who possesses rights of noninterference from the state or other individuals or groups. This form of liberalism provides the foundation for what is sometimes called *libertarianism*, the notion that individuals are entitled to what they justly possess and that they have a right to be free from interference from others. Other forms, emphasizing the equality of moral worth of individuals, attempt to develop a role for the society to offset inequalities of fortune. In health care, this more progressive version of liberalism provides a foundation for the affirmation of a universal right to at least certain forms of health care.

Liberalism is often associated with the use of the language of *rights*. These can be either legal or moral rights, which are not always coterminous. They each come in two forms. What are sometimes called negative rights, or rights of noninterference, are more closely associated with the first version of liberalism. Positive rights, or entitlement rights of access to certain social goods and services, are more closely associated with the second version.

These themes of liberty and equality are conspicuously absent from the Hippocratic tradition of medical ethics as well as some more traditional and authoritarian forms of religious medical ethics. Together they provide a dramatic challenge to the paternalism and laissez-faire indifference to more social concerns of the Hippocratic tradition.

The readings in this chapter provide examples of some of the major secular alternatives to the Hippocratic tradition in the Anglo-American and European West.

LIBERALISM: THE BASIC CONCEPT

Just Doctoring: Medical Ethics in the Liberal State

Troyen A. Brennan

──────────────INTRODUCTION TO READING──────────────

Since about 1970, various challenges to the traditional Hippocratic ethic of medicine have emerged in the public and scholarly debate. These have surfaced in legislation and court cases, philosophical literature and even from within the health professions. In secular thought, the most sustained challenge has come from liberal political philosophy.

In the following excerpt from his book *Just Doctoring*, Harvard physician and policy analyst Troyan Brennan describes the central features of liberalism and why they are incompatible with the more traditional Hippocratic ethic. Brennan summarizes an often-made distinction between classic liberalism, with its emphasis on the right of noninterference, and what he calls modern liberalism, with its emphasis on more positive rights associated with concern about equality.

What about liberalism? Webster's relates that liberalism is "a political philosophy based in belief in progress, the essential goodness of man, and the autonomy of the individual and standing for the protection of political and civil liberties." That sounds like it has a lot to do with law, justice, and morality; it also sounds like a decent description of the political philosophy that guides the United States, Canada, and Great Britain, to name a few of what I refer to as liberal states. Given the relationship of medical ethics to moral-political concerns in our liberal state, a firm grasp of liberalism must be central to the enterprise of this book. If we can understand what the liberal state is all about, it will be much easier to understand why issues of law and justice are and should be an increasingly important part of medical ethics.

The Core of Liberalism: Negative Freedom

What, then, are the core values of liberalism? Although there is no easy answer, one can probably safely say that liberals believe individuals should be able to make choices, and that the state should be impartial to these choices. Thus liberalism requires an area of noninterference for the individual, or freedom from interference. Isaiah Berlin has called this the sphere of negative freedom and his discussion can help elucidate the essence of the liberal state.[1] Berlin notes that there are two senses of freedom in political discussion. They are as follows:

> The first of these political senses of freedom . . . which I shall call the negative sense, is involved in the question, "What is the area within which the subject—a person or group of persons—is or should be left to do or be what he wants to do or be without interference by other persons?" The second, which I shall call the positive sense, is involved with the answer to the question, "What or who is the source of control of interference, that can determine someone to do or be one thing rather than another?"[2]

Berlin thus constructs two opposing senses of the word *freedom*. One centers on the individual's sphere of action. This sphere is to be quite large and the individual is to be left, to a large extent, unbridled. The other type of freedom, the positive type, is totally different. It involves the use of power or coercion by some in society, or the state itself, to help perfect or improve other individuals. The purpose of this coercion is to allow the citizen to live in accordance with his true self.

Negative freedom operates on the assumption that personal choice affirms one's humanity. Individual action possesses a value incommensurable with other types of action:

> There ought to exist a certain minimum area of personal freedom which can on no account be violated, for, if it is overstepped, the individual will find himself in an area too narrow for even that minimum development of his natural faculties which alone makes it possible to pursue, and even to conceive, the various ends which mankind holds good or right or sacred.[3]

These views reflect what I will call "classic liberalism." The classic liberal sense of freedom demands that the individual be left alone with her own projects. The exercise of free choice and pursuit of individual projects are what give life meaning, according to the liberal. Berlin here is echoing John Stuart Mill's conception of society and individual good. As Mill stated, this conception is embodied in "one very simple principle: That principle is that the sole end for which mankind are warranted individually or collectively, in interfering with the liberty of action of any of their number, is self-protection."[4] Of course, this negative freedom, or liberty, is protected by one's political rights.

Mill himself justified the liberal emphasis on negative freedom protected by rights on the bedrock of utilitarianism. His assertion that individual freedom guarantees the maximization of utility rested on his ultimate belief in the greatest good of individual thought. Mill was quite sure that the good of individual thought and action is a far more important consideration than the reasons for limiting individual freedom.

Berlin's rendition of negative freedom certainly concurs with this. Berlin and others do, nonetheless, take a step beyond Mill in their refusal to treat negative freedom and rights as instrumental values, simply justified by the ends served.[5] They argue instead that rights and the liberty or negative freedom that rights preserve are intrinsically good. The individual's liberty cannot be weighed against other goods. Thus liberal philosophers oppose positive freedom, or any form of coercion of the individual in an obdurate fashion. The nature of this opposition further illuminates the content of the liberal state.

According to Berlin, positive freedom issues from a different set of assumptions about what is valuable in society. The adherent of positive freedom sees herself and other human beings as imperfect, yet perfectible. Some human action must therefore be curtailed in order that more perfect arrangements and attitudes can come about in the future. Positive freedom asserts that in order that all may advance, some must be bridled.

Berlin, as a classic liberal, will not accept this. He is a proponent of negative freedom, which he believes is the only true freedom. He argues that societal decisions about the common good are given to misinterpretation and are fraught with the potential for tyranny of the majority, or even dictatorship by a few: "For it is this—the positive concept of liberty: not freedom from, but freedom to, which adherents of the 'negative' notion represent as being, at times, no better than a specious disguise for brutal tyranny."[6] Berlin thus fears positive freedom and seeks to contain it with the concept of personal liberty, or negative freedom.

In medicine today, we are often reminded of the negative freedom of the patient. The patient's freedom from interference comes through most strongly in situations in which patients request that their care be limited. The courts, including the Supreme Court in the recent case of *Cruzan v. Missouri Department of Human Services* have consistently reiterated that when a patient decides that he does not want heroic or lifesaving measures, and the patient is competent, then physicians cannot insist on further therapy. In the court analysis, a physician's insistence on therapy would be a violation of the patient's negative freedom, a freedom to refuse further invasive care. Physicians who argue that competent patients cannot understand the importance of their decision to limit their care are seeking, perhaps, to impose their own conception of what is good and to force the patient to accept further care. The courts usually reject this physician assertion of power and reiterate that the patient's negative freedom, or liberty, should be sacrosanct.

Negative freedom can provide the basis for a theory of justice when one links it to an unfettered right to property, the freedom to dispose of what is one's own. Classic liberal philosophy entails that one is free to do whatever one wants with one's possessions. One is free to paint one's own car. One has a right to paint it. One does not lose the freedom to paint one's own car simply because one has no paint. No paint does not mean no rights. Rights are characterized here as formal guarantees, not as material benefits of some sort.

As might be expected, the classic liberal thinks little of positive freedom, which he characterizes as an end-state theory. In this view, although the liberal values a certain, usually egalitarian, pattern of the distribution of goods in society, he also believes that "any distributional patterns with any egalitarian component is overturnable by the voluntary actions of individual people over time."[7] Thus inequality is the natural outcome of rights that guarantee liberties, and the classic liberal accepts this outcome. His belief is that as long as one respects others' rights, then we have no reason to blame him or her for getting wealthier.

Consider Robert Nozick's example of Wilt Chamberlain's ascendancy to fame and fortune. Nozick argues that Chamberlain is not to blame for his own abilities and resultant wealth and that those who would deny him his salary would be constantly trespassing on the personal life of the basketball player. In effect, this means that one can have liberty or equality but not both. Nozick would opt for the former, and he would use the rhetoric of rights to buttress his position. From this argument, it follows that institutions are just only insofar as they promote no interference. In the liberal view, the Internal Revenue Service's interest in Chamberlain's salary, or even the salary caps negotiated by the National Basketball Association with the Player's Association, are unjust.

This position itself represents an evolution of classic liberalism. I will call it "conservatism." A conservative like Nozick or Bertrand de Jouvenal[8] believes that redistribution is ethically wrong because it undermines and weakens notions of personal responsibility. Moreover, conservatives cast doubt on the ability of redistributionist policies to produce the good they intend. In essence, they deny that a central authority can possibly bring about a better pattern of distribution than will free citizens in the market.[9]

The conservative position has been questioned, especially by socialists, but even by other liberals. For instance, some argue that it ignores the impediments that stand in the way of some members of society simply because of the situation into which they were born.[10] Certain members of society will be unable to exercise those liberties granted them because they were born into a deprived setting. While admitting that each citizen may be granted a formal set of liberties outlining a sphere of activity within which he or she can operate, those opposed to conservatism point out that this set remains merely formal so long as people lack the substantive means to realize the potential of their own autonomy and humanity. The idea that formal liberty often fails to become substantive is the outstanding criticism of both classic liberalism and its progeny, conservatism.

There are several other grounds on which to challenge the conservative. Countering his assumption that inequality just happens, that it should be viewed as a natural occurrence, like the weather or volcanic eruptions, some would maintain that it is impossible to generate large amounts of inequality between individuals unless there are significant inequalities of power in a society. This argument is in turn supported by two other propositions. First, people are not all that different in the basic, or if you like, natural level of talents they have and can offer. Second, inequality is not a result of freedom of choice, but rather of some taking advantage of others. Thus inequality only occurs when some take advantage of inequity of power to use others as means to ends. In this view, liberty and the impartiality of liberalism simply support the appropriation of the means of production by the powerful and the resulting subversion of others.

One need not go to Marxist extremes, however, to fault the conservative for failing to take into account the value of equality, and for overvaluing pure liberty. The conservative statement that rights exist, that they are good, that they should be defended by just institutions, and that the outcome of such a polity is not a concern of justice cannot be logically sustained. It is, quite simply, wrong. Inequality is a result of the set of rights that are allowed in a society, and the inequality is in effect condoned by that set of rights.

The conservative's failure is his lack of consideration for the ways that economic or contractual claims that may legitimately be made by favored individuals in the type of society he values are not available to all its citizens, given a heritage of unequal wealth, education, and health care. This inequality is unjust, and the state must deal with it, not dismiss it as natural. As Albert Jonsen and Andre Hellegers have stated:

> When benefits and burdens can be so distributed, the problem of justice arises. Some who will benefit will not bear costs; some who will bear costs will not benefit. When the situation depends not on chance, but on planned and conscious decisions about the structure of the institution, it is necessary to ask, "Why should anyone benefit at the apparent cost to another?" These are the questions at the heart of . . . justice.[11]

Consider, for instance, the newborn child of a mother who has no health insurance and is not eligible for government relief programs. This mother, as a result of her exclusion from such programs, might have received substandard prenatal care for herself and her unborn child. Say that because of this lack of care, the child has suffered some intrauterine growth retardation, resulting in the sort of neurological deficits that good prenatal care is designed to avoid. Thus the existence of inequalities in society has created a situation in which one individual will be unable to take advantage of opportunities theoretically available to every member of the society because he was born with certain neurological problems. An advocate of egalitarianism would argue that this child represents a failure of conservatism, for the enshrinement of negative freedom has failed to guarantee him the enjoyment of life, at least, from the point of view of classic liberalism.

While conservativism is a natural evolution of classic liberalism, there are other offshoots. The most prominent is what I will call "modern liberalism," so as to distinguish it from classic liberalism and conservatism. Modern liberals recognize the arguments made by those who point out the importance of egalitarian programs. They realize equality must be balanced with liberty in the modern liberal state. It can be said that conservatives see themselves as defenders of liberty, while modern liberals are more concerned with equality.

The modern liberal realizes that granting greater liberty by placing an emphasis on rights allows for more inequality within a society and also realizes that liberty can bring rewards only if the material means to pursue that liberty are available. Modern liberals, while still valuing liberty, envision a society that can establish greater equality. In pursuit of this end, they would not balk at interference with certain individual liberties if a larger proportion of the society would benefit as a result.

Liberty, Equality, and Market Impartiality

Classic liberalism gives rise to a number of different moral-political philosophies, in particular, conservativism and modern liberalism. The core of liberalism, whether classic or modern, concerns liberty and impartiality. The concept of liberty guarantees the individual a sphere that is his or her own. Liberty provides an area in which one can operate unencumbered by the strictures of the society within which one lives. The state remains impartial to the individual's choices in this sphere: it guarantees liberty.

Given this core, how does modern liberalism address inequality? Liberal notions of equality celebrate the belief that all people are the same in their humanness, that no matter what physical and mental differences exist between us, society accepts each and every member as beings of incomparable worth. Thus, the concepts of both liberty and equality can represent the optimistic belief in perfectibility that characterizes liberalism of all flavors. Yet, as noted above, classic liberals and especially their conservative offspring might see some conflict between the values of liberty and equality. To understand this potential conflict, let us define liberalism more closely.

In the liberal state, an individual's liberty is primary, and the individual enjoys and utilizes his "freedom from" interference to develop his notion of a good life. This liberty is guaranteed by rights. Each citizen, in a model liberal polity, has an equal set of rights that includes an equal right to opportunities. The individual's liberty should not be, or should only minimally be, hampered by the policies of the state. The classic liberal conception assumes that a free market will provide the means for maximizing an individual's free choice. The government tends to stand aside and let the market order societal relations, allowing its citizens to take advantage of their liberty.

The classic liberal state is therefore fundamentally impartial. It allows the citizen to formulate her own notions of goodness, and to pursue them with little interference. As John Rawls notes, the liberal citizen need possess only two moral powers, a sense of justice and a notion of the good.[12] There are no special notions of virtue that underpin liberalism. Rather, liberalism encourages pluralism. Each citizen is allowed to develop and pursue her own sense of morality in the ideal liberal state. The government stands by impartially, making sure that the free market economy remains in place.

Of course, as modern liberals recognize, this state is only an ideal. The impartiality of liberalism does not empty the society of its sense of community. The liberal state is a polity, and its citizens realize they must live together, and so there are constraints on liberty. Instead of a formal impartiality and rampant pluralism of moral ideals, the modern liberal state features what Rawls calls an "overlapping consensus."[13] So long as there is some degree of consensus, the liberal state is a place where many views are tolerated. Certain views of moral behavior, such as those that call for racial purification, are excluded. Every Nazi or white supremacist cannot be allowed to take action based on his own sense of morality. While the liberal state does not preclude any view of society, it does exclude putting some into effect. Absolute liberty is thus diminished for the sake of the community. The modern liberal state is accomplished only through a series of compromises with the traditional liberal ideal compromises between equality and liberty.

The classic liberal ideal overlooks the fact that natural differences between persons are unavoidable. To bring about equality, it is thus sometimes necessary to have the state interfere in the pursuit of individual projects. Notions of equality thus tend to restrict liberties; in particular they restrict free choice in the market.

The liberal state, then, must carefully weigh the competing values of liberty and equality. Rights often act as the operators within this negotiation. The nature of the rights to which a citizen is entitled tends to outline the compromise between equality and liberty that has been reached within a society. On the one hand, a society that creates a right to health care that requires a great deal of government subsidy to realize it, will probably sanction a more than modest interference with liberty. On the other hand, a society that sanctions a fundamental right to personal property and that prohibits takings by the government will probably largely prohibit interference with liberty.

...

In summary, the central problem of the doctor-patient relationship is the inequality of knowledge, and thus of power. The doctor understands the complicated biological events that cause ill health; the patient who lacks the doctor's specialist training, cannot. The patient may also be emotionally weakened by ill health.

To resolve this inequality and create a relationship in which the patient can talk freely and openly with the doctor, a particular medical morality has developed. The physician is duty bound to treat the patient with greatest respect. The physician must maintain a loyalty to the patient and engender the patient's trust. The patient must "come first" even if this requires some self-effacement and sacrifice on the part of the physician, although in fact, "the patient comes first" ethic is synonymous with physician authority. Other concerns should not intrude on this relationship. The moral code of beneficence works best if it is isolated from the usual concerns of the liberal state, especially the competitive market. The doctor's moral code, not civil law, provides the foundation for the doctor-patient relationship. The dutiful doctor can withstand the pressures of moral hazard because of his ethical commitment. Other possible players in a medical care market would not be as immunized from profit. Thus fee-for-service dominates, and only conditionless insurance is allowed.

As a result, medical morality is estranged from the public morality that guides the liberal state. The notion of patient liberties and the justice provided by the public morality through law had little impact on medical morality. The patient's negative freedom is rather unimportant in the healing process described by Parsons and others. Contractual models of the doctor-patient relationship are overruled. A true market cannot operate.

The ethical theory of medicine was thus integral to, and sustained by, the economic and political structure of medical practice. Government officials and other professionals were excluded from the care of patients. The regulation of doctors was confined to the medical profession itself. A system of third-party payers was allowed so that economic constraints would not play a role in doctors' care of patients. In short, the doctor-patient relationship was insulated from the constraints of the market, the chief arbiter in the liberal state. Medical institutions thus meshed neatly with the ideology of medical ethics.

The notion of the symbiotic relationship of medical ethics and the medical enterprise is largely conceptual. There are a number of other possible explanations for the growth of institutions of medical care. The symbiotic relationship also assumes that certain aspects of the social morality (for instance, medical ethics) can remain relatively detached from the public morality of the liberal state. In the next chapter, we will look at some of the competing explanations for the peculiar structure of medical care, review the changes of the past fifteen years in that structure, and suggest that the public morality of the liberal state has asserted itself and, with changes in the nature of the medical enterprise, made the "patient comes first" brand of medical morality obsolete.

Medicine in the Liberal State

In the last chapter, I suggested that medical ethics has been conceptually at odds with liberalism. In this chapter, we further explore this conceptual dissonance, and the changes that have brought the medical enterprise more in step with our market-based, pluralist society.

Much of the discussion necessarily will proceed at a rather theoretical level. Physician behavior itself does not overtly evince many of the moral overtones we discuss here. Indeed, observers have noted that the typical practitioner pays little attention to the role of an ethical code in his daily work. Freidson's empirical study led him to the following conclusion:

> Curiously enough, we could raise little interest among physicians by interview questions about the problem of ethics in medical work. Ethics seemed to be unproblematic to them and rather less related to being a

doctor than to being a properly brought up (middle-class) human being. Ethicality was "pretty much common sense," . . . was learned "when you are brought up by your mother." . . . To most physicians the word seemed to refer to the norms of decency and honesty that were expected of all proper middle-class people and that had not and need not [have] been taught to students in medical school.[14]

Nonetheless, for the moment, a certain theoretical purity must be maintained to illustrate medical ethics in the liberal state.[15]

Medical Ethics and Paternalism

The central theme of medical ethics, from the perspective of the beneficence model, is the doctor and patient partnership. The physician is in a sense a friend who has a commitment, a duty, to the patient and is bound to treat the patient as an end in himself and, if necessary, to make sacrifices to help the patient return to health. The doctor and patient thus work together, but under the physician's leadership, for mutual ends. More accurately, the physician uses her specialized knowledge on behalf of the patient.

The problem with this model of medical ethics is that it overlooks pluralism, one of the primary virtues of the liberal state. Alasdair MacIntyre has argued quite convincingly that the liberal state allows and encourages a number of different moral points of view.[16] This pluralism creates the diversity that enriches the social morality. But it also eliminates the grounds one would use to justify action on behalf of another.

As MacIntyre relates, previous societies did not celebrate pluralism; rather, they encouraged conformity with a single moral point of view. But our society eschews such shared values. Instead we have only the minimal glue provided by the public morality of liberalism. More important, that public morality emphasizes the importance of individual choice and negative freedom, not shared values. Pluralism makes no effort to shape shared assumptions.

The medical ethics of "the patient comes first" model assumes that physicians can act on behalf of the patient simply because the physician is duty bound to help the patient place his welfare first. The problem for such a theory is that in a liberal state only the individual can define his or her own personal welfare. Thus the "patient comes first" model must conflict with liberalism. Specifically, the liberal state cannot accept the paternalism inherent in medical ethics.

Paternalism can be defined as interference with or failure to respect affairs normally designated as matters within an individual's sphere of liberty for the sake of that individual. Dworkin offers a more technical definition of paternalism as "roughly the interference with a person's liberty of action justified by reasons referring exclusively to the welfare, food, happiness, needs, interests or values of the person being coerced."[17] Paternalism thus represents a decrease in personal liberty by interfering with another's behavior, choice, or opportunity for choice for that person's well-being, though that interference need not be actual or physical, and indeed may simply be a failure to seek consent.

While that interference may be justified on the basis of a higher good, it is viewed in the liberal state with a great deal of suspicion. The liberal state maximizes the amount of negative freedom granted individuals so as to minimize the possibility of the abuses that can occur under the name of positive freedom. Liberalism assumes that the individual citizen typically knows what is best for himself; thus the rationale for paternalism is undercut, and individual autonomy is accorded the widest respect possible.

Times and situations occur even in the most liberal of states in which paternalism may be justified. For example, in our society parents are allowed and encouraged to restrict their children's freedom and to make decisions on their behalf. The close, affective ties between parents and children are the justification for paternalism. We do not fear, as a rule, that parents will take advantage of paternalism and exploit their children because parents usually behave in a dutiful and self-effacing manner. The ends of child welfare then are central to parental decision making.

To a certain degree, the analysis of the "patient comes first" medical ethics is analogous to familial love, in which the doctor (the parent) and the patient (the child) work together for a common good—the patient's welfare. This commitment justifies the doctor's decisions on behalf of the patient, and also justifies an institutional framework that isolates doctor and patient from the oversight of the liberal state. To the extent that these institutions flourish, we can assume that society is convinced that the medical profession's paternalism is not exploitive.

Others have taken a narrower position that paternalism is justified "only when the person's choice is different from what it would be given his or her normal character and decision-making abilities, and more specifically, only when the impairments in these abilities are such that they result in the person withholding consent to paternalistic interference to which he or she would have given consent."[18] By twisting or exaggerating the notion of impairments, however, a physician could justify paternalism every time her patient disagrees with a prescribed course of therapy (which leads Childress to argue that medical paternalism is much broader than mere coercion[19]). Believing that the expert knows best, the physician pushes ahead with a program of her own design in order to benefit the patient. Medical institutions nurture this endeavor, protecting the doctor's decisions from public judgment.

In a liberal state, in particular our liberal state, however, such broad physician prerogatives cannot be sustained. The medical enterprise, and the overly broad paternalism it sanctions, inevitably must be addressed. That is what occurred around 1970 when the American public perception of medicine began to change. In a variety of ways, the public became convinced that physician paternalism was really physician exploitation and that medicine was set up not to nurture the patient but to benefit the physician. This led to an assertion of patient autonomy and liberty and restriction of physician power. In the following section, we will review evidence of how the American liberal state began to rein in the powers of the medical profession and to reintegrate it with the principles of liberalism. In the process, physician paternalism was limited and the "patient comes first" ethic was discredited.

Notes

1. Isaiah Berlin, *Four Essays on Liberty* (London: Oxford University, Press, 1969).

2. Ibid., 24.

3. John Stuart Mill, *On Liberty* (Northbrook, Ill.: AHM Publishing,1947),

4. Ibid., 35.

5. Charles Fried, *Right and Wrong* (Cambridge: Harvard University Press, 1978).

6. Berlin, *Four Essays on Liberty*, 38.

7. Robert Nozick, *Anarchy, State and Utopia* (New York: Basic Books, 1974), 164.

8. Bertrand de Jouvenal, *The Ethics of Redistribution* (Indianapolis: Liberty Press, 1990).

9. Of course, some theorists whom I would call conservatives might see themselves as true liberals, and might refer to my modern liberalism as socialism. For instance, H. Tristram Engelhardt, in developing a theory of bioethics, refers to the linchpin of public authority as a matter of peaceable, mutual negotiation. This is a liberal view, but I would understand Engelhardt as a classic liberal or perhaps a conservative. See H. Tristram Engelhardt, *The Foundations of Bioethics* (New York: Oxford University Press, 1986), 44.

10. See, for example, C. B. McPherson, "Maximization of Democracy," in *Philosophy, Politics, and Society*, ed. P. Laslett and W. G. Runciman (New York: Barnes and Noble, 1967).

11. A. Hellegers and A. Jonsen, "Conceptual Foundations for an Ethic of Medical Care," in *Ethics and Health Policy*, ed. R. Branson and R. Veatch (Cambridge, Mass.: Ballinger Publishers Company, 1976), 38.

12. John Rawls, "Justice as Fairness: Political, Not Metaphysical," *Philosophy and Public Affairs* 14(1985): 223–251.

13. See John Rawls, "The Idea of an Overlapping Consensus," *Oxford Journal of Legal Studies*, 7, no. 1 (1986): 1. Rawls reiterates that the overlapping consensus is not a mere modus vivendi, but substantive and constitutive of morality. See also John Rawls, "The Domain of the Political and the Overlapping Consensus," *New York University Law Review* 64 (May 1989): 233–255.

14. See Freidson, *Doctoring Together*, 125

15. In subsequent chapters [in the book from which this reading is taken], we will return to more realistic encounters

16. Alasdair MacIntyre, *After Virtue: A Study in Moral Theory* (Notre Dame, Ind.: University of Notre Dame Press, 1981).

17. G. Dworkin, "Paternalism," In *Morality and the Law*, ed. R.A. Wasserstrom (Belmont, Calif.: Wadsworth, 1971), 108.

18. D.W. Brock, "Paternalism and Autonomy," *Ethics* 98 (1988): 550–566.

19. James Childress, *Who Should Decide? Paternalism in Health Care* (New York: Oxford University Press, 1982).

RESPECT FOR PERSONS

One of the central features of liberal political philosophy is its commitment to respect for the dignity of persons. From this perspective it is not sufficient morally to strive to do good for patients or others and to attempt to protect them from harm. Sometimes doing so can come at the price of infringing on the dignity of the individual. If it does, then, according to the tenets of liberal political philosophy, it is not necessarily morally right to do good for people in such cases. The prior concern—the side constraint on doing good for people— is that they are respected.

For example, there have been cases in which physicians have believed that they could benefit their patient by breaching the promise of confidentiality without the patient's approval. There have been cases in which they have attempted to protect patients from harm by refusing to disclose the truth of a bleak prognosis. There have been times when patients were forced to undergo medical treatment against their will because the physician believed it was for the patient's benefit. All of these are examples in which the Hippocratic ethic of benefitting the patient conflicts with the liberal ethic of showing respect.

These concerns about respect for persons are often expressed as general principles. The three examples just given can be placed under the general principles of fidelity to promises, veracity, and respect for autonomy There are other principles sometimes associated with this liberal philosophical perspective, but these three have been particularly important in the evolution of liberal medical ethics. In addition, the concern for treating people as equals is often associated with the moral principle of justice. In the following section, readings examine autonomy, one of these principles that form elements of the notion of respect for persons, and the issues of informed consent that derive from the concern about respecting autonomy. In the following section, the principle of justice and its implications for allocating scarce medical resources are addressed.

AUTONOMY

Autonomy

James Childress

──────────INTRODUCTION TO READING──────────

In addition to the principles of promise-keeping and veracity mentioned in the introduction to this section, an additional characteristic of action that many now consider to be inherently right-making is respect for another

person's autonomy. According to this view, even if one is certain that interfering with another's autonomous choices will do more good for that
person than respecting them, there is still some moral reason to forego
intervening. Some people consider respect for autonomy along with
fidelity to promises and honesty to be aspects of a broader principle of
respect for persons while others see them as more independent. The
following excerpt from James Childress's volume on paternalism spells out
what is meant by autonomy.

One aspect of respecting persons is respecting their *autonomy*; this is an implication of respecting persons as independent ends in themselves. Etymologically,
"autonomy" is compounded of *autos* (self) and *nomos* (law or rule). *Autonomia*
originally was used to indicate the independence of Greek city-states from
outside control, perhaps from a conqueror, and their determination of their
own laws. The notions of independence, self-rule, and self-determination recur
in explications of "autonomy," and their analysis is essential if we are to understand "what is essentially a metaphor."

It is customary to contrast "autonomy" and "heteronomy," "autonomy"
referring to self-rule and "heteronomy" referring to rule by other objects or
persons. Heteronomous persons, for example, might have surrendered their
judgment-making and decision-making to the state or to the church; their
actions would be heteronomous because they would be determined by what
the state or the church dictates. But although such persons may fall short of the
ideal of autonomy (which will be discussed later), they may have exercised and
even continued to exercise autonomy in the choice of the state or the church as
the source of their judgments and decisions. Thus, there is an important
distinction between *first-order* and *second-order* autonomy.[1] Persons who are
subservient to state or church would lack first-order autonomy, i.e., self-determination regarding the content of decisions and choices, because of their exercise of second-order autonomy, i.e., selection of the institution to which they
are subordinate. In other situations, first-order choices and actions such as the
use of some drugs may appear to be under inner compulsion or addiction. But
these agents retain some second-order autonomy: when they are made aware
of their condition, they may choose to seek help or to remain under compulsion or addiction because they want to. As Gerald Dworkin contends, a person
who is a drug addict and cannot break his physiological dependence on the
drug, and yet who wants to be under this compulsion, is autonomous at least in
this *second-order* sense, for he identifies with his addiction.[2]

Autonomy does not imply that an individual's life plan is his or her own
creation and that it excludes interest in others. The first implication focuses on
the source, the second on the object of autonomy.[3] Neither implication holds.
Autonomy simply means that a person chooses and acts freely and rationally
out of her own life plan, however ill-defined. That this life plan is her own does
not imply that she created it de novo or that it was not decisively influenced by
various factors such as family and friends. Some existentialists who use the

language of autonomy suggest that if an individual does not create his own life plan, or at least an independent series of choices, he is guilty of "bad faith." Recall Jean-Paul Sartre's advice to the young man who was trying to decide whether to join the Free French Forces or to remain to help his mother: "You're free, choose, that is, invent."[4] More satisfactory interpretations of autonomy recognize that it may be rooted in both society and history. The source of an individual's life plan may well be, for example, a religious tradition with which he identifies and which he appropriates. An example is a Jehovah's Witness' life plan which gives everlasting life priority over earthly life if the latter can be maintained only by blood transfusions. Thus, personal autonomy does not imply on asocial or ahistorical approach to life plans. It only means that whatever the life plan, and whatever its source, an individual takes it as his own.

Likewise, the object of autonomous life plans and choices is not limited to the individual himself or herself but may include various principles and values such as altruistic beneficence. Autonomy does not presuppose that the individual is uninterested in the positive or negative impact on others. For example, some discussions of autonomous suicide seem to suppose that the agent is acting autonomously only if she is uninterested in an impact on others. But the agent may view the act of suicide primarily as expression and communication. This was certainly true of Jo Roman, who committed suicide in order to create "on [her] own terms the final stroke of [her] life's canvas". A 62-year-old artist, she had originally planned to commit suicide on her seventy-fifth birthday but acted earlier because of her breast cancer. In addition, she carefully staged her suicide in order to have a public impact, particularly to convince others that "life can be transformed into art."[5] Her desire for expression and communication did not, however, make her act less autonomous. It is a distortion of autonomy to limit the object to the agent's own self. Both points can be summarized: in terms of input and output, autonomy is not asocial or ahistorical. Both communication and influence occur both ways.

Does this analysis of autonomy imply the "separateness of persons," a conception that undergirds several recent critiques of utilitarianism? According to these criticisms, utilitarianism tends to view separate individuals as having only instrumental, not intrinsic, value as either depositors or depositories of good. Against utilitarianism, they emphasize either the separateness of agents or the separateness of recipients or patients (i.e., those acted upon). In the former, the emphasis will be on the patient's rights.[6] But because the separateness of persons tends to suggest an atomistic individualism, it is better to focus on the distinctiveness of persons, while recognizing that both their sources and their objects may be social.

Respect for persons who are autonomous may differ from respect for persons who are not autonomous. Formal equality, sometimes referred to as the formal principle of justice, demands that similar cases be treated similarly and that equals be treated equally. But because it does not specify relevant similarities or dissimilarities, it is formal and thus empty until it receives material content from other sources. My interpretation of the principle of respect for persons identifies autonomy as one relevant similarity. When persons are autonomous, respect for them requires (or prohibits) certain actions that may not be required (or prohibited) in relation to nonautonomous persons. Several principles, particularly nonmaleficence, may establish minimum standards of conduct, such as noninfliction of harm in relation to all persons whatever their degree of autonomy. But what the principle of respect requires (and prohibits) in relation to autonomous persons will differ. Thus Kant excluded children and the insane from his discussion of the principle of respect of persons and Mill applied his discussion of liberty only to those who are in "The maturity of their faculties."[7] I will examine some aspects or criteria of autonomy before considering some specific requirements of respect for autonomous persons.

Two essential features of autonomy are (1) acting freely and (2) deliberating rationally. I will provide only a brief statement of these features which will be discussed in more detail in subsequent chapters. First, what is the relationship between competence and these two features of autonomy? Logically competence might be viewed as a precondition of deliberating rationally and acting freely or as a summary term for these two (and perhaps other) conditions. A person suffering from mental defects, for example, that would preclude either acting freely or deliberating rationally would be incompetent to make decisions. Competence is not an all or nothing matter. It may vary over time and from situation to situation. A person may be competent part of the time but incompetent the rest of the time; this will be called intermittent competence. And a person may be competent to act in X (e.g., to drive a car) but not in Y (e.g., to make decisions in a large family-operated business); this will be called limited competence.[8] One difficult question that will occupy out attention in later chapters is which way to err in borderline cases of competence.

Acting Freely

To act freely is, in part, to be outside the control of others. This point is implied by independence, and it excludes coercion, duress, undue influence, and manipulation. If a person is coerced—"your money or your life"—she is not acting freely even though she is deliberating rationally and acting intentionally. But, as we have seen, a person may exercise second-order autonomy by freely choosing to become dependent on a religious community for moral guidance. For example, a woman may decide not to have an abortion to save her life because she freely accepts the authority of the Catholic Church. To act freely also involves the absence of certain internal constraints such as compulsion and drug addiction. A person's action can be seriously encumbered or limited by either internal or external constraints that he or she cannot be said to be autonomous.

Indeed, internal constraints, for example, may be so severe that we do not hold the agent responsible for what he does. In some cases although the agent was causally responsible for what occurred, we do not hold him morally or legally responsible because he lacked the capacity for responsibility. Nonetheless a general use of the language of disease to discount responsibility for wrongful conduct is a sign of disrespect for persons:

> A *total* reinterpretation of wrong doing in terms of disease amounts to a denial of personal responsibility altogether. It *insults* the wrongdoer under the guise of *safeguarding* his interests. It treats him as though he were *not* a person, and falls foul accordingly of the very principle of respect to which it appeals. This is the element of vital truth in the doctrine which to many has seemed merely a bad joke, that a man has a *right* to be punished.[9]

Deliberating Rationally

Deliberation is "an imaginative rehearsal of various courses of action."[10] It can be encumbered or limited in various ways, particularly by a person's inability to reason because of mental illness or to reason fully because of inadequate or incomplete information about various courses of action and their consequences. It is possible in some cases to judge that a person's deliberation is irrational without calling into question the life plans, values, and ends on which the deliberation is based and without calling into question the weighting of the alternatives and their consequences. For example, a person may seek incompatible ends (such as preservation of a gangrenous leg) or choose ineffective means to his ends.[11] Suppose two patients refuse amputations of gangrenous feet, one because she wants to die and the other because she does not believe that the condition is fatal. In the latter case there may be grounds for holding that the patient is not deliberating rationally and thus is not autonomous. Nevertheless, as Bruce Miller reminds us, it is not always possible to separate factual and valuative errors in nonrational deliberation.

> A patient may refuse treatment because of its pain and inconvenience, e.g. Kidney dialysis, and choose to run the risk of serious illness and death. To say that such a patient has the relevant knowledge, if all other alternatives and their likely consequences have been explained, but that nonrational assignment of priorities has been made is much too simple. A good accurate characterization may be that the patient misappreciates certain aspects of the alternatives. The patient may be cognitively aware of the pain and inconvenience of the treatment, but because he or she has not experienced them, the assessment of their severity may be too great. If the patient has begun dialysis, assessment of the pain and inconvenience may not take into account the possibilities that the patient will adapt to them or that they may be reduced by adjustments in the treatment. Misappreciating the consequences of treatment in this way is not a lack of knowledge, nor is it simply a non-rational weighting; it involves matters of fact and value.[12]

In addition, even when it is possible to identify errors in factual beliefs, it may be difficult to determine that the person is not autonomous.

Several philosophers have used the notion of authenticity to explicate autonomy. For example, Gerald Dworkin views autonomy as authenticity plus independence, while Bruce Miller identifies four aspects of autonomy as free action, authenticity, effective deliberation and moral reflection. For Dworkin, authenticity is a person's identification with the determinants of his behavior so that they become his own. For Miller, it means that "an action is consistent with the attitudes, values, dispositions and life plans of the person."[13] The intuitive idea of authenticity is "acting in character." We wonder whether actions are autonomous if they are not consistent with what we know about a person (e.g., a sudden and unexpected decision to discontinue dialysis by a man who had displayed considerable courage and zest for life despite his years of disability). If they are in character (e.g., a Jehovah's Witness' refusal of a blood transfusion), we are less likely to suspect that they do not represent genuine autonomy. In addition, the notion of authenticity captures our sense that selves develop over time with persistent and enduring patterns; they are not simply collections of choices and acts. And yet it would be a mistake to make authenticity a criterion of autonomy. At most authenticity alerts us to relevant questions. If it is not satisfied, if the choice or action (such as refusal of treatment) is inconsistent with what we know of the person and his character, then we should seek justifications or explanations, some of which may indicate that the action is not autonomous (perhaps because it was under inner compulsion). We should also consider whether the person has experienced a change or even conversion in basic values and life plan and even whether we really knew the person as well as we previously thought. Actions apparently out of character and inauthentic can be caution flags that alert others to press for justifications and explanations in order to determine whether the actions are autonomous. By contrast, actions that are not free cannot count as autonomous.

An important distinction, drawn from Robert Nozick, may help to clarify the meaning of the principle of respect for persons: (1) autonomy as an end state or goal and (2) autonomy as a side constraint.[14] Frequently debates about paternalism are confused because all parties appeal to autonomy to justify their proposals without attending to differences that result from viewing autonomy as an end state as opposed to a side constraint. If autonomy is a side constraint, it limits the pursuit of goals such as health and survival; it even limits the pursuit of the goal of the preservation and restoration of autonomy itself. In pursuing goals for ourselves or for others we are not permitted to violate others' autonomy. Because what we do, not merely what happens is morally important, or nonviolation of autonomy is required. Whether autonomy is an absolute limit would depend on the moral theory; perhaps it could be violated in order to prevent a catastrophe. In contrast, when autonomy is viewed as an end state to be realized, its function in moral argument is very different. Autonomy is a condition, not a constraint, and the goal might be to minimize damage to autonomy whether that damage results from nature, disease, or other persons. In this view, some violations of autonomy (such as some decisions to reject patients' refusals of treatment) might be justified because overall more autonomy would result, and that is the desirable end state.

Eric Cassell, a strong proponent of autonomy, views it mainly as an end state rather that as a side constraint. He contends that autonomy (for which he uses Gerald Dworkin's formula, autonomy = authenticity + independence) is seriously compromised by illness, "the most important thief of autonomy," and that the primary function of medicine is to preserve, to repair, and to restore the patient's autonomy. When we are sick, our autonomy is greatly diminished because we are not "ourselves," our freedom of choice is limited, our knowledge is incomplete, and our reason is impaired. Although Cassell emphasizes the importance of relationships with family, friends, and physicians, he affirms that the best way to restore autonomy is "to cure the patient of the disease that impairs autonomy and return him to his normal life."[15]

To be sure, autonomy is an important end state of health care that professionals should pursue for their patients in order to benefit them. But it is an end state that individuals may autonomously choose not to pursue. By expanding the notion of autonomy to include freedom from the effects of disease,[16] and by conceiving it as a goal rather that as a right, Cassell fails to address the most important and difficult question: Can autonomy as a goal override autonomy as a right? Or does autonomy as a side constraint preclude its violation even to achieve the end state of restored or increased autonomy? The principle of respect for persons requires that autonomy be conceived as a side constraint and as a right, rather than as an end state, even if it does not establish an absolute limit (an issue that I will consider later). Pursuit of another's autonomy as an end state may be an important goal of altruistic beneficence, but the patient, rather that the agent, should determine how important it is.

The *ideal* of autonomy, especially moral autonomy, is neither a presupposition nor an implication of the principle of respect for persons, however much we admire persons who realize or approximate this ideal, so widely praised in the tradition of Western individualism. Recognition of this ideal and praise for the "autonomous person" would require additional premises that are not required for a defense of autonomy as a side constraint without denying the burden of autonomy for individuals and the importance of community and tradition. Gerald Dworkin argues that the ideal of moral autonomy

> represents a particular conception of morality—one that, among other features, places a heavy emphasis on rules and principles rather than virtues and practices. Considered purely internally there are conceptual, moral, and empirical difficulties in defining and elaborating a conception of autonomy which is coherent and provides us with an ideal worthy of pursuit. It is only through a more adequate understanding of notions such as tradition, authority, commitment, and loyalty, and of the forms of human community in which these have their roots, that we shall be able to develop a conception of autonomy free from paradox and worthy of admiration.[17]

My argument is that the principle of respect for persons requires that we construe autonomy as a constraint upon our pursuit of goals for ourselves or for others' wishes, choices, and actions in that they constrain and limit our pursuit of goals, whether these goals are for them, for others, or for ourselves, without committing ourselves to the goal of promoting autonomy or to the ideal of autonomous existence.

Notes

1. Dworkin, Gerald. "Autonomy and Behavior Control," *Hastings Center Report* 6:23, February 1976; for an important discussion, see Harry G. Frankfurt. "Freedom of the Will and the Concept of a Person." *Journal of Philosophy* 58:5–20, 14 January 1971. Frankfurt argues that "it is having second-order violations [when one wants a certain desire to be his will], and not having second-order desires generally that I regard as essential to being a person" (p. 10). Yet reason is presupposed because it is "only in virtue of his rational capacities that a person is capable of becoming critically aware of his own will and of forming volitions of the second order" (p. 12).

2. Dworkin, "Autonomy and Behavior Control," p. 25.

3. For use of this distinction between source and object in relation to ethical individualism, see Lukes, Steven. *Individualism.* New York: Harper & Row, 1973, Chap. 15.

4. Sartre, Jean-Paul. "Existentialism." In *Existentialism and Human Relations.* New York: Philosophical Library, 1957, pp. 24f

5. See "'Rational Suicide'?" *Newsweek,* 2 July 1979, 87; Laurie Johnston, "Artist Ends Her Life. . . ." *The New York Times,* 17 June 1979; and *Choosing Suicide,* a Documentary on PBS, 16 June 1980.

6. As a matter of emphasis, Bernard Williams represents the former, while Robert Nozick represents the latter. Also, see the illuminating discussion of the debate about the separateness of persons by Hart, H. L. A. "Between Utility and Rights." in *The Idea of Freedom: Essays in Honour of Isaiah Berlin,* edited by Alan Ryan, 77–98. Oxford: Oxford University Press, 1979.

7. See Kant, *The Doctrine of Virtue,* p. 122; and Mill, *On Liberty,* edited by Gertrude Himmelfarb. Harmondsworth, Eng.: Penguin, 1976. For an argument that paternalistic treatment is not necessarily incompatible with a concern to respect moral autonomy, see Husak, Douglas N. "Paternalism and Autonomy." *Philosophy and Public Affairs* 10:27–46, Winter 1981.

8. For a fuller discussion of competence, including these terms, see Beauchamp, Tom L. and James F. Childress. *Principles of Biomedical Ethics.* New York: Oxford University Press, 1979, Chapter 3. I do not treat competence as merely or primarily a legal matter, although the law has much to say about it.

9. Maclagan. "Respect for Persons as a Moral Principle," p. 301.

10. Dewey, John. *Theory of the Moral Life.* New York: Holt, Rinehart & Winston, 1960, p.135.

11. Mabbott, J. B. "Reason and Desire." *Philosophy* 28:113–123, 1953.

12. Miller. "Autonomy and the Refusal of Life-Saving Treatment." *Hastings Center Report* 11:22–28, August 1981.

13. Dworkin, G. "Autonomy and Behavior Control"; and Miller. "Autonomy and the Refusal of Life-Saving Treatment."

14. This distinction is developed by Nozick, Robert. *Anarchy, State, and Utopia.* New York: Basic Books, 1974, pp. 28–35. I use it for analytical purposes without accepting his normative theory.

15. I have drawn this statement of Cassell's position from his article "The Function of Medicine." *Hastings Center Report* 7:16–19, December 1977. See also his *The Healers*

Art: A New Approach to the Doctor-Patient Relationship. Philadelphia: Lippincott, 1976. Elsewhere he also considers cases of chronic care: "Naturally, autonomy is best served by a return to health. Increasingly, however, success in medicine does not mean a return to normalcy as it did with the infectious diseases. Rather, we are successful when patients requiring continuing care are able to function and live their lives with the least possible interference from their diseases or their medical care." Cassell. "Autonomy and Ethics in Action." *New England Journal of Medicine* 297:333–334, 11 August 1977. His discussion of cases sometimes expresses appreciation of autonomy as a side constraint, which is usually absent from his more theoretical statements.

16. This sort of expansion shifts the argument away from human interactions to conditions and goals: people are less autonomous when they are sick. While it is true that people are affected in various ways when they are sick, including having their options more severely limited, they can still be self-determining within these conditions. That is the important point, sometimes obscured by Cassell's contention that a sick person is not simply a person with a disease added on but a "sick person." See *The Healer's Art.*

17. Dworkin, Gerald. "Moral Autonomy." in *Morals, Science and Sociality*, Vol. III of *The Foundations of Ethics and Its Relationship to Science*, edited by H. Tristram Engelhardt, Jr., and Daniel Callahan, 170. Hastings-on-Hudson, N.Y.: The Hastings Center, 1978. p. 170.

Canterbury v. Spence

United States Court of Appeals, District of Columbia Circuit, 1972

───────────INTRODUCTION TO READING───────────

The most important practical, medical, ethical, and legal application of the principle of autonomy occurs in the doctrine of informed consent. While Hippocratic medical ethics would, upon occasion, inform patients of the potential risks of a medical procedure and give patients choices, this occurred only when the physician believed it was in the patient's interest. Often Hippocratic physicians believed that too much information was upsetting and confusing to patients and that, if given choices about treatment, patients would choose foolishly. There is no inherent right of patients to consent to treatment in Hippocratic medical ethics.

Throughout the twentieth century the doctrine of informed consent has evolved from its tepid Hippocratic basis to a more robust right grounded in the moral principle of autonomy and the legal right of self-determination. The most critical issue has been whether a physician should follow the "professional standard," disclosing only what colleagues similarly situated would disclose (regardless of whether that provides enough information for the patient to make an informed choice) or should follow the "reasonable person standard," disclosing whatever a reasonable person in the patient's situation would need to know to make an adequately informed choice. The American courts began addressing this issue in the late 1950s. The controversy came to a head in the early 1970s when several cases, including the one excerpted here, led to the adoption of the reasonable person standard grounded in liberal political philosophy and the overturning of the more paternalistic Hippocratic professional standard.

The record we review tells a depressing tale. A youth troubled only by back pain submitted to an operation without being informed of a risk of paralysis incidental thereto. A day after the operation he fell from his hospital bed after having been left without assistance while voiding. A few hours after the fall, the lower half of his body was paralyzed, and he had to be operated on again. Despite extensive medical care, he has never been what he was before. Instead of the back pain, even years later, he hobbled about on crutches, a victim of paralysis of the bowels and urinary incontinence. In a very real sense this lawsuit is an understandable search for reasons.

...

In December, 1958, he began to experience severe pain between his shoulder blades. . . . Appellant secured an appointment with Dr. Spence, who is a neurosurgeon. . . . [After a minor procedure to determine the cause of pain,] Dr. Spence told appellant that he would have to undergo a laminectomy—the excision of the posterior arch of the vertebra—to correct what he suspected was a ruptured disc. Appellant did not raise any objection to the proposed operation nor did he probe into its exact nature. . . .

For approximately the first day after the operation appellant recuperated normally, but then suffered a fall and an almost immediate setback. . . . Several hours later, appellant began to complain that he could not move his legs and that he was having trouble breathing; paralysis seems to have been virtually total from the waist down . . . and appellant was again taken into the operating room. . . .

Appellant's control over his muscles improved somewhat after the second operation but he was unable to void properly. . . . For several years after his discharge he was under the care of several specialists, and at all times was under the care of a urologist. At the time of the trial in April, 1968, appellant required crutches to walk, still suffered from urinal incontinence and paralysis of the bowels, and wore a penile clamp. . . .

Appellant filed suit in the District Court on March 7, 1963, four years after the laminectomy and approximately two years after he attained his majority. The complaint stated several causes of action against each defendant. Against Dr. Spence it alleged, among other things, negligence in the performance of the laminectomy and failure to inform him beforehand of the risk involved. Against the hospital the complaint charged negligent post-operative care in permitting appellant to remain unattended after the laminectomy, in failing to provide a nurse or orderly to assist him at the time of his fall, and in failing to maintain a side rail on his bed. The answers denied the allegations of negligence and defended on the ground that the suit was barred by the statute of limitations. . . .

Dr. Spence further testified that even without trauma paralysis can be anticipated "somewhere in the nature of one percent" of the laminectomies performed, a risk he termed "a very slight possibility." He felt that communication of that risk to the patient is not good medical practice because it might deter patients from undergoing needed surgery and might produce adverse psychological reactions which could preclude the success of the operation.

At the close of appellant's case in chief, each defendant moved for a directed verdict and the trial judge granted both motions. The basis of the ruling, he explained, was that appellant had failed to produce any medical evidence indicating negligence on Dr. Spence's part in diagnosing appellant's malady or in performing the laminectomy. . . .The judge did not allude specifically to the alleged breach of duty by Dr. Spence to divulge the possible consequences of the laminectomy.

We reverse. The testimony of appellant and his mother that Dr. Spence did not reveal the risk of paralysis from the laminectomy made out a prima facie case of violation of the physician's duty to disclose , which Dr. Spence's explanation did not negate as a matter of law. . . . Elucidation of our reasoning necessitates elaboration on a number of points. In Part V we investigate the scope of the disclosure requirement and in Part VI the physician's privileges not to disclose. In Part VII we examine the role of causality. . . .

Suits charging failure by a physician adequately to disclose the risks and alternatives of proposed treatment are not innovations in American law. They date back a good half-century, and in the last decade they have multiplied rapidly. There is, nonetheless, disagreement among the courts and the commentators on many major questions, and there is no precedent of our own directly in point. For the tools enabling resolution of the issues on this appeal, we are forced to begin at the first principles.

The root premise is the concept, fundamental in American jurisprudence, that "[e]very human being of adult years and sound mind has a right to determine what shall be done with his own body. . . ." True consent to what happens to one's self is the informed exercise of a choice, and that entails an opportunity to evaluate knowledgeably the options available and the risks attendant upon each. The average patient has little or no understanding of the medical arts, and ordinarily has only his physician to whom he can look for enlightenment with which to reach an intelligent decision. From these almost axiomatic considerations springs the need, and in turn the requirement, of a reasonable divulgence by physician to patient to make such a decision possible. . . .

The cases demonstrate that the physician is under an obligation to communicate specific information to the patient when the exigencies of reasonable care call for it. . . . Just as plainly, due care normally demands that the physician warn the patient of any risks to his well-being which contemplated therapy may involve.

The context in which the duty of risk-disclosure arises is invariably the occasion for decision as to whether a particular treatment procedure is to be undertaken. To the physician, whose training enables a self-satisfying evaluation, the answer may seem clear, but it is the prerogative of the patient, not the physician, to determine for himself the direction in which his interests seem to lie. To enable the patient to chart his course understandably, some familiarity with the therapeutic alternatives and their hazards becomes essential. . . .

We now find, as a part of the physician's overall obligation to the patient, a similar duty of reasonable disclosure of the choices with respect to proposed therapy and the dangers inherently and potentially involved.

This disclosure requirement, on analysis, reflects much more of a change in doctrinal emphasis than a substantive addition to malpractice law. . . .

Duty to disclose has gained recognition in a large number of American jurisdictions, but more largely on a different rationale. The majority of courts dealing with the problem have made the duty depend on whether it was the custom of physicians practicing in the community to make the particular disclosure to the patient. If so, the physician may be held liable for an unreasonable and injurious failure to divulge, but there can be no recovery unless the omission forsakes a practice prevalent in the profession. We agree that the physician's noncompliance with a professional custom to reveal, like any other departure from prevailing medical practice, may give rise to liability to the patient. We do not agree that the patient's cause of action is dependent upon the existence and nonperformance of a relevant professional tradition.

There are, in our view, formidable obstacles to acceptance of the notion that the physician's obligation to disclose is either germinated or limited by medical practice. To begin with, the reality of any discernible custom reflecting a professional consensus on communication of option and risk information to patients is open to serious doubt. We sense the danger that what in fact is no custom at all may be taken as an affirmative custom to maintain silence, and that physician-witnesses to the so-called custom may state merely their personal opinions as to what they or others would do under given conditions. We cannot gloss over the inconsistency between reliance on a general practice respecting divulgence and, on the other hand, realization that the myriad of variables among patients makes each case so different that its omission can rationally be justified only by the effect of its individual circumstances. Nor can we ignore the fact that to bind the disclosure obligation to medical usage is to arrogate the decision on revelation to the physician alone. Respect for the patient's right of self-determination on particular therapy demands a standard set by law for physicians rather than one which physicians may or may not impose upon themselves. . . .

Once the circumstances give rise to a duty on the physician's part to inform his patient, the next inquiry is the scope of the disclosure the physician is legally obliged to make. The courts have frequently confronted this problem but no uniform standard defining the adequacy of the divulgence emerges from the decisions. Some have said "full" disclosure, a norm we are unwilling to adopt literally. It seems obviously prohibitive and unrealistic to expect physicians to discuss with their patients every risk of proposed treatment—no matter how small or remote—and generally unnecessary from the patient's viewpoint as well. Indeed, the cases speaking in terms of "full" disclosure appear to envision something less than total disclosure, leaving unanswered the question of just how much.

The larger number of courts, as might be expected, have applied tests framed with reference to prevailing fashion within the medical profession. Some have measured the disclosure by "good medical practice," others by what a reasonable practitioner would have bared under the circumstances, and still others by what medical custom in the community would demand. We have explored this rather considerable body of law but are unprepared to follow it. The duty to disclose, we have reasoned, arises from phenomena apart from medical custom and practice. The latter, we think, should no more establish the scope of the duty than its existence. Any definition of scope in terms purely of a professional standard is at odds with the patient's prerogative to decide on projected therapy himself. That prerogative, we have said, is at the very foundation of the duty to disclose, and both the patient's right to know and the physician's correlative obligation to tell him are diluted to the extent that its compass is dictated by the medical profession.

In our view, the patient's right of self-decision shapes the boundaries of the duty to reveal. That right can be effectively exercised only if the patient possesses enough information to enable an intelligent choice. The scope of the physician's communications to the patient, then, must be measured by the patient's need, and that need is the information material to the decision. Thus the test for determining whether a particular peril must be divulged is its materiality to the patient's decision: all risks potentially affecting the decision must be unmasked. And to safeguard the patient's interest in achieving his own determination on treatment, the law must itself set the standard for adequate disclosure.

Optimally for the patient, exposure of a risk would be mandatory whenever the patient would deem it significant to his decision, either singly or in combination with other risks. Such a requirement, however, would summon the physician to second-guess the patient, whose ideas on materiality could hardly be known to the physician. That would make an undue demand upon medical practitioners, whose conduct, like that of others, is to be measured in terms of reasonableness. Consonantly with orthodox negligence doctrine, the physician's liability for nondisclosure is to be determined on the basis of foresight, not hindsight; no less than any other aspect of negligence, the issue on nondisclosure must be approached from the viewpoint of the reasonableness of the physician's divulgence in terms of what he knows or should know to be the patient's informational needs. If, but only if, the fact-finder can say that the physician's communication was unreasonably inadequate is an imposition of liability legally or morally justified.

Of necessity, the content of the disclosure rests in the first instance with the physician. Ordinarily it is only he who is in position to identify particular dangers; always he must make a judgment, in terms of materiality, as to whether and to what extent revelation to the patient is called for. He cannot know with complete exactitude what the patient would consider important to his decision, but on the basis of his medical training and experience he can sense how the average, reasonable patient expectably would react. Indeed, with knowledge of, or ability to learn, his patient's background and current condition, he is in a position superior to that of most others—attorneys, for example—who are called upon to make judgments on pain of liability in damages for unreasonable miscalculation.

From these considerations we derive the breadth of the disclosure of risks legally to be required. The scope of the standard is not subjective as to either the physician or the patient; it remains objective with due regard for the patient's informational needs and with suitable leeway for the physician's situation. In broad outline, we agree that "[a] risk is thus material when a reasonable person in what the physician knows or should know to be the patient's position, would be likely to attach significance to the risk or cluster of risks in deciding whether or not to forego the proposed therapy."

The topics importantly demanding a communication of information are the inherent and potential hazards of the proposed treatment, the alternatives to that treatment, if any, and the results likely if the patient remains untreated. The factors contributing significance to the dangerousness of a medical technique are, of course, the incidence of injury and the degree of the harm threatened. A very small chance of death or serious disablement may well be significant; a potential disability which dramatically outweighs the potential benefit of the therapy or the detriments of the existing malady may summons discussion with the patient. . . .

Two exceptions to the general rule of disclosure have been noted by the courts. Each is in the nature of a physician's privilege not to disclose, and the reasoning underlying them is appealing. Each, indeed, is but a recognition that, as important as is the patient's right to know, it is greatly outweighed by the magnitudinous circumstances giving rise to the privilege. The first comes into play when the patient is unconscious or otherwise incapable of consenting, and harm from a failure to treat is imminent and outweighs any harm threatened by the proposed treatment. When a genuine emergency of that sort arises, it is settled that the impracticality of conferring with the patient dispenses with need for it. Even in situations of that character the physician should, as current law requires, attempt to secure a relative's consent if possible. But if time is too short to accommodate discussion, obviously the physician should proceed with the treatment.

The second exception obtains when risk-disclosure poses such a threat of detriment to the patient as to become unfeasible or contraindicated from a medical point of view. It is recognized that patients occasionally become so ill or emotionally distraught on disclosure as to foreclose a rational decision, or complicate or hinder the treatment, or perhaps even pose psychological damage to the patient. Where that is so, the cases have generally held that the physician is armed with a privilege to keep the information from the patient, and we think it clear that portents of that type may justify the physician in action he deems medically warranted. The critical inquiry is whether the physician responded to a sound medical judgment that communication of the risk information would present a threat to the patient's well-being.

The physician's privilege to withhold information for therapeutic reasons must be carefully circumscribed, however, for otherwise it might devour the disclosure rule itself. The privilege does not accept the paternalistic notion that the physician may remain silent simply because divulgence might prompt the patient to forego therapy the physician feels the patient really needs. That attitude presumes instability or perversity for even the normal patient, and runs counter to the foundation principle that the patient should and ordinarily can make the choice for himself. Nor does the privilege contemplate operation save where the patient's reaction to risk information, as reasonable foreseen by the physician, is menacing. And even in a situation of that kind, disclosure to a close relative with a view to securing consent to the proposed treatment may be the only alternative open to the physician.

No more than breach of any other legal duty does nonfulfillment of the physician's obligation to disclose alone establish liability to the patient. An unrevealed risk that should have been made known must materialize, for otherwise the omission, however unpardonable, is legally without consequence. Occurrence of the risk must be harmful to the patient, for negligence unrelated to injury is nonactionable. And, as in malpractice actions generally, there must be a causal relationship between the physician's failure to adequately divulge and damage to the patient. . . .

Reversed and remanded for a new trial.

JUSTICE

Justice: A Philosophical Review

Allen Buchanan

──────────────INTRODUCTION TO READING──────────────

In the essay that follows Allen Buchanan sets out the major options for answering the question of how health-care resources ought to be distributed. He identifies three major options. The first, utilitarianism, is related to the Hippocratic ethical principle in that it focuses on the production of benefits. While the Hippocratic ethic, however, limits attention solely to the individual patient, utilitarianism expands the horizon to count as morally relevant all possible benefits and harms to all persons. Buchanan makes clear that there are varieties within utilitarianism. Some forms consider the consequences of actions directly; others assess the consequences of moral rules. Some assess aggregate utility; others average benefits.

Buchanan then introduces John Rawls as a major proponent of a non-utilitarian theory of distribution. In this system—the only one in which justice is really an independent principle unrelated to other, previously considered moral principles such as beneficence and autonomy—social practices (such as health-care systems) ought to be arranged so that inequalities benefit the least well-off in the community. This often, but not always, amounts to making people more equal. It would not lead to equality in cases where inequalities actually help those least well-off (such as perhaps by paying large salaries to talented physicians in order to get them to help sick people). Thus a variant on the Rawlsian distribution would be an even more radical egalitarianism whereby people are held to have a right to equality even if inequalities produce more benefit for persons on the bottom.

Finally, Buchanan introduces libertarianism, derived from a more exclusive emphasis on liberty or autonomy as a moral principle, and then examines the health care implications of all of these options.

Introduction

The past decade has seen the burgeoning of bioethics and the resurgence of theorizing about justice. Yet until now these two developments have not been as mutually enriching as one might have hoped. Bioethicists have tended to concentrate on micro issues (moral problems of individual or small group decision making), ignoring fundamental moral questions about the macro structure within which the micro issues arise. Theorists of justice have advanced very general principles but have typically neglected to show how they can illuminate the particular problems we face in health care and other urgent areas.

Micro problems do not exist in an institutional vacuum. The parents of a severely impaired newborn and the attending neonatologist are faced with the decision of whether to treat the infant aggressively or to allow it to die because neonatal intensive care units now exist which make it possible to preserve the lives of infants who previously would have died. Neonatal intensive care units exist because certain policy decisions have been made which allocated certain social resources to the development of technology for sustaining defective newborns rather than for preventing birth defects. Limiting moral inquiry to the micro issues supports an unreasoned conservatism by failing to examine the health care institutions within which micro problems arise and by not investigating the larger array of institutions of which the health care sector is only one part. Since not only particular actions but also policies and institutions may be just or unjust, serious theorizing about justice forces us to expand the narrow focus of the micro approach by raising fundamental queries about the background: social, economic, and political institutions from which micro problems emerge.

On the other hand, the attention to individual cases which dominates contemporary bioethics can provide a much needed concrete focus for refining and assessing competing theories of justice. The adequacy or inadequacy of a moral theory cannot be determined by inspecting the principles which constitute it. Instead, rational assessment requires an on-going process in which general principles are revised and refined through confrontation with the rich complexity of our considered judgments about particular cases, while our judgments about particular cases are gradually structured and modified by our provisional acceptance of general principles. Since our considered judgments about particular cases may often be more sensitive and sure than our assessments of abstract principles, careful attention to accurately described, concrete moral situations is essential for theorizing about justice.

Further, it is not just that the problems of bioethics provide one class of test cases for theories of justice among others: the problems of bioethics are among the most difficult and pressing issues with which a theory of justice must cope. It appears, then, that the continued development of both bioethics and of theorizing about justice in general requires us to explore the problems of justice in health care. In this essay I hope to contribute to that enterprise by first providing a sketch of three major theories of justice and by then attempting to ascertain some of their implications for moral problems in health care.

Theories of Justice

Utilitarianism

Utilitarianism purports to be a comprehensive moral theory, of which a utilitarian theory of justice is only one part. There are two main types of comprehensive utilitarian theory: Act and Rule Utilitarianism. Act Utilitarianism defines rightness with respect to particular acts: an act is right if and only if it maximizes utility. Rule Utilitarianism defines rights with respect to rules of action and makes the rightness of particular acts depend upon the rules under which those acts fall. A rule is right if and only if general compliance with that rule (or with a set of rules of which it is an element) maximizes utility, and a particular action is right if and only if it falls under such a rule.

Both Act and Rule Utilitarianism may be versions of either Classic or Average Utilitarianism. Classic Utilitarianism defines the rightness of acts or rules as maximization of aggregate utility; Average Utilitarianism defines rightness as maximization of utility per capita. The aggregate utility produced by an act or by general compliance with a rule is the sum of the utility produced for each individual affected. Average utility is the aggregate utility divided by the number of individuals affected. 'Utility' is defined as pleasure, satisfaction, happiness, or as the realization of preferences, as the latter are revealed through individuals' choices.

The distinction between Act and Rule Utilitarianism is important for a utilitarian theory of justice, since the latter must include an account of when institutions are just. Thus, institutional rules may maximize utility even though those rules do not direct individuals as individuals or as occupants of institutional positions to maximize utility in a case by case fashion. For example, it may be that a judicial system which maximizes utility will do so by including rules which prohibit judges from deciding a case according to their estimates of what would maximize utility in that particular case. Thus the utilitarian justification of a particular action or decision may not be that it maximizes utility, but rather that it falls under some rule of an institution or set of institutions which maximizes utility.[1]

Some utilitarians, such as John Stuart Mill, hold that principles of justice are the most basic moral principles because the utility of adherence to them is especially great. According to this view, utilitarian principles of justice are those utilitarian moral principles which are of such importance that they may be enforced, if necessary. Some utilitarians, including Mill perhaps, also hold that among the utilitarian principles of justice are principles specifying individual rights, whether the latter are thought of as enforceable claims which take precedence over appeals to what would maximize utility in the particular case. Indeed, some contemporary rights theorists such as Ronald Dworkin define a (justified) right claim as one which takes precedence over mere appeals to what would maximize utility.

A utilitarian moral theory, then, can include rights principles which themselves prohibit appeals to utility maximization, so long as the justification of those principles is that they are part of an institutional system which maximizes utility. In cases where two or more rights principles conflict, considerations of utility may be invoked to determine which rights principles are to be given priority. Utilitarianism is incompatible with rights only if rights exclude appeals to utility maximization at all levels of justification, including the most basic institutional level. Rights founded ultimately on considerations of utility may be called derivative, to distinguish them from rights in the strict sense.

Utilitarianism is the most influential version of teleological moral theory. A moral theory is teleological if and only if it defines the good independently of the right and defines the right as that which maximizes the good. Utilitarianism defines the good as happiness (satisfaction, etc.), independently of any account of what is morally right, and then defines the right as that which maximizes the good (either in the particular case or at the institutional level).

A moral theory is deontological if and only if it is not a teleological theory, i.e., if and only if it either does not define the good independently of the right or does not define the right as that which maximizes the good. Both the second and third theories of justice we shall consider are deontological theories.

John Rawls's Theory: Justice as Fairness

In *A Theory of Justice* Rawls pursues two main goals. The first is to set out a small but powerful set of principles of justice which underlie and explain the considered moral judgments we make about particular actions, policies, laws, and institutions. The second is to offer a theory of justice superior to Utilitarianism. These two goals are intimately related for Rawls because he believes that the theory which does a better job of supporting and accounting for our considered judgments is the better theory, other things being equal. The principles of justice Rawls offers are as follows:

1. The principle of greatest equal liberty:
   Each person is to have an equal right to the most extensive system of equal basic liberties compatible with a similar system of liberty for all ([6], pp. 60, 201–205).
2. The principle of equality of fair opportunity:
   Offices and positions are to be open to all under conditions of equality of fair opportunity-persons with similar abilities and skills are to have equal access to offices and positions ([6], pp. 60, 73, 83–89).[2]
3. The difference principle:
   Social and economic institutions are to be arranged so as to benefit maximally the worst off ([6], pp. 60, 75–83).[3]

The basic liberties referred to in (1) include freedom of speech, freedom of conscience, freedom from arbitrary arrest, the right to hold personal property, and freedom of political participation (the right to vote, to run for office, etc.). Since the demands of these principles may conflict, some way of ordering them is needed. According to Rawls, (1) is *lexically prior* to (2) and (2) is *lexically prior* to (3). A principle 'P' is lexically prior to a principle 'Q' if and only if we are first to satisfy the requirements of 'P' before going on to satisfy the requirements of 'Q.' Lexical priority allows no trade-offs between the demands of conflicting principles: the lexically prior principle takes absolute priority.

Rawls notes that "many kinds of things are said to be just or unjust: not only laws, institutions, and social systems, but also particular actions . . . decisions, judgments and imputations. . . ." ([6], p. 7). But he insists that the primary subject of justice is the *basic structure* of society because it exerts a pervasive and profound influence on individuals' life prospects. The basic structure is the entire set of major political, legal, economic, and social institutions. In our society the basic structure includes the Constitution, private ownership of the means of production, competitive markets, and the monogamous family. The basic structure plays a large role in distributing the burdens and benefits of cooperation among members of society.

If the primary subject of justice is the basic structure, then the primary problem of justice is to formulate and justify a set of principles which a just basic structure must satisfy. These principles will specify how the basic structure is to distribute prospects of what Rawls calls *primary goods*. They include the basic liberties (listed above under (2), as well as powers, authority, opportunities, income, and wealth. Rawls says that primary goods are things that every rational person is presumed to want, because they normally have a use, whatever a person's rational plan of life ([6], p. 62). Principle (1) regulates the distribution of prospects of basic liberties; (2) regulates the distribution of prospects of powers and authority, so far as these are attached to institutional offices and positions, and (3) regulates the distribution of prospects of the other primary goods, including wealth and income. Though the first and second principles require equality, the difference principle allows inequalities so long as the total system of institutions of which they are a part maximizes the prospects of the worst off to the primary goods in question.

Rawls advances three distinct types of justification for his principles of justice. Two appeal to our considered judgments, while the third is based on what he calls the Kantian interpretation of his theory.

The first type of justification rests on the idea, mentioned earlier, that if a set of principles provides the best account of our considered judgments about what is just or unjust, then that is a reason for accepting those principles. A set of principles accounts for our judgments only if those judgments can be derived from the principles, granted the relevant facts for their application.

Rawls's second type of justification maintains that if a set of principles would be chosen under conditions which, according to our considered judgments, are appropriate conditions for choosing principles of justice, then this is a reason for accepting those principles. The second type of justification includes three parts: (1) A set of conditions for choosing principles of justice must be specified. Rawls labels the complete set of conditions the 'original position.' (2) It must be shown that the conditions specified are (according to our considered judgments) the appropriate conditions of choice. (3) It must be shown that Rawls's principles are indeed the principles which would be chosen under those conditions.

Rawls construes the choice of principles of justice as an ideal social contract. "The principles of justice for the basic structure of society are the principles that free and rational persons . . . would accept in an initial situation of equality as defining the fundamental terms of their association" ([6], p. 11). The idea of a social contract has several advantages. First, it allows us to view principles of justice as the object of a *rational collective choice*. Second, the idea of *contractual obligation* is used to emphasize that the choice expresses a basic commitment and that the principles agreed on may be rightly enforced. Third, the idea of a contract as a *voluntary agreement* which set terms for mutual advantage suggests that the principles of justice should be "such as to draw forth the "willing cooperation" ([6], p. 15) of all members of society, including those who are worse off.

The most important elements of the original position or our purposes are a) the characterization of the parties to the contract as individuals who desire to pursue their own life plans effectively and who "have a highest-order interest in how . . . their interests . . . are shaped and regulated by social institutions" ([8], p. 64); b) the 'veil of ignorance,' which is a constraint on the information the parties are able to utilize in choosing principles of justice; and c) the requirement that the principles are to be chosen on the assumption that they will be complied with by all (the universalizability condition) ([61], p. 132).

The parties are characterized as desiring to maximize their shares of primary goods, because these goods enable one to implement effectively the widest range of life plans and because at least some of them, such as freedom of speech and of conscience, facilitate one's freedom to choose and revise one's life plan or conception of the good. The parties are to choose "from behind a veil of ignorance" so that information about their own particular characteristics or social positions will not lead to bias in the choice of principles. Thus they are described as not knowing their race, sex, socioeconomic, or political status, or even the nature of their particular conceptions of the good. The informational restriction also helps to insure that the principles chosen will not place avoidable restrictions on the individual's freedom to choose and revise his or her life plan.[4]

Though Rawls offers several arguments to show that his principles would be chosen in the original position, the most striking is the *maximin* argument. According to this argument, the rational strategy in the original position is to choose that set of principles whose implementation will maximize the minimum share of primary goods which one can receive as a member of society, and principles (1), (2), and (3) will insure the greatest minimal share. Rawls's claim is that because these principles protect one's basic liberties and opportunities and insure an adequate minimum of goods such as wealth and income (even if one should turn out to be among the worst off) the rational thing is to choose them, rather than to gamble with one's life prospects by opting for alternative principles. In particular, Rawls contends that it would be irrational to reject his principles and allow one's life prospect to be determined by what would maximize utility, since utility maximization might allow severe deprivation or even slavery for some, so long as this contributed sufficiently to the welfare of others.

Rawls raises an important question about this second mode of justification when he notes that this original position is purely hypothetical. Granted that the agreement is never actually entered into, why should we regard the principles as binding? The answer, according to Rawls, is that we do in fact accept the conditions embodied in the original position ([6], p. 21). The following qualification, which Rawls adds immediately after claiming that the conditions which constitute the original position are appropriate for the choice of principles of justice according to our considered judgments, introduces his third type of justification: "Or if we do not [accept the conditions of the original position as appropriate for choosing principles of justice] *then perhaps we can be persuaded to do so by the philosophical* reflections" (emphasis added [6], p. 21). In the

Kantian interpretation section of *A Theory of Justice*, Rawls sketches a certain kind of philosophical justification for the conditions which make up the original position (based on Kant's conception of the 'noumenal self' or autonomous agent).

For Kant an autonomous agent's will is determined by rational principles and rational principles are those which can serve as principles for all rational beings, not just for this or that agent, depending upon whether or not he has some particular desire which other rational beings may not have. Rawls invites us to think of the original position as the perspective from which autonomous agents see the world. The original position provides a "procedural interpretation" of Kant's idea of a Realm of Ends or community of "free and equal rational beings". We express our nature as autonomous agents when we act from principles that would be chosen in conditions which reflect that nature ([6], p. 252).

Rawls concludes that, when persons such as you and I accept those principles that would be chosen in the original position, we express our nature as autonomous agents, i.e., we act autonomously. There are three main grounds for this thesis, corresponding to the three features of the original position cited earlier. First, since the veil of ignorance excludes information about any particular desires which a rational agent may or may not have, the choice of principles is not determined by any particular desire. Second, since the parties strive to maximize their share of primary goods, and since primary goods are attractive to them because they facilitate freedom in choosing and revising life plans and because they are flexible means not tied to any particular ends, this is another respect in which their choice is not determined by particular desires. Third, the original position includes the requirement that they will be principles of rational agents in general and not just for agents who happen to have this or that particular desire.

In the *Foundation of the Metaphysics of Morals* Kant advances a moral philosophy which identifies autonomy with rationality [4]. Hence for Kant the question "Why should one express our nature as autonomous agents?" is answered by the thesis that rationality requires it. Thus if Rawls's third type of justification succeeds in showing that we best express our autonomy when we accept those principles in the belief that they would be chosen from the original position, and if Kant's identification of autonomy with rationality is successful, the result will be a justification of Rawls's principles which is distinct from both the first and second modes of justification. So far as this third type of justification does not make the acceptance of Rawls's principles hinge on whether the principles themselves or the conditions from which they would be chosen match our considered judgments, it is not directly vulnerable either to the charge that Rawls has misconstrued our considered judgments or that congruence with considered judgments, like the appeal to mere consensus, has no justificatory force.

It is important to see that Rawls understands his principles of justice as principles which *generate rights* in what I have called the strict sense. Claims based upon the three principles are to take precedence over considerations of utility and the principles themselves are not justified on the grounds that a basic structure which satisfies them will maximize utility. Moreover, Rawls's theory is not a teleological theory of any kind because it does not define the right as that which maximizes the good, where the good is defined independently of the right. Instead it is perhaps the most influential current instance of a deontological theory.

Nozick's Libertarian Theory

There are many versions of libertarian theory, but their characteristic doctrine is that coercion may only be used to prevent or punish physical harm, theft, and fraud, and to enforce contracts. Perhaps the most influential and systematic recent instance of Libertarianism is the theory presented by Robert Nozick in *Anarchy, State, and Utopia* [5]. In Nozick's theory of justice, as in libertarian theories generally, the right to private property is fundamental and determines both the legitimate role of the state and the most basic principles of individual conduct.

Nozick contends that individuals have a property right in their persons and in whatever 'holdings' they come to have through actions which conform to (1) "the principle of justice in [initial] acquisition" and (2) "the principle of justice in transfer" ([5], p. 151). The first principle specifies the ways in which an individual may come to own hitherto unowned things without violating anyone else's rights. Here Nozick largely follows John Locke's famous account of how one makes natural objects one's own by "mixing one's labor" with them or improving them through one's labor. Though Nozick does not actually formulate a principle of justice in (initial) acquisition, he does argue that whatever the appropriate formulation is it must include a 'Lockean Proviso', which places a constraint on the holdings which one may acquire through one's labor. Nozick maintains that one may appropriate as much of an unowned item as one desires so long as (a) one's appropriation does not worsen the conditions of others in a special way, namely, by creating a situation in which others are "no longer . . . able to use freely [without exclusively appropriating] what [they] . . . previously could" or (b) one properly compensates those whose condition is worsened by one's appropriation in the way specified in (a) ([5], pp. 178–179). Nozick emphasizes that the Proviso only picks out one way in which one's appropriation may worsen the condition of others; it does not forbid appropriation or require compensation in cases in which one's appropriation of an unowned thing worsens another's condition merely by limiting his opportunities to appropriate (rather than merely use) that thing, i.e., to make it his property.

The second principle states that one may justly transfer one's legitimate holdings to another through sale, trade, gift or bequest and that one is entitled to whatever one receives in any of these ways, so long as the person from whom one receives it was entitled to that which he transferred to you. The right to property which Nozick advances is the right to exclusive control over anything one can get through initial appropriation (subject to the Lockean Proviso) or through voluntary exchanges with others entitled to what they transfer. Nozick concludes that a distribution is just if and only if it arose from another just distribution by legitimate means. The principle of justice in initial acquisition specifies the legitimate 'first moves,' while the principle of justice in transfers specifies the legitimate ways of moving from one distribution to another: "Whatever arises from a just situation by just steps is itself just" ([5], p. 151).

Since not all existing holdings arose through the 'just steps' specified by the principles of justice in acquisition and transfer, there will be a need for a *principle of rectification* of past injustices. Though Nozick does not attempt to formulate such a principle he thinks that it might well require significant redistribution of holdings.

Apart from the case of rectifying past violations of the principles of acquisition and transfer, however, Nozick's theory is strikingly anti-redistributive. Nozick contends that attempts to force anyone to contribute any part of his legitimate holdings to the welfare of others is a violation of that person's property rights, whether it is undertaken by private individuals or the state. On this view, coercively backed taxation to raise funds for welfare programs of any kind is literally theft. Thus, a large proportion of the activities now engaged in by the government involve gross injustices.

After stating his theory of rights, Nozick tries to show that the state is legitimate so long as it limits its activities to the enforcement of these rights and eschews redistributive functions. To do this he employs an 'invisible hand explanation,' which purports to show how the minimal state could arise as an unintended consequence of a series of voluntary transactions which violate no one's rights. The phrase 'invisible hand explanation' is chosen to stress that the process by which the minimal state could emerge fits Adam Smith's famous account of how individuals freely pursuing their own private ends in the market collectively produce benefits which are not the aim of anyone.

The process by which the minimal state could arise without violating anyone's rights is said to include four main steps ([5], pp. 10–25).[5] First, individuals in a 'state of nature' in which (Libertarian) moral principles are generally respected would form a plurality of 'protective agencies' to enforce their libertarian rights, since individual efforts at enforcement would be inefficient and liable to abuse. Second, through competition for clients, a 'dominant protective agency' would eventually emerge in given geographical area. Third, such an agency would eventually become a 'minimal state' by asserting a claim of monopoly over protective services in order to prevent less reliable efforts at enforcement which might endanger its clients: it would forbid 'independents' (those who refused to purchase its services) from seeking other forms of enforcement. Fourth, again assuming that correct moral principles are generally followed, those belonging to the dominant protective agency would compensate the 'independents,' presumably by providing them with free or partially subsidized protection services. With the exception of taxing its clients to provide compensation for the independents, the minimal state would act only to protect persons against physical injury, theft, fraud, and violations of contracts.

It is striking that Nozick does not attempt to provide any systematic *justification* for the Lockean rights principles he advocates. In this respect he departs radically from Rawls. Instead, Nozick assumes the correctness of the Lockean principles and then, on the basis of that assumption, argues that the minimal state and only the minimal stated is compatible with the rights those principles specify.

He does, however, offer some arguments against the more-than-minimal state which purport to be independent of that particular theory of property rights which he assumes. These arguments may provide indirect support for his principles insofar as they are designed to make alternative principles, such as Rawls's, unattractive. Perhaps most important of these is an argument designed to show that any principle of justice which demands a certain distributive end state or pattern of holdings will require frequent and gross disruptions of individuals' holdings for the sake of maintaining that end state or pattern. Nozick supports this general conclusion by a vivid example. He asks us to suppose that there is some distribution of holdings 'D_1' which is required by some end-state or patterned theory of justice and that 'D_1' is achieved at time 'T.' Now suppose that Wilt Chamberlain, the renowned basketball player, signs a contract stipulating that he is to receive twenty-five cents from the price of each ticket to the home games in which he performs, and suppose that he nets $250,000, from this arrangement. We now have a new distribution 'D_2'. Is 'D_2' unjust? Notice that by hypothesis those who paid the price of admission were entitled to control over the resources they held in 'D_1' (as were Chamberlain and the team's owners). The new distribution arose through voluntary exchanges of legitimate holdings, so it is difficult to see how it could be unjust, even if it does diverge from 'D_1'. From this and like examples, Nozick concludes that attempts to maintain any end-state or patterned distributive principle would require continuous interference in peoples' lives ([5], pp. 161–163).

As in the cases of Utilitarianism and Rawls's theory, Nozick and libertarians generally do not limit morality to justice. Thus, Nozick and others emphasize that a libertarian theory of individual rights is to be supplemented by a libertarian theory of virtues which recognizes that not all moral principles are suitable objects of enforcement and that moral life includes more than the nonviolation of rights. Libertarians invoke the distinction between justice and charity to reply to those who complain that a Lockean theory of property rights legitimizes crushing poverty for millions. They stress that while justice demands that we not be forced to contribute to the well-being of others, charity requires that we help even those who have no right to our aid.[6]

Implications for Health Care

Now that we have a grasp of the main ideas of three major theories of justice, we can explore briefly some of their implications for health care. To do this we may confront the theories with four questions:

1. Is there a right to health care? (If so, what is its basis and what is its content?)
2. How, in order of priority, is health care related to other goods, or how are health care needs related to other needs? (If there is a right to health care, how is it related to other rights?)
3. How, in order of priority, are various forms of health care related to one another?
4. What can we conclude about the justice or injustice of the current health care system?

In some cases, as we shall see, the theories will provide opposing answers to the same question; in others, the theories may be unhelpfully silent.

We have already seen that the Utilitarian position on rights in general is complex. If by a right we mean a right in the strict sense, i.e., a claim which takes precedence over mere appeals to utility at all levels, including the most basic institutional level, then Utilitarianism denies the existence of rights in general, including the right to health care. If, on the other hand, we mean by right a claim that takes precedence over mere appeals to utility at the level of particular actions or at some institutional level short of the most basic, but which is justified ultimately by appeal to the utility of the total set of institutions, then Utilitarianism does not exclude, and indeed may even require rights, including a right to health care. Whether or not the total institutional array which maximizes utility will include a right to health care will depend upon a wealth of *empirical facts* not deducible from the principle of utility itself. The nature and complexity of the relevant facts can best be appreciated by considering briefly the bearing of Utilitarianism on questions (2) and (3). A utilitarian system of (derivative) rights will pick out certain goods as those which make an especially large contribution to the maximumization of utility. It is reasonable to assume, on the basis of empirical data, that health care, or at least certain forms of health care, is among them. Consider, for example, prenatal care, broadly conceived as including genetic screening and counseling (at least for special risk groups), prenatal nutritional care and medical examinations for expectant mothers, medical care during delivery, and basic pediatric services in the crucial months after birth. If empirical research indicates (1) that a system of institutional arrangements which maximizes utility would include such services and (2) that such services can best be assured if they are accorded the status of a right, with all that this implies, including the use of coercive sanctions where necessary, then according to Utilitarianism there is such a (derivative) right. The strength and content of this right relative to other (derivative) rights will be determined by the utility of health care as compared with other kinds of goods.

It is crucial to note that, for the utilitarian, empirical research must determine not only whether certain health care services are to be provided as a matter of rights but also whether the right in question is to be an equal right enjoyed by all persons. No commitment to equality of rights is included in the utilitarian principle itself, nor is there any commitment to equal distribution of any kind. Utilitarianism is egalitarian only in the sense that in calculating what will maximize utility each person's welfare is to be included.

Utilitarian arguments, sometimes based on empirical data, have been advanced to show that providing health care free of charge as a matter of right would encourage wasteful use of scarce and costly resources because the individual would have no incentive to restrain his 'consumption' of health care. The cumulative result, it is said, would be quite disutilitarian: a breakdown of the health care system or a disastrous curtailment of other basic services to cover the spiraling costs of health care. In contrast (proponents of this argument continue) a market in health care encourages 'consumers' to use resources wisely because the costs of the services an individual receives are borne by that individual.

On the other side of the utilitarian ledger, empirical evidence may be marshalled to show that the benefits of a right to health care outweigh the costs, including the costs of possible overuse, and that a market in health care would not maximize utility because those who need health care the most may not be able to afford it.

Similarly, even if there is a utilitarian justification for a right to health care, empirical evidence must again be presented to show that it should be an equal right. For it is certainly conceivable that, under certain circumstances at least, utility could be maximized by providing extensive health care only for some groups, perhaps even a minority, rather than for all persons.

Utilitarians who advocate a right to health care often argue that this right, like other basic rights, should be equal, on the basis of the assumption of diminishing marginal utility. The idea, roughly, is that with respect to many goods, including health care, there is a finite upper bound to the satisfaction a person can gain from being provided with additional amounts of the goods in question. Hence, if in general we are all subject to the phenomenon of diminishing marginal utility in the case of health care and if the threshold of diminishing marginal utility is in general sufficiently low, then there are sound utilitarian reasons for distributing health care equally.

Finally, it should be clear that for the utilitarian the issue of priorities within health care, as well as that of priorities between health care and other goods, must again be settled by empirical research. If, as seems likely, utility maximization requires more resources for prevention and health maintenance rather than for curative intervention after pathology has already developed, then this will be reflected in the content of the utilitarian right to health care. If, as many writers have contended, the current emphasis in the U.S. on high technology intervention produces less utility than would a system which stresses prevention and health maintenance (for example through stricter control of pollution and other environmental determinants of disease), then the utilitarian may conclude that the current system is unjust in this respect. Empirical data would also be needed to ascertain whether more social resources should be devoted to high- or low-technology intervention: for example, neonatal intensive care units versus 'well-baby clinics.' These examples are intended merely to illustrate the breadth and complexity of the empirical research needed to apply Utilitarianism to crucial issues in health care.

Libertarian theories such as Nozick's rely much less heavily upon empirical premises for answers to questions (1)–(4). Since the libertarian is interested only in preventing violations of libertarian rights, and since the latter are rights against certain sorts of interferences rather than rights to be provided with anything, the question of what will maximize utility is irrelevant. Further, any effort to implement any right to health care whatsoever is an injustice, according to the libertarian.

There are only two points at which empirical data are relevant for Nozick. First, whether or not any current case of appropriation of hitherto unheld things satisfies the Lockean Proviso is a matter of fact to be ascertained by empirical methods. Second, empirical historical research is needed to determine what sort of redistribution for the sake of rectifying past injustices is necessary. If, for example, physicians' higher incomes are due in part to government policies which violate libertarian rights, then rectificatory redistribution may be required. And indeed libertarians have argued that two basic features of the current health care system do involve gross violations of libertarian rights. First, compulsory taxation to provide equipment, hospital facilities, research funds, and educational subsidies for medical personnel is literally theft. Second, some argue that government enforced occupational licensing laws which prohibit all but the established forms of medical practice violate the right to freedom of contract (3). Those who raise this second objection also usually argue that the function of such laws is to secure a monopoly for the medical establishment while sharply limiting the supply of doctors so as to keep medical fees artificially high. Whether or not such arguments are sound it is important to note that Libertarianism is not to be confused with Conservatism. A theory which would institute a free market in medical services, abolish government subsidies, and reduce government regulation of medical practice to the prevention of injury and fraud and the enforcement of contracts has radical implications for changing the current system.

Libertarianism offers straightforward answers to questions (2) and (3). Even if it can be shown that health care in general, and certain forms of health care more than others, are especially important for the happiness or even the freedom of most persons, this fact is quite irrelevant from the perspective of a libertarian theory of justice, though it is no doubt significant for the libertarian concerned with charity or other virtues which exceed the requirements of justice. Nozick and other libertarians recognize that a free market in medical services may in fact produce severe inequalities and that there is no assurance that all or even most will be able to afford adequate medical care. Though the humane libertarian will find this condition unfortunate and will aid those in need and encourage others to do likewise voluntarily, he remains adamant that no one has a right to health care and that hence none may rightly be forced to aid another.

According to Rawls, the most basic questions about health care are not to be decided either by consideration of utility nor by market processes. Instead they are to be settled ultimately by appeal to those principles of justice which would be chosen in the original position. As we shall see, however, the implications of Rawls's principles for health care are far from clear.[7]

No principle explicitly specifying a right to health care is included among Rawls's principle of justice. Further, since those principles are intended to regulate the basic structure of society as a whole, they are not themselves intended to guide the decisions individuals make in particular health care situations, nor are they themselves to be applied directly to health care institutions. We are not to assume that either individual physicians or administrators of particular policies or programs are to attempt to allocate health care so as to maximize the prospects of the worse off. In Rawls's theory, as in Utilitarianism, the rightness or wrongness of particular actions or policies depends ultimately upon the nature of the entire institutional structure within which they exist. Hence, Rawls's theory can provide us with fruitful answers at the micro level only if its implications at the macro level are adequately developed.

If Rawls's theory includes a right to health care, it must be a right which is in some way derivative upon the basic rights laid down by the Principle of Greatest Equal Liberty, the Principle of Equality of Fair Opportunity, and the Difference Principle. And if there is to be such a derivative right to health care, then health care must either be among the primary goods covered by the three principles or it must be importantly connected with some of those goods. Now at least some forms of health care (such as broad services for prevention and health maintenance, including mental health) seem to share the earmarks of Rawlsian primary goods: they facilitate the effective pursuit of ends in general and may also enhance our ability to criticize and revise our conceptions of the good. Nonetheless, Rawls does not explicitly list health care among the social primary goods included under the three principles. However, he does include wealth under the Difference Principle and defines it so broadly that it might be thought to include access to health care services. In "Fairness to Goodness" Rawls defines wealth as virtually any legally exchangeable social asset; this would cover health care 'vouchers' if they could be cashed or exchanged for other goods ([7], p. 540).

Let us suppose that health care is either itself a primary good covered by the Difference Principle or that health care may be purchased with income or some other form of wealth which is included under the Difference Principle. In the former case, depending upon various empirical conditions, it might turn out that the best way to insure that the basic structure satisfies the Difference Principle is to establish a state-enforced right to health care. But whether maximizing the prospects of the worst off will require such a right and what the content of the right will be will depend upon what weight is to be assigned to health care relative to other primary goods included under the Difference Principle. Similarly, a weighting must also be assigned if we are to determine whether the share of wealth one receives under the Difference Principle would be sufficient both for health care needs and for other ends. Unfortunately, though Rawls acknowledges that a weighted index of primary goods is needed if we are to be able to determine what would maximize the prospects of the worst off, he offers no account of how the weighting is to be achieved.

The problem is especially acute in the case of health care, because some forms of health care are so costly that an unrestrained commitment to them would undercut any serious commitment to providing other important goods. Thus, it appears that until we have some solution to the weighting problem Rawls's theory can shed only a limited light upon the question of priority relations between health care and other goods and among various forms of health care. Rawls's conception of primary goods may explain what distinguishes health care from those things that are not primary goods, but this is clearly not sufficient.

Perhaps because he is aware of the exorbitant demands which certain health care needs may place upon social resources, Rawls stipulates that the parties in the original position are to choose principles of justice on the assumption that their needs fall within the 'normal range' ([9], pp. 9–10). His ideal may be that the satisfaction of extremely costly special needs for health care may not be a matter of justice but rather of *charity*. If some reasonable way of drawing the line between 'normal' needs which fall within the gambit of principles of justice and 'special' needs which are the proper object of the virtue of charity could be developed, then this would be a step towards solving the priority problems mentioned above.

It has been suggested that the Principle of Equality of Fair Opportunity, rather than the Difference Principle, might provide the basis for a Rawlsian right to health care ([2], pp. 16–18). While I cannot accord this proposal the consideration it deserves here, I wish to point out that there are four difficulties which make it problematic. First, priority problems still remain. For now we are faced with the task of assigning a weight to health care relative to those other factors (such as education) which are also determinants of opportunity. Further, since the Principle of Equality of Fair Opportunity is lexically prior to the Difference Principle, we must again face the prospect that commitment to the former principle might swallow up social resource needed for providing important goods included under the latter.

Second, because it refers only to opportunities for occupying social *positions and offices*, rather than to opportunities in general, the Principle of Equality of Fair Opportunity might be thought too narrow to provide an adequate foundation for a right to health care. Rawls might respond either by defining 'position' rather broadly or by arguing that opportunities for attaining positions and offices are related to opportunities in general in such a way that equality in the former insures equality in the latter.

Third, and more importantly, Rawls's Principle of Equality of Fair Opportunity take 'abilities' and 'skills' as given, requiring only that persons with equal or similar abilities and skills are to have equal prospects of attaining social positions and offices. Yet clearly inequalities in health care can produce severe inequalities in abilities and skills. For example, poor nutrition and medical care during gestation can result in mental retardation, and many health problems hinder the development of skills and abilities. Hence it might be argued that if the Principle of Opportunity is to provide an adequate basis for a right to health care it must be reformulated to capture the crucial influence of health care or the lack of it upon individual development.

Each of the theories of justice under consideration offers a theoretical basis for answering some basic questions concerning justice in health care. We have seen, however, that none of them provides unambiguous answers to all of the questions and that each depends for its application upon a wealth of empirical premises, many of which may not now be available. Each theory does at least rule out some answers and each supplies us with a perspective from which to pursue issues which we cannot ignore. Nonetheless, almost all of the work in developing an account of justice in health care remains to be done.[8]

Notes

1. In this essay I shall be concerned for the most part with utilitarianism at the institutional level, and I shall proceed on the assumption that a set of institutions which maximizes utility will include rules which bar other direct applications of the principle of utility itself. Consequently, I will mainly be concerned with Rule Utilitarianism, rather than Act Utilitarianism (the latter being the view that the rightness or wrongness of a given act depends solely upon whether it maximizes utility). For an original and interesting attempt to show that Act Utilitarianism is compatible with social norms that bar direct appeals to utility, see [10].

2. Rawls sometimes refers to the "Principle of Equality of Fair Opportunity" and sometimes to the "Principle of Fair Equality of Opportunity." For convenience I will stay with the former label.

3. The phrase "worst off " refers to those who are worst off with respect to prospects of the social primary goods regulated by the Difference Principle.

4. For a detailed elaboration of this point, see [1].

5. For a fundamental objection to Nozick's invisible hand explanation, see [11].

6. P. Singer [12], expanding an argument developed earlier by R. Titmuss, argues that the existence of markets for certain goods may in fact undermine the motivation for charity.

7. See [2].

8. I would like to thank Earl Shelp and William Hanson for their very helpful comments on an earlier draft of this paper.

References

1. Buchanan, A. "Revisability and Rational Choice." *Canadian Journal of Philosophy* 5:395–408, 1975.
2. Daniels, N. "Rights to Health Care and Distributive Justice: Programmatic Worries." *Journal of Medicine and Philosoph* 4:174–191, 1979.
3. Friedman, M. *Capitalism and Freedom.* Chicago: University of Chicago Press, 1962, pp. 137–160.
4. Kant, I. *Foundations of the Metaphysics of Morals* (transl. by L. W. Beck), New York: Bobbs- Merrill, 1959, Part III.
5. Nozick, R. *Anarchy, State and Utopia.* New York: Basic Books, 1974.
6. Rawls, J. A *Theory of Justice.* Cambridge, Mass.: Harvard University Press, 1971.
7. Rawls, J. "Fairness to Goodness." *Philosophical Review* 84:536–554, 1975.
8. Rawls, J. "Reply to Alexander and Musgrave." *Quarterly Journal of Economics* 88:633–655, November 1974.
9. Rawls, J. "Responsibility for Ends." Stanford University, Unpublished Lecture, 1979.
10. Sartorius, R. *Individual Conduct and Social Norms.* Encino, Calif.: Dickenson Publishing, 1975.

11. Sartorius, R. "The Limits of Libertarianism." In *Liberty and the Rule of Law*, edited by R.L. Cunningham, 87–131. College Station, Texas: Texas A and M University Press, 1979.
12. Singer, P. "Rights and the Market." In *Justice and Economic Distribution*, edited by J. Arthur and W. Shaw, pp. 207–221. Englewood Cliffs, NJ.: Prentice-Hall, 1978.

Medical Care as a Right: A Refutation

Robert M. Sade

────────────────INTRODUCTION TO READING────────────────

In order to see how one of these principles, the principle of liberty, might be developed into a formula for allocating resources, we turn to an essay of Robert M. Sade, a physician who interprets rights to refer exclusively to freedom of action or liberty. Beginning with a fundamental right to one's life, he derives a right to act on one's own values, and to dispose of resources as one sees fit. In reading this essay one should focus on what it is Sade claims people own and the extent to which it can be deemed to belong to them. Does, for instance, knowledge belong to individuals or is it common property? Under what circumstances could persons be expected to agree, perhaps in advance, that they will acquire knowledge under the condition that it will be used in particular ways?

─────────────────────────────────

The current debate on health care in the United States is of the first order of importance to the health professions, and of no less importance to the political future of the nation, for precedents are now being set that will be applied to the rest of American society in the future. In the enormous volume of verbiage that has poured forth, certain fundamental issues have been so often misrepresented that they have now become commonly accepted fallacies. This paper will be concerned with the most important of these misconceptions, that health care is a right, as well as a brief consideration of some of its corollary fallacies.

Rights—Morality and Politics

The concept of rights has its roots in the moral nature of man and its practical expression in the political system that he creates. Both morality and politics must be discussed before the relation between political rights and health care can be appreciated.

A "right" defines a freedom of action. For instance, a right to a material object is the uncoerced choice of the use to which the object will be put; a right to a specific action, such as free speech, is the freedom to engage in that activity without forceful repression. The moral foundation of the rights of man begins with the fact that he is a living creature: he has the right to his own life. All other rights are corollaries of this primary one; without the right to life, there can be no others, and the concept of rights itself becomes meaningless.

The freedom to live, however, does not automatically ensure life. For man, a specific course of action is required to sustain his life, a course of action that must be guided by reason and reality and has as its goal the creation or acquisition of material values, such as food and clothing, and intellectual values, such as self-esteem and integrity. His moral system is the means by which he is able to select the values that will support his life and achieve his happiness.

Man must maintain a rather delicate homeostasis in a highly demanding and threatening environment, but has at his disposal a unique and efficient mechanism for dealing with it: his mind. His mind is able to perceive, to identify precepts, to integrate them into concepts, and to use those concepts in choosing actions suitable to the maintenance of his life. The rational function of mind is volitional, however; a man must choose to think, to be aware, to evaluate, to make conscious decisions. The extent to which he is able to achieve his goals will be directly proportional to his commitment to reason seeking them.

The right to life implies three corollaries: the right to select the values that one deems necessary to sustain one's own life; the right to exercise one's own judgment of the best course of action to achieve the chosen values; and the right to dispose of those values, once gained, in any way one chooses, without coercion by other men. The denial of any one of these corollaries severely compromises or destroys the right to life itself. A man who is not allowed to choose his own goals, is prevented from setting his own course in achieving those goals and is not free to dispose of the values he has earned is no less than a slave to those who usurp those rights. The right to private property, therefore, is essential and indispensable to maintaining free men in a free society.

Thus, it is the nature of man as a living, thinking being that determines his rights—his "natural rights." The concept of natural rights was slow in dawning on human civilization. The first political expression of that concept had its beginnings in 17th and 18th century England through such exponents as John Locke and Edmund Burke, but came to its brilliant debut as a form of government after the American Revolution. Under the leadership of such men as Thomas Paine and Thomas Jefferson, the concept of man as a being sovereign unto himself, rather than a subdivision of the sovereignty of a king, emperor or state, was incorporated into the formal structure of government for the first time. Protection of the lives and property of individual citizens was the salient characteristic of the Constitution of 1787. Ayn Rand has pointed out that the principle of protection of the individual against the coercive force of government made the United States the first moral society in history.[1]

In a free society, man exercises his right to sustain his own life by producing economic values in the form of goods and services that he is, or should be, free to exchange with other men who are similarly free to trade with him or not. The economic values produced, however, are not given as gifts by nature, but exist only by virtue of the thought and effort of individual men. Goods and services are thus owned as a consequence of the right to sustain life by one's own physical and mental effort.

If the chain of natural rights is interrupted, and the right to a loaf of bread, for example, is proclaimed as primary (avoiding the necessity of earning it), every man owns a loaf of bread, regardless of who produced it. Since ownership is the power of disposal,[2] every man may take his loaf from the baker and dispose of it as he wishes with or without the baker's permission. Another element has thus been introduced into the relation between men: the use of force. It is crucial to observe who has initiated the use of force: it is the man who demands unearned bread as a right, not the man who produced it. At the level of an unstructured society it is clear who is moral and who immoral. The man who acted rationally by producing food to support his own life is moral. The man who expropriated the bread by force is immoral.

To protect this basic right to provide for the support of one's own life, men band together for their mutual protection and form governments. This is the only proper function of government: to provide for the defense of individuals against those who would take their lives or property by force. The state is the repository for retaliatory force in a just society wherein the only actions prohibited to individuals are those of physical harm or the threat of physical harm to other men. The closest that man has ever come to achieving this ideal of government was in this country after its War of Independence.

When a government ignores the progression of natural rights arising from the right to life, and agrees with a man, a group of men, or even a majority of its citizens, that every man has a right to a loaf of bread, it must protect that right by the passage of laws ensuring that everyone gets his loaf in the process depriving the baker of the freedom to dispose of his own product. If the baker disobeys the law, asserting the priority of his right to support himself by his own rational disposition of the fruits of his mental and physical labor, he will be taken to court by force or threat of force where he will have more property forcibly taken from him (by fine) or have his liberty taken away (by incarceration). Now the initiator of violence is the government itself. The degree to which a government exercises its monopoly on the retaliatory use of force by asserting a claim to the lives and property of its citizens is the degree to which it has eroded its own legitimacy. It is a frequently overlooked fact that behind every law is a policemen's gun or a soldier's bayonet. When that gun and bayonet are used to initiate violence, to take property or to restrict liberty by force, there are no longer any rights, for the lives of the citizens belong to the state. In a just society with a moral government, it is clear that the only "right" to the bread belongs to the baker, and that a claim by any other man to that right is unjustified and can be enforced only by violence or the threat of violence.

Rights—Politics and Medicine

The concept of medical care as the patient's right is immoral because it denies the most fundamental of all rights, that of a man to his own life and the freedom of action to support it. Medical care is neither a right nor a privilege: it is a service that is provided by doctors and others to people who wish to purchase it. It is the provision of this service that a doctor depends upon for his livelihood, and is his means of supporting his own life. If the right to health care belongs to the patient, he starts out owning the services of a doctor without the necessity of either earning them or receiving them as a gift from the only man who has the right to give them: the doctor himself. In the narrative above substitute "doctor" for "baker" and "medical service" for "bread." American medicine is now at the point in the story where the state has proclaimed the nonexistent "right" to medical care as a fact of public policy, and has begun to pass the laws to enforce it. The doctor finds himself less and less his own master and more and more controlled by forces outside of his own judgment.

For instance, under the proposed Kennedy-Griffiths bill,[3] there will be a "Health Security Board," which will be responsible for administering the new controls to be imposed on doctors, hospitals and other "providers" of health care (Sec. 121). Specialized services, such as major surgery, will be done by "qualified specialists" [Sec. 22(b) (2)], such qualifications being determined by the Board (Sec. 42). Furthermore, the patient can no longer exercise his own initiative in finding a specialist to do his operation, since he must be referred to the specialist by a nonspecialist—i.e., a general practitioner or family doctor [Sec. 22(b)]. Licensure by his own state will not be enough to be a qualified practitioner; physicians will also be subject to a second set of standards, those established by the Board [Sec. 42(a)]. Doctors will no longer be considered competent to determine their own needs for continuing education, but must meet requirements established by the Board [Sec. 42(c)]. The professional staff of a hospital will no longer be able to determine which of its members are qualified to perform which kinds of major surgery; specialty-board certification or eligibility will be required, with certain exceptions that include meeting standards established by the Board [Sec. 42(d)].

Control of doctors through control of the hospitals in which they practice will also be exercised by the Board by way of a list of requirements, the last of which is a "sleeper" that will by its vagueness allow the Board almost any regulation of the hospital: The hospital must meet "such other requirements as the Board finds necessary in the interest of quality of care and the safety of patients in the institution" [Sec. 43(i)]. Hospitals will also not be allowed to undertake construction without higher approval by a state agency or by the Board (Sec. 52).

In the name of better organization and coordination of services, hospitals, nursing homes and other providers will be further controlled through the Board's power to issue directives forcing the provider to furnish services selected by the Board [Sec. 131(a)(1),(2)] at a place selected by the Board [Sec. 131(a)(3)]. The Board can also direct these providers to form associations with one another of various sorts, including "making available to one provider the professional and technical skills of another" [Sec. 131(a)(B)], and such other linkages as the Board thinks best [Sec. 131(a)(4)(C)].

These are only a few of the bill's controls of the health-care industry. It is difficult to believe that such patent subjugation of an entire profession could ever be considered a fit topic for discussion in any but the darkest corner of a country founded on the principles of life and liberty. Yet the Kennedy-Griffiths bill is being seriously debated today in the Congress of the United States.

The irony of this bill is that, on the basis of the philosophic premises of its authors, it does provide a rationally organized system for attempting to fulfill its goals, such as "making health services available to all residents of the United States." If the government is to spend tens of billions of dollars on health services, it must assure in some way that the money is not being wasted. Every bill currently before the national legislature does, should, and must provide some such controls. The Kennedy-Griffiths bill is the closest we have yet come to the logical conclusion and inevitable consequence of two fundamental fallacies: that health care is a right, and that doctors and other health workers will function as efficiently serving as chattels of the state as they will living as sovereign human beings. It is not, and they will not.

Any act of force is anti-mind. It is a confession of the failure of persuasion, the failure of reason. When politicians say that the health system must be forced into a mold of their own design, they are admitting their inability to persuade doctors and patients to use the plan voluntarily; they are proclaiming the supremacy of the state's logic over the judgments of the individual minds of all concerned with health care. Statists throughout history have never learned that compulsion and reason are contradictory, that a forced mind cannot think effectively and, by extension, that a regimented profession will eventually choke and stagnate from its own lack of freedom. A persuasive example of this is the moribund condition of medicine as a profession is Sweden, a country that has enjoyed socialized medicine since 1955. Werkö, a Swedish physician, has stated: "The details and the complicated working schedule have not yet been determined in all hospitals and districts, but the general feeling of belonging to a free profession, free to decide—at least in principle—how to organize its work has been lost. Many hospital-based physicians regard their work now with an apathy previously unknown."[4] One wonders how American legislators will like having their myocardial infarctions treated by apathetic internists, their mitral valves replaced by apathetic surgeons, their wives' tumors removed by apathetic gynecologists. They will find it very difficult to legislate self-esteem, integrity and competence into the doctors whose minds and judgments they have throttled.

If anyone doubts that health legislation involves the use of force, a dramatic demonstration of the practical political meaning of the "right to health care" was acted out in Quebec in the closing months of 1970.[5] In that unprecedented threat of violence by a modern Western government against a group of its citizens, the doctors of Quebec were literally imprisoned in the province by Bill 41, possibly the most repressive piece of legislation ever enacted against the medical profession, and far more worthy of the Soviet Union or Red China than a Western democracy. Doctors objecting to a new Medicare law were forced to continue working under penalty of jail sentence and fines of up to $500 a day away from their practices. Those who spoke out publicly against the bill were subject to jail sentences of up to a year and fines of up to $50,000 a day. The facts that the doctors did return to work and that no one was therefore jailed or fined do not mitigate the nature or implications of the passage of Bill 41. Although the dispute between the Quebec physicians and their government was not one of principle but of the details of compensation, the reaction of the state to resistance against coercive professional regulation was a classic example of the naked force that lies behind every act of social legislation.

Any doctor who is forced by law to join a group or a hospital he does not choose, or is prevented by law from prescribing a drug he thinks is best for his patient, or is compelled by law to make any decisions he would not otherwise have made, is being forced to act against his own mind, which means forced to act against his own life. He is also being forced to violate his most fundamental professional commitment, that of using his own best judgment at all times for the greatest benefit of his patient. It is remarkable that this principle has never been identified by a public voice in the medical profession, and that the vast majority of doctors in this country are being led down the path to civil servitude, never knowing that their feelings of uneasy foreboding have a profoundly moral origin, and never recognizing that the main issues at stake are not those being formulated in Washington, but are their own honor, integrity and freedom, and their own survival as sovereign human beings.

Some Corollaries

The basic fallacy that health care is a right has led to several corollary fallacies, among them the following:

That health is primarily a community or social rather than individual concern.[6] A simple calculation from American mortality statistics[7] quickly corrects that false concept: 67 per cent of deaths in 1967 were due to diseases known to be caused or exacerbated by alcohol, tobacco smoking or over-eating, or were due to accidents. Each of those factors is either largely or wholly correctable by individual action. Although no statistics are available, it is likely that morbidity, with the exception of common respiratory infections, has a relation like that of mortality to personal habits and excesses.

That state medicine has worked better in other countries than free enterprise has worked here. There is no evidence to support that contention, other than anecdotal testimonials and the spurious citation of infant mortality and longevity statistics. There is, on the other hand, a good deal of evidence to the contrary.[8,9]

That the provision of medical care somehow lies outside the laws of supply and demand, and that government-controlled health care will be free care. In fact, no service or commodity lies outside the economic laws. Regarding health care, market demand, individual want, and medical need are entirely different things, and have a very complex relation with the cost and the total supply of available care, as recently discussed and clarified by Jeffery et al.[10] They point out that "'health is purchaseable,' meaning that somebody has to pay for it, individually or collectively, at the expense of foregoing the current or future consumption of other things." The question is whether the decision of how to allocate the consumer's dollar should belong to the consumer or to the state. It has already been shown that the choice of how a doctor's services should be rendered belongs only to the doctor: in the same way the choice of whether to buy a doctor's service rather than some other commodity or service belongs to the consumer as a logical consequence of the right to his own life.

That opposition to national health legislation is tantamount to opposition to progress in health care. Progress is made by the free interaction of free minds developing new ideas in an atmosphere conducive to experimentation and trial. If group practice really is better than solo, we will find out because the success of groups will result in more groups (which has, in fact, been happening); if prepaid comprehensive care really is the best form of practice, it will succeed and the health industry will swell with new Kaiser-Permanente plans. But let one of these or any other form of practice become the law, and the system is in a straightjacket that will stifle progress. Progress requires freedom of action, and that is precisely what national health legislation aims at restricting.

That doctors should help design the legislation for a national health system, since they must live with and within whatever legislation is enacted. To accept this concept is to concede to the opposition its philosophic premises, and thus to lose the battle. The means by which nonproducers and hangers-on throughout history have been able to expropriate material and intellectual values from the producers has been identified only relatively recently: the sanction of the victim.[11] Historically, few people have lost their freedom and their rights without some degree of complicity in the plunder. If the American medical profession accepts the concept of health care as the right of the patient, it will have earned the Kennedy-Griffiths bill by default. The alternative for any health professional is to withhold his sanction and make clear who is being victimized. Any physician can say to those who would shackle his judgment and control his profession: I do not recognize your right to my life and my mind, which belong to me and me alone; I will not participate in any legislated solution to any health problem.

In the face of the raw power that lies behind government programs, nonparticipation is the only way in which personal values can be maintained. And it is only with the attainment of the highest of those values—integrity, honesty and self-esteem—that the physician can achieve his most important professional value, the absolute priority of the welfare of his patients.

The preceding discussion should not be interpreted as proposing that there are no problems in the delivery of medical care. Problems such as high cost, few doctors, low quantity of available care in economically depressed areas may be real, but it is naive to believe that governmental solutions through coercive legislation can be anything but shortsighted and formulated on the basis of political expediency. The only long-range plan that can hope to provide for the day after tomorrow is a "nonsystem"—that is, a system that proscribes the imposition by force (legislation) of any one group's conception of the best forms of medical care. We must identify our problems and seek to solve them by experimentation and trial in an atmosphere of freedom from compulsion. Our sanction of anything less will mean the loss of our personal values, the death of our profession, and a heavy blow to political liberty.

Notes

1. Rand, A. *Man's Rights, Capitalism: The Unknown Ideal.* New York: New American Library, 1967, pp. 320–329.

2. Von Mises, L. *Socialism: An Economic and Sociological Analysis.* New Haven, Conn.: Yale University Press, 1951, pp. 37–55.

3. Kennedy, E. M. "Introduction of the Health Security Act." *Congressional Record* 116:S 14338–S 14361, 1970.

4. Werkö, L. "Swedish Medical Care in Transition. " *New England Journal of Medicine* 284:360-366, 1971.

5. "Quebec Medicare and Medical Services Withdrawal." Toronto: Canadian Medical Association, 19 October 1970.

6. Millis, J. S. "Wisdom? Health? Can Society Guarantee Them?" *New England Journal of Medicine* 283:260–261, 1970.

7. Department of Health, Education, and Welfare, Public Health Service. *Vital Statistics of the United States 1967. Vol. II, Mortality Part A.* Washington, D.C. Government Printing Office, 1969. pp. 1–7.

8. *Financing Medical Care: An Appraisal of Foreign Programs,* edited by H. Shoeck. Caldwell, Idaho: Caxton Printers, 1962.

9. Lynch, M. J., and S. S. Raphael. *Medicine and the State.* Springfield, Ill.: Charles C Thomas, 1963.

10. Jeffers, J. R., M. F. Bognanno, and J. C. Bartlett. "On the Demand Versus Need for Medical Services and the Concept of Shortage. " *American Journal of Public Health* 61:46–63, 1971.

11. Rand, A. *Atlas Shrugged.* New York: Random House, 1957, p. 1066.

Securing Access to Health Care: *President's Commission for the Study of Ethical Problems in Medicine and Biomedical and Behavioral Research*

──────── INTRODUCTION TO READING ────────

Many people recognize alternatives to a system of allocating resources based solely on individual liberty. The President's Commission for the Study of Ethical Problems in Medicine and Biomedical and Behavioral Research, a national body charged with assessing biomedical ethical and policy issues, asserts in a 1983 report that equitable access to health care means that all citizens are able to secure an adequate level of care without excessive burdens. This concept of equitable access incorporates considerations of both efficiency in maximizing benefits and fair distribution that focuses on the rights of the least well-off. The following excerpt from its report explains its notion of equitable access.

The Concept of Equitable Access to Health Care

The special nature of health care helps explain why it ought to be accessible, in a fair fashion, to all.[1] But if this ethical conclusion is to provide a basis for evaluating current patterns of access to health care and proposed health policies, the meaning of fairness or equity in this context must be clarified. The concept of equitable access needs definition in its two main aspects: the level of care that ought to be available to all and the extent to which burdens can be imposed on those who obtain these services.

Access to What?

"Equitable access" could be interpreted in a number of ways: equality of access, access to whatever an individual needs or would benefit from, or access to an adequate level of care.

Equity as Equality. It has been suggested that equity is achieved either when everyone is assured of receiving an equal quantity of health care dollars or when people enjoy equal health. The most common characterization of equity as equality, however, is as providing everyone with the same level of health care. In this view, it follows that if a given level of care is available to one individual it must be available to all. If the initial standard is set high, by reference to the highest level of care presently received, an enormous drain would result on the resources needed to provide other goods. Alternatively, if the standard is set low in order to avoid an excessive use of resources, some beneficial services would have to be withheld from people who wished to purchase them. In other words, none would be allowed access to more services or services of higher quality than those available to everyone else, even if he or she were willing to pay for those services from his or her personal resources.

As long as significant inequalities in income and wealth persist, inequalities in the use of health care can be expected beyond those created by differences in need. Given people with the same pattern of preferences and equal health care needs, those with greater financial resources will purchase more health care. Conversely, given equal financial resources, the different patterns of health care preferences that typically exist in any population will result in a different use of health services by people with equal health needs. Trying to prevent such inequalities would require interfering with people's liberty to use their income to purchase an important good like health care while leaving them free to use it for frivolous or inessential ends. Prohibiting people with higher incomes or stronger preferences for health care from purchasing more care than everyone else gets would not be feasible, and would probably result in a black market for health care.

Equity as Access Solely According to Benefit or Need. Interpreting equitable access to mean that everyone must receive all health care that is of any benefit to them also has unacceptable implications. Unless health is the only good or resources are unlimited, it would be irrational for a society—as for an individual—to make a commitment to provide whatever health care might be beneficial regardless of cost. Although health care is of special importance, it is surely not all that is important to people. Pushed to an extreme, this criterion might swallow up all of society's resources, since there is virtually no end to the fund that could be devoted to possibly beneficial care for diseases and disabilities and to their prevention.

Equitable access to health care must take into account not only the benefits of care but also the cost in comparison with other goods and services to which those resources might be allocated. Society will reasonably devote some resources to health care but reserve most resources for other goals. This, in turn, will mean that some health services (even of a lifesaving sort) will not be developed or employed because they would produce too few benefits in relation to their costs and to other ways the resources for them might be used.

It might be argued that the notion of "need" provides a way to limit access to only that care that confers especially important benefits. In this view, equity as access according to need would place less severe demands on social resources than equity according to benefit would. There are, however, difficulties with the notion of need in this context. On the one hand, medical need is often not narrowly defined but refers to any condition for which medical treatment might be effective. Thus, "equity as access according to need" collapses into "access according to whatever is of benefit."

On the other hand, "need" could be even more expansive in scope than "benefit." Philosophical and economic writings do not provide any clear distinction between "needs" and "wants" or "preferences." Since the term means different things to different people, "access according to need" could become "access to any health services a person wants." Conversely, need could be interpreted very narrowly to encompass only a very minimal level of services—for example, those "necessary to prevent death."[2]

Equity as an Adequate Level of Health Care. Although neither "everything needed" nor "everything beneficial" nor "everything that anyone else is getting" are defensible ways of understanding equitable access, the special nature of health care dictates that everyone have access to some level of care: enough care to achieve sufficient welfare, opportunity, information, and evidence of interpersonal concern to facilitate a reasonably full and satisfying life. That level can be termed "an adequate level of health care." The difficulty of sharpening this amorphous notion in a workable foundation for health policy is a major problem in the United States today. This concept is not new; it is implicit in the public debate over policy in this country. . . .

Understanding equitable access to health care to mean that everyone should be able to secure an adequate level of care has several strengths. Because an adequate level of care may be less than "all beneficial care" and because it does not require that all needs be satisfied, it acknowledges the need for setting priorities with health care and signals a clear recognition that society's resources are limited and that there are other goods besides health. Thus, interpreting equity as access to adequate care does not generate an open-ended obligation. One of the chief dangers of interpretations of equity that require virtually unlimited resources for health care is that they encourage the view that equitable access is an impossible ideal. Defining equity as an adequate level of care for all avoids an impossible commitment of resources without falling into the opposite error of abandoning the enterprise of seeking to ensure that health care is in fact available for everyone.

In addition, since providing an adequate level of care is a limited moral requirement, this definition also avoids the unacceptable restriction on individual liberty entailed by the view that equity requires equality. Provided that an adequate level is available to all, those who prefer to use their resources to obtain care that exceeds that level do not offend any ethical principle in doing so. Finally, the concept of adequacy, as the Commission understands it, is society-relative. The content of adequate care will depend upon the overall resources available in a given society, and can take into account a consensus of expectations about what is adequate in a particular society at a particular time in its historical development. This permits the definition of adequacy to be altered as societal resources and expectations change.[3]

With What Burdens?

It is not enough to focus on the care that individuals receive; attention must be paid to the burdens they must bear in order to obtain it—waiting and travel time, the cost and availability of transport, the financial cost of the care itself. Equity requires not only that adequate care be available to all, but also that these burdens not be excessive.

If individuals must travel unreasonably long distances, wait for unreasonably long hours, or spend most of their financial resources to obtain care, some will be deterred from obtaining adequate care, with adverse effects on their health and well-being. Others may bear the burdens, but only at the expense of their ability to meet other important needs. If one of the main reasons for providing adequate care is that health care increases welfare and opportunity, then a system that required large numbers of individuals to forego food, shelter, or educational advancement in order to obtain care would be self-defeating and irrational.

The concept of acceptable burdens in obtaining care, as opposed to excessive ones, parallels in some respects the concept of adequacy. Just as equity does not require equal access, neither must the burdens of obtaining adequate care be equal for all persons. What is crucial is that the variations in burdens fall within an acceptable range. As in determining an adequate level of care, there is no simple formula for ascertaining when the burdens of obtaining care fall within such a range. Yet some guidelines can be formulated. To illustrate, since a given financial outlay represents a greater sacrifice to a poor person than to a rich person, "excessive" must be understood in relation to income. Obviously everyone cannot live the same distance from a health facility, and some individuals choose to locate in remote and sparsely populated areas. Concern about an inequitable burden would be appropriate, however, when identifiable groups must travel a great distance or long time to receive care—though people may appropriately be expected to travel farther to get specialized care, for example, than to obtain primary or emergency care.

Although differences in the burdens individuals must bear to obtain care do not necessarily represent inequities, they may trigger concern for two reasons. Such discrepancies may indicate that some people are, in fact, bearing excessive burdens, just as some differences in the use of care may indicate that some lack adequate care. Also, certain patterns of differences may indicate racial or ethnic discrimination.

Whether any such discrepancies actually constitute an inequitable distribution of burdens ultimately depends upon the role these differences play in the larger system under which the overall burdens of providing an adequate level of care are distributed among the citizens of this country. It may be permissible, for example, for some individuals to bear greater burdens in the form of out-of-pocket expenses for care if this is offset by a lower bill for taxes devoted to health care. Whether such differences in the distribution of burdens are acceptable cannot be determined by looking at a particular burden in isolation.

A Societal Obligation

Society has a moral obligation to ensure that everyone has access to adequate care without being subject to excessive burdens. In speaking of a societal obligation the Commission makes reference to society in the broadest sense—the collective American community. The community is made up of individuals, who are in turn members of many other, overlapping groups, both public and private: local, state, regional, and national units; professional and workplace organizations; religious, educational and charitable organizations; and family, kinship, and ethnic groups. All these entities play a role in discharging societal obligations.

The Commission believes it is important to distinguish between society, in this inclusive sense, and government as one institution among others in society. Thus the recognition of a collective or societal obligation does not imply that government should be the only or even the primary institution involved in the complex of making health care available. It is the Commission's view that the societal obligation to ensure equitable access for everyone may best be fulfilled in this country by a pluralistic approach that relies upon the coordinated contributions of actions by both the private and public sectors.

Securing equitable access is a societal rather than a merely private or individual responsibility for several reasons. First, while health is of special importance for human beings, health care—especially scientific health care—is a social product requiring the skills and efforts of many individuals; it is not something that individuals can provide for themselves solely through their own efforts. Second, because the need for health care is both unevenly distributed among persons and highly unpredictable and because the cost of securing care may be great, few individuals could secure adequate care without relying on some social mechanism for sharing the costs. Third, if persons generally deserved their health conditions or if the need for health care were fully within the individual's control, the fact that some lack adequate care would not be viewed as an inequity. But differences in health status, and hence differences in health care needs, are largely undeserved because they are, for the most part, not within the individual's control.

Uneven and Unpredictable Health Needs

While requirements for other basic necessities, such as adequate food and shelter, vary among people within a relatively limited range, the need for health care is distributed very unevenly and its occurrence at any particular time is highly unpredictable. One study shows 50% of all hospital billings are for only 13% of the patients, the seriously chronically ill.[4]

Moreover, health care needs may be minor or overwhelming, in their personal as well as financial impact. Some people go through their entire lives seldom requiring health care, while others face medical expenses that would exceed the resources of all but the wealthiest. Moreover, because the need for care cannot be predicted, it is difficult to provide for it by personal savings from income. Under the major program that pays for care for the elderly, 40% of aged enrollees had no payments at all in 1977 and 37% fell into a low payment group (averaging $129 per year), while 8.8% averaged $7011 in annual expenditures.[5]

Responsibility for Differences in Health Status

Were someone responsible for (and hence deserving of) his or her need for health care, then access to the necessary health care might be viewed as merely an individual concern. But the differences among people's needs for health care are for the most part not within their control, and thus are not something for which they should be held accountable. Different needs for care are largely a matter of good or bad fortune—that is, a consequence of a natural and social lottery that no one chooses to play.

In a very real sense, people pay for the consequences of the actions that cause them illness or disability—through the suffering and loss of opportunity they experience. The issue here is a narrower one: to what extent is the societal responsibility to secure health care for the sick and injured limited by personal responsibility for the need for health care? It seems reasonable for people to bear the foreseeable consequences (in terms of health care needs) of their informed and voluntary choices. Indeed, as an ethical matter, the principle of self-determination implies as a corollary the responsibility of individuals for their choices.

However, to apply the notion of personal responsibility in a fair way in setting health care policy would be a complex and perhaps impossible task. First, identifying those people whose informed, voluntary choices have caused them foreseeable harm would be practically as well as theoretically very difficult. It is often not possible to determine the degree to which an individual's behavior is fully informed regarding the health consequences of the behavior. Efforts to educate the public about the effects of life-style on health are desirable, but it must also be acknowledged that today people who conscientiously strive to adopt a healthy life-style find themselves inundated with an enormous amount of sometimes contradictory information about what is healthful. Voluntariness is also especially problematic regarding certain behaviors that cause some people ill health, such as smoking and alcohol abuse.[6] Moreover, there are great difficulties in determining the extent of the causal role of particular behavior on an individual's health status. For many behaviors, consequences appear only over long periods of time, during which many other elements besides the particular behavior have entered into the causal process that produces a disease or disability. For example, the largely unknown role of genetic predispositions for many diseases makes it difficult to designate particular behaviors as their "cause."

Second, even if one knew who should be held responsible for what aspects of their own ill health, policies aimed at institutionalizing financial accountability for "unhealthy behavior" or at denying the necessary health care for those who have "misbehaved" are likely to involve significant injustices and other undesirable consequences. Leaving people free to engage in health-risky behavior only if they can afford to pay for its consequences is fair only if the existing patterns of income distribution are fair, and if the payment required fully accounts for all the costs to society for the ill health and its treatment. Moreover, since some unhealthy behavior can be monitored more easily than others, problems of discrimination would inevitably arise; even when feasible, monitoring such behavior would raise serious concerns about the invasion of privacy. Finally, the ultimate sanction—turning away from the hospital door people who are responsible for their own ill health—would reverberate in unwanted and perhaps very harmful ways in the community at large. The Commission concludes that within programs to secure equitable access to health care, serious practical and ethical difficulties would follow attempts to single out the consequences of behavior and to make individuals of health-risky behavior solely responsible for those consequences.

However, even if it is inappropriate to hold people responsible for their health status, it is appropriate to hold them responsible for a fair share of the cost of their own health care. Society's moral obligation to provide equitable access for all and the individual responsibility for bearing a share of the costs of achieving equity rest on the same considerations of fairness. Individuals who—because they know that others will come to their aid—fail to take reasonable steps to provide for their own health care when they could do so without excessive burdens would be guilty of exploiting the generosity of their fellow citizens. The societal obligation is therefore balanced by corresponding individual obligations. In light of the special importance of health care, the largely undeserved character of differences in health status, and the uneven distribution and unpredictability of health care needs, society has a moral obligation to ensure adequate care for all. Saying that the obligation is societal (rather than merely individual) stops short, however, of identifying who has the ultimate responsibility for ensuring that the obligation is successfully met.

Notes

1. For a discussion of other important factors, the uneven distribution of need, and its largely undeserved nature, see pp. 23–25 of *Securing Access to Health Care*.

2. The Federal government employed this criterion in the mid-1970s when it dropped requirements providing dental care for adult public program beneficiaries under Medicaid. It claimed that dental services were not services whose absence could be considered as "life-threatening."

3. There are practical as well as ethical reasons for a nation like the United States, which possesses resources to provide a high level of services, not to take a narrow view of "adequacy." A lesser level of care would make it extremely difficult to establish a desirable mix of services; narrow limits would foster intense competition among different types of care and possibly skew the adequate level toward life-threatening care to the exclusion of other very beneficial forms of care such as preventive medicine. An inadequate level, accompanied by a private market alternative treatment, would generate

inequities by encouraging the flight of resources (as is now the case with physicians who choose to serve privately insured patients to the exclusion of noninsured and publicly insured individuals).

4. Zook, C.J., and F. D. Moore. "High Cost Users of Medical Care." *New England Journal of Medicine* 302:996, 1982.

5. Davis, Karen. *Medicare Reconsidered.* Duke University Medical Center Private Sector Conference, Durham, N.C., 15–16 March 1982.

6. Wikler, Daniel. "Persuasion and Coercion for Health." *Milbank Memorial Fund Quarterly/Health & Society* 56:303, 1978.

RIGHTS-BASED CODES

A Patient's Bill of Rights

American Hospital Association

──────────────INTRODUCTION TO READING──────────────

One of the most important manifestations of the emphasis on rights in medical ethics is the American Hospital Association's statement articulating a bill of rights for patients. It demonstrates the shift to the perspective of Western liberal political philosophy. Note that rights are taken primarily as "liberty rights," that is the right to non interference or "entitlement rights" focusing on non-economic issues such as the right to considerate and respectful care. This rights focus does not yet address the more entitlement rights claims with more direct economic implications, the claims summarized in the phrase "the right to health care." The "Bill of Rights" was originally adopted in 1973. The version presented here is the revision adopted by the American Hospital Association's Board of Trustees, October 21, 1992.

Introduction

Effective health care requires collaboration between patients and physicians and other health care professionals. Open and honest communication, respect for personal and professional values, and sensitivity to differences are integral to optimal patient care. As the setting for the provision of health services, hospitals must provide a foundation for understanding and respecting the rights and responsibilities of patients, their families, physicians, and other care-givers. Hospitals must ensure a health care ethic that respects the role of patients in decision making about treatment choices and other aspects of their care. Hospitals must be sensitive to cultural, racial, linguistic, religious, age, gender, and other differences as well as the needs of persons with disabilities.

The American Hospital Association presents *A Patient's Bill of Rights* with the expectation that it will contribute to more effective patient care and be supported by the hospital on behalf of the institution, its medical staff, employ-ees, and patients. The American Hospital Association encourages health care institutions to tailor this bill of rights to their patient community by translating and/or simplifying the language of this bill of rights as may be necessary to ensure that patients and their families understand their rights and responsible titles.

Bill of Rights

1. The patient has the right to considerate and respectful care.
2. The patient has the right to and is encouraged to obtain from physi-cians and other direct caregivers relevant, current, and understandable infor-mation concerning diagnosis, treatment, and prognosis.

Except in emergencies when the patient lacks decision-making capacity and the need for treatment is urgent, the patient is entitled to the opportunity to discuss and request information related to the specific proce-dures and/or treatments, the risks involved, the possible length of recupera-tion, and the medically reasonable alternatives and their accompanying risks and benefits.

Patients have the right to know the identity of physicians, nurses, and others involved in their care, as well as when those involved are students, resi-dents, or other trainees. The patient also has the right to know the immediate and long-term financial implications of treatment choices, insofar as they are known.

3. The patient has the right to make decisions about the plan of care prior to and during the course of treatment and to refuse a recommended treatment or plan of care to the extent permitted by law and hospital policy and to be informed of the medical consequences of this action. In case of such refusal, the patient is entitled to other appropriate care and services that the hospital provides or transfer to another hospital. The hospital should notify patients of any policy that might affect patient choice within the institution.

4. The patient has the right to have an advance directive (such as a living will, health care proxy, or durable power of attorney for health care) concern-ing treatment or designating a surrogate decision maker with the expectation that the hospital will honor the intent of that directive to the extent permitted by law and hospital policy.

Health care institutions must advise patients of their rights under state law and hospital policy to make informed medical choices, ask if the patient has an advance directive, and include that information in patient records. The patient has the right to timely information about hospital policy that may limit its ability to implement fully a legally valid advance directive.

5. The patient has the right to every consideration of privacy. Case discussion, consultation, examination, and treatment should be conducted so as to protect each patient's privacy.

6. The patient has the right to expect that all communications and records pertaining to his/her care will be treated as confidential by the hospital, except in cases such as suspected abuse and public health hazards when reporting is permitted or required by law. The patient has the right to expect that the hospital will emphasize the confidentiality of this information when it releases it to any other parties entitled to review information in those records.

7. The patient has the right to review the records pertaining to his/her medical care and to have the information explained or interpreted as necessary, except when restricted by law.

8. The patient has the right to expect that, within its capacity and policies, a hospital will make reasonable response to the request of a patient for appropriate and medically indicated care and services. The hospital must provide evaluation, service and/or referral as indicated by the urgency of the case. When medically appropriate and legally permissible, or when a patient has so requested, a patient may be transferred to another facility. The institution to which the patient is to be transferred must first have accepted the patient for transfer. The patient must also have the benefit of complete information and explanation concerning the need for, risks. benefits, and alternatives to such a transfer.

9. The patient has the right to ask and be informed of the existence of business relationships among the hospital, educational institutions, other health care providers, or payers that may influence the patient's treatment and care.

10. The patient has the right to consent to or decline to participate in proposed research studies or human experimentation affecting care and treatment of requiring direct patient involvement, and to have those studies fully explained prior to consent. A patient who declines to participate in research or experimentation is entitled to the most effective care that the hospital can otherwise provide.

11. The patient has the right to expect reasonable continuity of care when appropriate and to be informed by physicians and other caregivers of available and realistic patient care options when hospital care is no longer appropriate.

12. The patient has the right to be informed of hospital policies and practices that relate to patient care, treatment, and responsibilities. The patient has the right to be informed of available resources for resolving disputes, grievances, and conflicts, such as ethics committees, patient representatives, or other mechanisms available in the institutions. The patient has the right to be informed of the hospital's charges for services and available payment methods.

The collaborative nature of health care requires that patients, or their families/surrogates, participate in their care. The effectiveness of care and patient satisfaction with the course of treatment depend, in part, on the patient fulfilling certain responsibilities. Patients are responsible for providing information about past illnesses, hospitalizations, medications, and other matters related to health status. To participate effectively in decision making, patients must be encouraged to take responsibility for requesting additional information or clarification about their health status or treatment when they do not fully understand information and instructions. Patients are also responsible for ensuring that the health care institution has a copy of their written advance directive if they have one. Patients are responsible for informing their physicians and other caregivers if they anticipate problems in following prescribed treatment. Patients should also be aware of the hospital's obligation to be reasonably efficient and equitable in providing care to other patients and the community. The hospital's rules and regulations are designed to help the hospital meet this obligation. Patients and their families are responsible for making reasonable accommodations to the needs of the hospital, other patients, medical staff, and hospital employees. Patients are responsible for providing necessary information for insurance claims and for working with the hospital to make payment arrangements, when necessary. A person's health depends on much more than health care services. Patients are responsible for recognizing the impact of their life-style on their personal health.

Conclusion

Hospitals have many functions to perform, including the enhancement of health status, health promotion, and the prevention and treatment of injury and disease; the immediate and ongoing care and rehabilitation of patients; the education of health professionals, patients, and the community; and research. All these activities must be conducted with an overriding concern for the values and dignity of patients.

Convention for Protection of Human Rights and Dignity of the Human Being with Regard to the Application of Biology and Biomedicine: Convention on Human Rights and Biomedicine

Council of Europe

─────────────INTRODUCTION TO READING─────────────

In 1997 member nations of the Council of Europe formally signed a Convention for Protection of Human Rights in biomedicine, often called the Bioethics Convention. Twenty-one of the forty member nations signed immediately indicating that they were initiating the formal ratification process. The convention is the first international, legally binding set of rules on human medical research, genetics, embryology, and transplantation. It also addresses human dignity in the practice of medicine, equitable access to health care, and informed consent, and formally declares the primacy of the individual over the interests of society and science. Notice that it relies heavily on the language of rights rather than the more traditional focus on benefits and harms. Only the future will tell whether the remaining countries sign on and whether they actually bring their domestic law into conformity with the convention's provisions.

Preamble

The Member States of the Council of Europe, the other States and the European Community Signatories hereto,

Bearing in mind the Universal Declaration of Human Rights proclaimed by the General Assembly of the United Nations on 10 December 1948;

Bearing in mind the Convention for the Protection of Human Rights and Fundamental Freedoms of 4 November 1950;

Bearing in mind the European Social Charter of 18 October 1961;

Bearing in mind the International Covenant on Civil and Political Rights and the International Covenant on Economic, Social and Cultural Rights of 16 December 1966;

Bearing in mind the Convention for the Protection of Individuals with regard to Automatic Processing of Personal Data of 28 January 1981;

Bearing in mind the Convention on the Rights of the Child of 20 November 1989;

Considering that the aim of the Council of Europe is the achievement of a greater unity between its members and that one of the methods by which that aim is to be pursued is the maintenance and further realisation of human rights and fundamental freedoms;

Conscious of the accelerating developments in biology and medicine;

Convinced of the need to respect the human being both as an individual and as a member of the human species and recognising the importance of ensuring the dignity of the human being;

Conscious that the misuse of biology and medicine may lead to acts endangering human dignity;

Affirming that progress in biology and medicine should be used for the benefit of present and future generations;

Stressing the need for international co-operation so that all humanity may enjoy the benefits of biology and medicine;

Recognising the importance of promoting a public debate on the questions posed by the application of biology and medicine and the responses to be given thereto;

Wishing to remind all members of society of their rights and responsibilities;

Taking account of the work of the Parliamentary Assembly in this field, including Recommendation 1160 (1991) on the preparation of a convention on bioethics;

Resolving to take such measures as are necessary to safeguard human dignity and the fundamental rights and freedoms of the individual with regard to the application of biology and medicine,

Have agreed as follows:

Chapter I—General Provisions

Article 1—Purpose and Object

Parties to this Convention shall protect the dignity and identity of all human beings and guarantee everyone, without discrimination, respect for their integrity and other rights and fundamental freedoms with regard to the application of biology and medicine.

Each Party shall take in its internal law the necessary measures to give effect to the provisions of this Convention.

Article 2—Primacy of the Human Being

The interests and welfare of the human being shall prevail over the sole interest of society or science.

Article 3—Equitable Access to Health Care

Parties, taking into account health needs and available resources, shall take appropriate measures with a view to providing, within their jurisdiction, equitable access to health care of appropriate quality.

Article 4—Professional Standards

Any intervention in the health field, including research, must be carried out in accordance with relevant professional obligations and standards.

Chapter II—Consent

Article 5—General Rule

An intervention in the health field may only be carried out after the person concerned has given free and informed consent to it.

This person shall beforehand be given appropriate information as to the purpose and nature of the intervention as well as on its consequences and risks.

The person concerned may freely withdraw consent at any time.

Article 6—Protection of Persons Not Able to Consent

1. Subject to Articles 17 and 20 below, an intervention may only be carried out on a person who does not have the capacity to consent, for his or her direct benefit.

2. Where, according to law, a minor does not have the capacity to consent to an intervention, the intervention may only be carried out with the authorisation of his or her representative or an authority or a person or body provided for by law.

The opinion of the minor shall be taken into consideration as an increasingly determining factor in proportion to his or her age and degree of maturity.

3. Where, according to law, an adult does not have the capacity to consent to an intervention because of a mental disability, a disease or for similar reasons, the intervention may only be carried out with the authorisation of his or her representative or an authority or a person or body provided for by law.

The individual concerned shall as far as possible take part in the authorisation procedure.

4. The representative, the authority, the person or the body mentioned in paragraphs 2 and 3 above shall be given, under the same conditions, the information referred to in Article 5.

5. The authorisation referred to in paragraphs 2 and 3 above may be withdrawn at any time in the best interests of the person concerned.

Article 7—Protection of Persons Who Have a Mental Disorder

Subject to protective conditions prescribed by law, including supervisory, control and appeal procedures, a person who has a mental disorder of a serious nature may be subjected, without his or her consent, to an intervention aimed at treating his or her mental disorder only where, without such treatment, serious harm is likely to result to his or her health.

Article 8—Emergency Situation

When because of an emergency situation the appropriate consent cannot be obtained, any medically necessary intervention may be carried out immediately for the benefit of the health of the individual concerned.

Article 9—Previously Expressed Wishes

The previously expressed wishes relating to a medical intervention by a patient who is not, at the time of the intervention, in a state to express his or her wishes shall be taken into account.

Chapter III—Private Life and Right to Information

Article 10—Private Life and Right to Information

1.   Everyone has the right to respect for private life in relation to information about his or her health.

2.   Everyone is entitled to know any information collected about his or her health. However, the wishes of individuals not to be so informed shall be observed.

3.   In exceptional cases, restrictions may be placed by law on the exercise of the rights contained in paragraph 2 in the interests of the patient.

Chapter IV—Human Genome

Article 11—Non-Discrimination

Any form of discrimination against a person on grounds of his or her genetic heritage is prohibited.

Article 12—Predictive Genetic Tests

Tests which are predictive of genetic diseases or which serve either to identify the subject as a carrier of a gene responsible for a disease or to detect a genetic predisposition or susceptibility to a disease may be performed only for health purposes or for scientific research linked to health purposes, and subject to appropriate genetic counselling.

Article 13—Interventions on the Human Genome

An intervention seeking to modify the human genome may only be undertaken for preventive, diagnostic or therapeutic purposes and only if its aim is not to introduce any modification in the genome of any descendants.

Article 14—Non-Selection of Sex

The use of techniques of medically assisted procreation shall not be allowed for the purpose of choosing a future child's sex, except where serious hereditary sex-related disease is to be avoided.

Chapter V—Scientific Research

Article 15—General Rule

Scientific research in the field of biology and medicine shall be carried out freely, subject to the provisions of this Convention and the other legal provisions ensuring the protection of the human being.

Article 16—Protection of Persons Undergoing Research

Research on a person may only be undertaken if all the following conditions are met:

    i. there is no alternative of comparable effectiveness to research on humans;

   ii. the risks which may be incurred by that person are not disproportionate to the potential benefits of the research;

  iii. the research project has been approved by the competent body after independent examination of its scientific merit, including assessment of the importance of the aim of the research, and multidisciplinary review of its ethical acceptability;

  iv. the persons undergoing research have been informed of their rights and the safeguards prescribed by law for their protection;

   v. the necessary consent as provided for under Article 5 has been given expressly, specifically and is documented. Such consent may be freely withdrawn at any time.

Article 17—Protection of Persons Not Able to Consent to Research

   1.   Research on a person without the capacity to consent as stipulated in Article 5 may be undertaken only if all the following conditions are met:

    i. the conditions laid down in Article 16, sub-paragraphs i to iv, are fulfilled;

   ii. the results of the research have the potential to produce real and direct benefit to his or her health;

  iii. research of comparable effectiveness cannot be carried out on individuals capable of giving consent;

  iv. the necessary authorisation provided for under Article 6 has been given specifically and in writing; and

   v. the person concerned does not object.

   2.   Exceptionally and under the protective conditions prescribed by law, where the research has not the potential to produce results of direct benefit to the health of the person concerned, such research may be authorised subject to the conditions laid down in paragraph 1, sub-paragraphs i, iii, iv and v above, and to the following additional conditions:

    i. the research has the aim of contributing, through significant improvement in the scientific understanding of the individual's condition, disease or disorder, to the ultimate attainment of results capable of conferring benefit to the person concerned or to other persons in the same age category or afflicted with the same disease or disorder or having the same condition;

ii. the research entails only minimal risk and minimal burden for the individual concerned.

Article 18—Research on Embryos in Vitro

1. Where the law allows research on embryos in vitro, it shall ensure adequate protection of the embryo.

2. The creation of human embryos for research purposes is prohibited.

Chapter VI—Organ and Tissue Removal from Living Donors for Transplantation Purposes

Article 19—General Rule

1. Removal of organs or tissue from a living person for transplantation purposes may be carried out solely for the therapeutic benefit of the recipient and where there is no suitable organ or tissue available from a deceased person and no other alternative therapeutic method of comparable effectiveness.

2. The necessary consent as provided for under Article 5 must have been given expressly and specifically either in written form or before an official body.

Article 20—Protection of Persons Not Able to Consent to Organ Removal

1. No organ or tissue removal may be carried out on a person who does not have the capacity to consent under Article 5.

2. Exceptionally and under the protective conditions prescribed by law, the removal of regenerative tissue from a person who does not have the capacity to consent may be authorised provided the following conditions are met:

i. there is no compatible donor available who has the capacity to consent;

ii. the recipient is a brother or sister of the donor;

iii. the donation must have the potential to be life-saving for the recipient;

iv. the authorisation provided for under paragraphs 2 and 3 of Article 6 has been given specifically and in writing in accordance with the law and with the approval of the competent body;

v. the potential donor concerned does not object.

Chapter VII—Prohibition of Financial Gain and Disposal of a Part of the Human Body

Article 21—Prohibition of Financial Gain

The human body and its parts shall not, as such, give rise to financial gain.

Article 22—Disposal of a Removed Part of the Human Body

When in the course of an intervention any part of a human body is removed, it may be stored and used for a purpose other than that for which it was removed, only if this is done in conformity with appropriate information and consent procedures.

Chapter VIII—Infringements of the Provisions of the Convention

Article 23—Infringement of the Rights or Principles

The Parties shall provide appropriate judicial protection to prevent or to put a stop to an unlawful infringement of the rights and principles set forth in this Convention at short notice.

Article 24—Compensation for Undue Damage

The person who has suffered undue damage resulting from an intervention is entitled to fair compensation according to the conditions and procedures prescribed by law.

Article 25—Sanctions

Parties shall provide for appropriate sanctions to be applied in the event of infringement of the provisions contained in this Convention.

Chapter IX—Relation between this Convention and Other Provisions

Article 26—Restrictions on the Exercise of the Rights

1. No restrictions shall be placed on the exercise of the rights and protective provisions contained in this Convention other than such as are prescribed by law and are necessary in a democratic society in the interest of public safety, for the prevention of crime, for the protection of public health or for the protection of the rights and freedoms of others.

2. The restrictions contemplated in the preceding paragraph may not be placed on Articles 11, 13, 14, 16, 17, 19, 20 and 21.

Article 27—Wider Protection

None of the provisions of this Convention shall be interpreted as limiting or otherwise affecting the possibility for a Party to grant a wider measure of protection with regard to the application of biology and medicine than is stipulated in this Convention.

Chapter X—Public Debate

Article 28—Public Debate

Parties to this Convention shall see to it that the fundamental questions raised by the developments of biology and medicine are the subject of appropriate public discussion in the light, in particular, of relevant medical, social, economic, ethical and legal implications, and that their possible application is made the subject of appropriate consultation.

Chapter XI—Interpretation and Follow-Up of the Convention

Article 29—Interpretation of the Convention

The European Court of Human Rights may give, without direct reference to any specific proceedings pending in a court, advisory opinions on legal questions concerning the interpretation of the present Convention at the request of:

— the Government of a Party, after having informed the other Parties;

— the Committee set up by Article 32, with membership restricted to the Representatives of the Parties to this Convention, by a decision adopted by a two-thirds majority of votes cast.

Article 30—Reports on the Application of the Convention

On receipt of a request from the Secretary General of the Council of Europe any Party shall furnish an explanation of the manner in which its internal law ensures the effective implementation of any of the provisions of the Convention.

Chapter XII—Protocols

Article 31—Protocols

Protocols may be concluded in pursuance of Article 32, with a view to developing, in specific fields, the principles contained in this Convention.

The Protocols shall be open for signature by Signatories of the Convention. They shall be subject to ratification, acceptance or approval. A Signatory may not ratify, accept or approve Protocols without previously or simultaneously ratifying, accepting or approving the Convention.

Chapter XIII—Amendments to the Convention

Article 32—Amendments to the Convention

1. The tasks assigned to "the Committee" in the present article and in Article 29 shall be carried out by the Steering Committee on Bioethics (CDBI), or by any other committee designated to do so by the Committee of Ministers.

2. Without prejudice to the specific provisions of Article 29, each member State of the Council of Europe, as well as each Party to the present Convention which is not a member of the Council of Europe, may be represented and have one vote in the Committee when the Committee carries out the tasks assigned to it by the present Convention.

3. Any State referred to in Article 33 or invited to accede to the Convention in accordance with the provisions of Article 34 which is not Party to this Convention may be represented on the Committee by an observer. If the European Community is not a Party it may be represented on the Committee by an observer.

4. In order to monitor scientific developments, the present Convention shall be examined within the Committee no later than five years from its entry into force and thereafter at such intervals as the Committee may determine.

5. Any proposal for an amendment to this Convention, and any proposal for a Protocol or for an amendment to a Protocol, presented by a Party, the Committee or the Committee of Ministers shall be communicated to the Secretary General of the Council of Europe and forwarded by him or her to the member States of the Council of Europe, to the European Community, to any Signatory, to any Party, to any State invited to sign this Convention in accordance with the provisions of Article 33 and to any State invited to accede to it in accordance with the provisions of Article 34.

6. The Committee shall examine the proposal not earlier than two months after it has been forwarded by the Secretary General in accordance with paragraph 5. The Committee shall submit the text adopted by a two-thirds majority of the votes cast to the Committee of Ministers for approval. After its approval, this text shall be forwarded to the Parties for ratification, acceptance or approval.

7. Any amendment shall enter into force, in respect of those Parties which have accepted it, on the first day of the month following the expiration of a period of one month after the date on which five Parties, including at least four member States of the Council of Europe, have informed the Secretary General that they have accepted it.

In respect of any Party which subsequently accepts it, the amendment shall enter into force on the first day of the month following the expiration of a period of one month after the date on which that Party has informed the Secretary General of its acceptance.

Chapter XIV—Final Clauses

Article 33—Signature, Ratification and Entry into Force

1. This Convention shall be open for signature by the member States of the Council of Europe, the non-member States which have participated in its elaboration and by the European Community.

2. This Convention is subject to ratification, acceptance or approval. Instruments of ratification, acceptance or approval shall be deposited with the Secretary General of the Council of Europe.

3. This Convention shall enter into force on the first day of the month following the expiration of a period of three months after the date on which five States, including at least four member States of the Council of Europe, have expressed their consent to be bound by the Convention in accordance with the provisions of paragraph 2 of the present article.

4. In respect of any Signatory which subsequently expresses its consent to be bound by it, the Convention shall enter into force on the first day of the month following the expiration of a period of three months after the date of the deposit of its instrument of ratification, acceptance or approval.

Article 34—Non-Member States

1. After the entry into force of this Convention, the Committee of Ministers of the Council of Europe may, after consultation of the Parties, invite any non-member State of the Council of Europe to accede to this Convention by a decision taken by the majority provided for in Article 20, paragraph d, of the Statute of the Council of Europe, and by the unanimous vote of the representatives of the Contracting States entitled to sit on the Committee of Ministers.

2. In respect of any acceding State, the Convention shall enter into force on the first day of the month following the expiration of a period of three months after the date of deposit of the instrument of accession with the Secretary General of the Council of Europe.

Article 35—Territories

1. Any Signatory may, at the time of signature or when depositing its instrument of ratification, acceptance or approval, specify the territory or territories to which this Convention shall apply. Any other State may formulate the same declaration when depositing its instrument of accession.

2. Any Party may, at any later date, by a declaration addressed to the Secretary General of the Council of Europe, extend the application of this Convention to any other territory specified in the declaration and for whose international relations it is responsible or on whose behalf it is authorised to give undertakings. In respect of such territory the Convention shall enter into force on the first day of the month following the expiration of a period of three months after the date of receipt of such declaration by the Secretary General.

3. Any declaration made under the two preceding paragraphs may, in respect of any territory specified in such declaration, be withdrawn by a notification addressed to the Secretary General. The withdrawal shall become effective on the first day of the month following the expiration of a period of three months after the date of receipt of such notification by the Secretary General.

Article 36—Reservations

1.   Any State and the European Community may, when signing this Convention or when depositing the instrument of ratification, acceptance, approval, or accession, make a reservation in respect of any particular provision of the Convention to the extent that any law then in force in its territory is not in conformity with the provision. Reservations of a general character shall not be permitted under this article.

2.   Any reservation made under this article shall contain a brief statement of the relevant law.

3.   Any Party which extends the application of this Convention to a territory mentioned in the declaration referred to in Article 35, paragraph 2, may, in respect of the territory concerned, make a reservation in accordance with the provisions of the preceding paragraphs.

4.   Any Party which has made the reservation mentioned in this article may withdraw it by means of a declaration addressed to the Secretary General of the Council of Europe. The withdrawal shall become effective on the first day of the month following the expiration of a period of one month after the date of its receipt by the Secretary General.

Article 37—Denunciation

1.   Any Party may at any time denounce this Convention by means of a notification addressed to the Secretary General of the Council of Europe.

2.   Such denunciation shall become effective on the first day of the month following the expiration of a period of three months after the date of receipt of the notification by the Secretary General.

Article 38—Notifications

The Secretary General of the Council of Europe shall notify the member States of the Council, the European Community, any Signatory, any Party and any other State which has been invited to accede to this Convention of:

    a. any signature;
    b. the deposit of any instrument of ratification, acceptance, approval or accession;
    c. any date of entry into force of this Convention in accordance with Articles 33 or 34;
    d. any amendment or Protocol adopted in accordance with Article 32, and the date on which such an amendment or Protocol enters into force;
    e. any declaration made under the provisions of Article 35;
    f. any reservation and withdrawal of reservation made in pursuance of the provisions of Article 36;
    g. any other act, notification or communication relating to this Convention.

In witness whereof the undersigned, being duly authorised thereto, have signed this Convention.

Done at Oviedo (Asturias), this 4th day of April 1997, in English and in French, both texts being equally authentic, in a single copy which shall be deposited in the archives of the Council of Europe. The Secretary General of the Council of Europe shall transmit certified copies to each member State of the Council of Europe, to the European Community, to the non-member States which have participated in the elaboration of this Convention, and to any State invited to accede to this Convention.

Consumer Bill of Rights and Responsibilities: Report to the President of the United States

Advisory Commission on Consumer Protection and Quality in the Health Care Industry, November 1997

──────────────INTRODUCTION TO READING──────────────

In 1997 President Clinton appointed The Advisory Commission on Consumer Protection and Quality in the Health Care Industry. Its mission was to "advise the President on changes occurring in the health care system and recommend measures as may be necessary to promote and assure health care quality and value, and protect consumers and workers in the health care system." As part of its work, the President asked the Commission to draft a "consumer bill of rights."

The Commission includes 34 members and is co-chaired by The Honorable Alexis M. Herman, Secretary of Labor, and The Honorable Donna E. Shalala, Secretary of Health and Human Services. Its members include individuals from a wide variety of backgrounds including consumers, business, labor, health care providers, health plans, state and local governments, and health care quality experts.

On February 20, 1998, President Clinton issued an Executive Memorandum directing all federal health plans including Medicare, Medicaid, the Departments of Defense and Labor, the Veterans' Health Programs, and the Federal Employees Health Benefits Program, to come into "substantial compliance" with the Bill of Rights. It also included a call for Congress to pass a patients' bill of rights that would apply to private health plans in the United States. What follows is the President's Advisory Commission on Consumer Protection and Quality in the Health Care Industry's executive summary of the eight areas of consumer rights and responsibilities contained in its Consumer Bill of Rights.

Executive Summary

I. Information Disclosure

Consumers have the right to receive accurate, easily understood information and some require assistance in making informed health care decisions about their health plans, professionals, and facilities.
This information should include:

- **Health plans:** Covered benefits, cost-sharing, and procedures for resolving complaints; licensure, certification, and accreditation status; comparable measures of quality and consumer satisfaction; provider network composition; the procedures that govern access to specialists and emergency services; and care management information.
- **Health professionals:** Education and board certification and recertification; years of practice; experience performing certain procedures; and comparable measures of quality and consumer satisfaction.
- **Health care facilities:** Experience in performing certain procedures and services; accreditation status; comparable measures of quality and worker and consumer satisfaction; procedures for resolving complaints; and community benefits provided.

Consumer assistance programs must be carefully structured to promote consumer confidence and to work cooperatively with health plans, providers, payers and regulators. Sponsorship that assures accountability to the interests of consumers and stable, adequate funding are desirable characteristics of such programs.

1. The term "health plans" is used throughout this report and refers broadly to indemnity insurers, managed care organizations (including health maintenance organizations and preferred provider organizations), self-funded employer-sponsored plans, Taft-Hartley trusts, church plans, association plans, state and local government employee programs, and public insurance programs (i.e., Medicare and Medicaid).

II. Choice of Providers and Plans

Consumers have the right to a choice of health care providers that is sufficient to ensure access to appropriate high-quality health care.
To ensure such choice, health plans should provide the following:

Provider Network Adequacy: All health plan networks should provide access to sufficient numbers and types of providers to assure that all covered services will be accessible without unreasonable delay—including access to emergency services 24 hours a day and seven days a week. If a health plan has an insufficient number or type of providers to provide a covered benefit with the appropriate degree of specialization, the plan should ensure that the consumer obtains the benefit outside the network at no greater cost than if the benefit were obtained from participating providers. Plans also should establish and maintain adequate arrangements to ensure reasonable proximity of providers to the business or personal residence of their members.

Access to Qualified Specialists for Women's Health Services: Women should be able to choose a qualified provider offered by a plan—such as gynecologists, certified nurse midwives, and other qualified health care providers—for the provision of covered care necessary to provide routine and preventative women's health care services.

Access to Specialists: Consumers with complex or serious medical conditions who require frequent specialty care should have direct access to a qualified specialist of their choice within a plan's network of providers. Authorizations, when required, should be for an adequate number of direct access visits under an approved treatment plan.

Transitional Care: Consumers who are undergoing a course of treatment for a chronic or disabling condition (or who are in the second or third trimester of a pregnancy) at the time they involuntarily change health plans or at a time when a provider is terminated by a plan for other than cause should be able to continue seeing their current specialty providers for up to 90 days (or through completion of postpartum care) to allow for transition of care. Providers who continue to treat such patients must accept the plan's rates as payment in full, provide all necessary information to the plan for quality assurance purposes, and promptly transfer all medical records with patient authorization during the transition period.

Public and private group purchasers should, wherever feasible, offer consumers a choice of high-quality health insurance products. Small employers should be provided with greater assistance in offering their workers and their families a choice of health plans and products.

III. Access to Emergency Services

Consumers have the right to access emergency health care services when and where the need arises. Health plans should provide payment when a consumer presents to an emergency department with acute symptoms of sufficient severity—including severe pain—such that a "prudent layperson" could reasonably expect the absence of medical attention to result in placing that consumer's health in serious jeopardy, serious impairment to bodily functions, or serious dysfunction of any bodily organ or part.

To ensure this right:

- Health plans should educate their members about the availability, location, and appropriate use of emergency and other medical services; cost-sharing provisions for emergency services; and the availability of care outside an emergency department.
- Health plans using a defined network of providers should cover emergency department screening and stabilization services both in network

and out of network without prior authorization for use consistent with the prudent layperson standard. Non-network providers and facilities should not bill patients for any charges in excess of health plans' routine payment arrangements.

- Emergency department personnel should contact a patient's primary care provider or health plan, as appropriate, as quickly as possible to discuss follow-up and post-stabilization care and promote continuity of care.

IV. Participation in Treatment Decisions

Consumers have the right and responsibility to fully participate in all decisions related to their health care. Consumers who are unable to fully participate in treatment decisions have the right to be represented by parents, guardians, family members, or other conservators.

In order to ensure consumers' right and ability to participate in treatment decisions, health care professionals should:

- Provide patients with easily understood information and opportunity to decide among treatment options consistent with the informed consent process. Specifically,
  - Discuss all treatment options with a patient in a culturally competent manner, including the option of no treatment at all.
  - Ensure that persons with disabilities have effective communications with members of the health system in making such decisions.
  - Discuss all current treatments a consumer may be undergoing, including those alternative treatments that are self-administered.
  - Discuss all risks, benefits, and consequences to treatment or nontreatment.
  - Give patients the opportunity to refuse treatment and to express preferences about future treatment decisions.
- Discuss the use of advance directives—both living wills and durable powers of attorney for health care—with patients and their designated family members.
- Abide by the decisions made by their patients and/or their designated representatives consistent with the informed consent process.

To facilitate greater communication between patients and providers, health care providers, facilities, and plans should:

- Disclose to consumers factors—such as methods of compensation, ownership of or interest in health care facilities, or matters of conscience—that could influence advice or treatment decisions.
- Ensure that provider contracts do not contain any so-called "gag clauses" or other contractual mechanisms that restrict health care providers' ability to communicate with and advise patients about medically necessary treatment options.
- Be prohibited from penalizing or seeking retribution against health care professionals or other health workers for advocating on behalf of their patients.

V. Respect and Nondiscrimination

Consumers have the right to considerate, respectful care from all members of the health care system at all times and under all circumstances. An environment of mutual respect is essential to maintain a quality health care system.

Consumers must not be discriminated against in the delivery of health care services consistent with the benefits covered in their policy or as required by law based on race, ethnicity, national origin, religion, sex, age, mental or physical disability, sexual orientation, genetic information, or source of payment.

Consumers who are eligible for coverage under the terms and conditions of a health plan or program or as required by law must not be discriminated against in marketing and enrollment practices based on race, ethnicity, national origin, religion, sex, age, mental or physical disability, sexual orientation, genetic information, or source of payment.

VI. Confidentiality of Health Information

Consumers have the right to communicate with health care providers in confidence and to have the confidentiality of their individually identifiable health care information protected. Consumers also have the right to review and copy their own medical records and request amendments to their records.

In order to ensure this right:

* With very few exceptions, individually identifiable health care information can be used without written consent for health purposes only, including the provision of health care, payment for services, peer review, health promotion, disease management, and quality assurance.
* In addition, disclosure of individually identifiable health care information without written consent should be permitted in very limited circumstances where there is a clear legal basis for doing so. Such reasons include: medical or health care research for which an institutional review board has determined anonymous records will not suffice, investigation of health care fraud, and public health reporting.
* To the maximum feasible extent in all situations, nonidentifiable health care information should be used unless the individual has consented to the disclosure of individually identifiable information. When disclosure is required, no greater amount of information should be disclosed than is necessary to achieve the specific purpose of the disclosure.

VII. Complaints and Appeals

All consumers have the right to a fair and efficient process for resolving differences with their health plans, health care providers, and the institutions that serve them, including a rigorous system of internal review and an independent system of external review.

Internal appeals systems should include:

- Timely written notification of a decision to deny, reduce, or terminate services or deny payment for services. Such notification should include an explanation of the reasons for the decisions and the procedures available for appealing them.
- Resolution of all appeals in a timely manner with expedited consideration for decisions involving emergency or urgent care consistent with time frames consistent with those required by Medicare (i.e., 72 hours).
- A claim review process conducted by health care professionals who are appropriately credentialed with respect to the treatment involved. Reviews should be conducted by individuals who were not involved in the initial decision.
- Written notification of the final determination by the plan of an internal appeal that includes information on the reason for the determination and how a consumer can appeal that decision to an external entity.
- Reasonable processes for resolving consumer complaints about such issues as waiting times, operating hours, the demeanor of health care personnel, and the adequacy of facilities.

External appeals systems should:

- Be available only after consumers have exhausted all internal processes (except in cases of urgently needed care).
- Apply to any decision by a health plan to deny, reduce, or terminate coverage or deny payment for services based on a determination that the treatment is either experimental or investigational in nature; apply when such a decision is based on a determination that such services are not medically necessary and the amount exceeds a significant threshold or the patient's life or health is jeopardized.
- Be conducted by health care professionals who are appropriately credentialed with respect to the treatment involved and subject to conflict-of-interest prohibitions. Reviews should be conducted by individuals who were not involved in the initial decision.
- Follow a standard of review that promotes evidence-based decision making and relies on objective evidence.
- Resolve all appeals in a timely manner with expedited consideration for decisions involving emergency or urgent care consistent with time frames consistent with those required by Medicare (i.e., 72 hours).

2.   The right to external appeals does not apply to denials, reductions, or terminations of coverage or denials of payment for services that are specifically excluded from the consumer's coverage as established by contract.

VIII. Consumer Responsibilities

In a health care system that protects consumers' rights, it is reasonable to expect and encourage consumers to assume reasonable responsibilities.

Greater individual involvement by consumers in their care increases the likelihood of achieving the best outcomes and helps support a quality improvement, cost-conscious environment. Such responsibilities include:

- Take responsibility for maximizing healthy habits, such as exercising, not smoking, and eating a healthy diet.
- Become involved in specific health care decisions.
- Work collaboratively with health care providers in developing and carrying out agreed-upon treatment plans.
- Disclose relevant information and clearly communicate wants and needs.
- Use the health plan's internal complaint and appeal processes to address concerns that may arise.
- Avoid knowingly spreading disease.
- Recognize the reality of risks and limits of the science of medical care and the human fallibility of the health care professional.
- Be aware of a health care provider's obligation to be reasonably efficient and equitable in providing care to other patients and the community.
- Become knowledgeable about his or her health plan coverage and health plan options (when available) including all covered benefits, limitations, and exclusions, rules regarding use of network providers, coverage and referral rules, appropriate processes to secure additional information, and the process to appeal coverage decisions.
- Show respect for other patients and health workers.
- Make a good-faith effort to meet financial obligations.
- Abide by administrative and operational procedures of health plans, health care providers, and government health benefit programs.
- Report wrongdoing and fraud to appropriate resources or legal authorities.

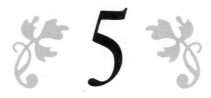

Medical Ethical
Theories Outside
Western Culture

Introduction

The religions of Judaism and Christianity and the secular thought of the political philosophy of liberalism in the Anglo-American West are not the only alternatives to a Hippocratic medical ethic. Outside of the Anglo-American West there are a number of religious and philosophical alternatives. Most of them build their medical ethics on a more general underlying philosophical or religious foundation. Some of the medical ethical expressions are only fragmentary. Others are quite richly developed systems.

Socialist countries have medical ethics that reflect the broad philosophical commitments of socialism. Some of these are manifest in the democratic socialist states of Western Europe. Others, such as those that existed in the Soviet Union and Eastern Europe and continue to exist in contemporary China, reflect the Marxism upon which those societies have been based. This chapter presents the Oath of the Soviet Physician as well as descriptions of medical ethics in Russia and China.

Another major alternative to Hippocratic ethics is found in the moral legal system of Islam. Having common roots with Judaism and Christianity, Islam grounds its ethics in the Quran, the book composed of writings of Muhammad

217

accepted by Muslims as the revelations of Allah. A detailed system of medical ethical positions is derived from the Quran. Presented here is a summary of Islamic medical ethics and the code of ethics for medical professionals of the Islamic Medical Association of the USA and Canada.

Eastern cultures have medical ethical systems closely related to and derived from the teachings of their major religious/philosophical traditions. Indian culture is dominated by the complex tradition of Hinduism. The ethics of the tradition reflects the important philosophical doctrines such as *karma*. A summary of the major positions together with one of the ancient Oaths, the Oath of Initiation from the Caraka Samhita, are presented here.

Chinese medical ethics draws on its major traditions as well: Confucianism, Buddhism, and Taoism. The dominant Confucian orthodoxy was challenged by Taoist and Buddhist variants. Tao Lee's summary reveals the interplay of these traditions.

In Japan Buddhist influences from China and Korea began to penetrate and intermix with indigenous Japanese beliefs (the system called Shintoism in Western scholarship). Space permits only one example of the product of that intermixing: a sixteenth-century code revealing strong Buddhist influence called the Seventeen Rules of Enjuin. The samples presented here only hint at the richness of the diversity of medical ethical systems in cultures outside the Anglo-American.

In addition to these grand and ancient Eastern traditions, there are other medical ethical systems of belief and value grounded in the cultures of perhaps every culture that has existed in the world. When the first edition of the book was prepared in the mid-1980s, it was apparent that two broad cultural traditions should be included that, due to lack of available primary and secondary materials, could not be. African and Hispanic cultures include diverse and rich groups. Fortunately, in the short time that has passed, an insightful literature on the medical ethics of these cultures is beginning to appear. In some ways they stand outside of Western culture and could be included in this chapter. African cultures predating European influence incorporate belief systems that have profound influence on medical beliefs and values. On the other hand, there is beginning to appear a literature on the unique African-American perspective on medical ethics. This incorporates influences from the West that have led placing this literature in a separate chapter that follows this one.

Likewise, while Hispanic culture incorporates Western philosophical thought and Roman Catholic moral theology, it is also profoundly distinct from the Anglo perspectives that dominate Chapters 2 and 3. At the same time, Hispanic thought in the Western Hemisphere also incorporates pre-Colombian influences that make it hard to simply add the material on Hispanic medical ethics to Chapters 2 and 3. Hence, as with the African and African-American medical ethical literature, a separate chapter will be devoted to Ibero-American medical ethical perspectives.

EASTERN EUROPE

The Oath of Soviet Physicians

─────────────── INTRODUCTION TO READING ───────────────

The commitment of the Hippocratic physician to focus solely on the welfare of the patient did not square with the ideology of the Communist countries whose ethics, grounded in Marxism, required a more social theory in which physicians were to serve the public and the Soviet state applying what it called the "principles of Communist morality."

In 1971 the Presidium of the Supreme Soviet adopted a new medical oath and ordered that all physicians and graduating medical students take it. It is of note that it is the state, rather than the medical profession, that is responsible for this requirement. Also worth noting is the focus on preventive medicine and public health, the commitment to practice wherever required by society, and the pledge of faithfulness to the people and the Soviet state.

Having received the high title of physician and beginning a career in the healing arts, I solemnly swear:

to dedicate all my knowledge and all my strength to the care and improvement of human health, to treatment and prevention of disease, and to work conscientiously wherever the interests of the society will require it;

to be always ready to administer medical aid, to treat the patient with care and interest, and to keep professional secrets;

to constantly improve my medical knowledge and diagnostic and therapeutic skill, and to further medical science and the practice of medicine by my own work;

to turn, if the interests of my patients will require it, to my professional colleagues for advice and consultation, and to never refuse myself to give advice or help;

to keep and to develop the beneficial traditions of medicine in my country, to conduct all my actions according to the principles of the Communistic morale, to always keep in mind the high calling of the Soviet physician, and the high responsibility I have to my people and to the Soviet government.

I swear to be faithful to this Oath all my life long.

Toward a Bioethics
in Post-Communist Russia

Pavel D. Tichtchenko and Boris G. Yudin

──────────────INTRODUCTION TO READING──────────────

With the collapse of the Soviet Union, the ethical commitment reflected in the Soviet Oath no longer seemed appropriate. The changes in health care and health care ethics were rapid and dramatic. The Russians adopted a new ethic patterned closely after the Hippocratic Oath, as was seen in the text in Chapter 1. The realities of Russian life have, however, become complex and the ethical positions adopted are similarly complex.

Two of the most important leaders in medical ethics in Russia both before and after the end of the Union are Pavel Tichtchenko and Boris Yudin, both of the Institute of Philosophy, Russian Academy of Science. In this reading they describe the changes in the health care system and outline contemporary Russian positions on key issues in bioethics. The post script was prepared in 1999 especially for this volume.

In the last 7 years, Russia has seen deep changes in all spheres of political and economic life. Some new realities have appeared in Russian medicine as well. This paper tells the story of how these changes came about, what kind of unusual situations were created, and how these situations are recognized in professional and public debates.

Modern Features of the Russian Healthcare System

At the beginning of the 1980s, the need for substantial changes in the healthcare system was widely recognized in the Soviet Union. The question of how a new system should be structured was opened to political and professional debates by Communist authorities. At first these debates were heavily influenced by Marxist-Leninist ideology, and all changes were directed toward modernization in an old-fashioned manner, i.e., to make direct State and Party control more effective.

The epoch of Gorbachev's "perestroika" gave birth to a fresh idea of pluralism in medical practice. Now we can see the combination of State, cooperative, and private medical institutions. Some central hospitals in Moscow and St. Petersburg have incorporated this kind of pluralism in their general structures. For example, there are maternity hospitals where in one department the service is free of charge and in another department, where conditions and services are much better, it is necessary to pay. As of January 1992, the payment for 4 days at the hospital is about 4,000 rubles (equal to the 4–month salary of a researcher in the Institute of Philosophy, half that of Gorbachev, and the same as a bus driver). Several private hospitals are now run by religious institutions. The professional squabble between advocates of free-market economy (minority) and advocates of socialization (majority) has little influence on everyday politics. Medical practitioners prefer to make their choices not on the grounds of ideological preferences but in a utilitarian manner, looking for individual or corporate benefits. Another feature of the modern Russian healthcare system is the gradual increase in the influence of the independent mass media. Today, healthcare providers are much more interested in having a good image expressed by newspapers and television programs.

On 28 June 1991 in the Russian Supreme Soviet, a law was passed that included regulations for a new insurance model in Russian medicine. The law will go into effect in 1993 and requires two kinds of medical insurance—obligatory (all citizens) and voluntary (individual or collective). The obligatory insurance is to cover the necessary minimum of medical services and the voluntary covers all other expenses. State, private, and other kinds of medical insurance companies will have equal opportunities. The main goal of this legal initiative was to make patients interested in preserving their health and physicians interested in the high quality of their work. Unfortunately, this law to some extent is only a kind of declaration of intentions of the new democratic authorities. A large number of necessary preliminary steps have not yet been performed. The old guard of the medical establishment preserved their power, and very often they only imitate reformist activity. Even the leaders of Soviet psychiatry who are personally responsible for the collaboration with the KGB are not yet retired.

Still, the process of change in the Russian healthcare system has started and, in combination with such new (for our country) phenomena as charity funds, independent organizations of patients (diabetic societies, clubs of asthmatic people, etc.), and invalids, is producing some of the necessary preconditions for the existence of bioethics.

1.   Healthcare political decision making, previously monopolized by State medical power, now is distributed among State committees, medical professional corporations, private capital, independent charitable funds and organizations, and the mass media.

2.   The multiplicity of independent actors in our healthcare system is correlated with legitimate multiplicity of moral values that those actors are ready to use in decision making.

   a.   A new role of the active patient is emerging.

   b.   Medical professionals are becoming more liberated from their usual dependency on the State.

   c.   Gradually, public discussions become the necessary social mechanism of justification for each kind of policy in the healthcare delivery system.

Ethics in general and bioethics in particular can exist only when people meet conflicts of moral values in their practice, when such differences are legitimized, and when people can and are ready to solve these conflicts by peaceful public moral discussion, looking for mutual benefits. These preconditions of bioethics are incorporated into a healthcare system that is now in a state of chaos and misery.

The part of Russia's GNP destined for medical needs is negligible. This problem is highlighted during strikes of healthcare professionals. Shortages of every kind of resource are dramatic. On February 4, 1992, a preliminary strike of the staff of Moscow Institute of Emergency Aid (Sklifosofsky Institute) took place. Among the slogans were "Hungry physicians are useless for patients." In 1992, the Russian Ministry of Healthcare has absolutely no funds to support the approximately 100 scientific research institutes that are at its disposal. According to some estimates the number of beds in Russian hospitals this year will be reduced 50% because of decreases in the real healthcare budget. The inability of the State to provide the necessary minimum healthcare for people stimulates further increases in commercialization of Russian medicine and provokes legal methods in the healthcare providers' struggle for survival.

Distributive Justice

The fair distribution of extremely limited resources and facilities is among the most important medical ethical issues facing post-Communist Russia. The new understanding of distributive justice can be explained by a single illustration. When Gorbachev, as President of the USSR, met the problem of distribution of Western humanitarian help during the winter season of 1990–91, he had subordinated the distributive mechanism to the KGB. However, in this winter, new democratic authorities decided to organize Regional Committees, which include statesmen, representatives of the Church and the political opposition, publicly recognized respectable persons, media people, etc. This change means an evident shift of decision making from the absolute monopoly of the State as the distributor of goods to some kind of equilibrium of State and public forces. Of course, a KGB officer could meet moral problems in his practice as distributor, but he had no *need for* public moral justification of his decisions. The practice of Regional Committees is based to a great extent on evaluation of principles of just distribution through moral public discussion and consensus. A new practice of public moral discourse has originated, which is a sign of hope for bioethics in our country.

Another change concerns the tactics of justification of inequality of distribution of social benefits, including access to healthcare. The principle of socialism "from each according to his (her) abilities, to each according to his (her) work" had been used to justify the existing inequality: a high-ranking Party boss had greater access to healthcare because his work had greater social value. New democratic authorities inherited such privileges with the presupposed model for justification.

In addition to this old sense of justice, a new one has emerged. Now there are a lot of advocates of the idea that inequality produced by fair competition in a market economy is also just. Those who produce more social goods should have the right to greater access to social benefits, including medical services. The beneficent and charitable practices of "newly rich" men are actively advertised. Increasing public justification of inequality becomes a very important moral balance to traditionally influential egalitarian feelings among Russian people.

Definition of Death and Transplantation of Organs

There is no ethical debate in Russia on the problem of the definition of death. Brain-oriented criteria did not cause any publicly articulated objections. The concept was legalized by temporary instructions of the Soviet Healthcare Ministry in 1985. In 1987, the permanent instruction was adopted. In this instruction, death is diagnosed by the irreversible cessation of brain stem function, or "brain death." The diagnostic tests do not differ from those used in other countries. In special applications, there was a complete enumeration of medical institutions (very limited) where the practical usage of this definition was permitted. The majority of hospitals and clinics had no necessary equipment for diagnostic tests or well-trained neurologists. The worst aspect of the situation is that diagnosis of brain death is usually made by doctors who are in close relationship with scientific teams responsible for organ transplantations.

Inadmissibility of this situation is well recognized by all involved parties. In December 1990, The Centre of Surgery of the USSR Academy of Medical Sciences organized a special meeting where ethical and legal problems of transplantology were discussed. Progress was made during a 3-day international meeting on Bioethics and Social Consequences of Biomedical Research organized on the initiative of UNESCO by the USSR Academy of Sciences' National Center for Human Science, the Institute of Philosophy, and The Centre of Surgery USSR Academy of Medical Sciences in May 1991. The special Declaration of Soviet Participants in the UNESCO international meeting was issued in view of the development of clinical transplantology. This Declaration calls upon:

1. the State and public organizations working for charity and beneficence to form an independent association for the development of clinical transplantology whose main task would be the implementation of economic, legal, and ethical decisions without which the development of clinical transplantology in our country is impossible;

2. the scientific academies, societies, and organizations that finance scientific research and clinical practices to organize independent committees to perform legal, ethical, and economic assessment of the projects to be financed;

3. the Committee for Public Education to include in school, college, and university curricula courses in bioethics that would prepare the future generations to meet extraordinary situations that will be created by new biomedical technologies.

Of course this action was only a declaration but it showed the readiness of medical authorities to collaborate with philosophers, clergy, lawyers, and the public to solve their professional problems, rather than trying to do so only within the professional community.

One of the most acute problems is financial. The State has not enough money to finance transplantology. New resources were found in joint ventures with Russian and foreign medical firms (for example, providing clinical testing of new drugs or medical equipment), in charity funds, in private charity donations, and in forms of cooperation with nonmedical institutions on a barter basis. The barter system is specific for modern Russia. For example, when one of the largest plants in Moscow helped one of the surgery hospitals with money and equipment, the plant workers received privileges on a "waiting list" for transplantation of kidneys. The same situation occurs with foreign patients who are ready to cover expenses in hard currency. There were some objections in the media against "illegal and amoral sale of Russian kidneys abroad." One of the influential members of the Commission on Healthcare Problems in the Moscow Soviet named this practice "The Satan business." But none of those critics made any useful recommendation for how to solve our financial problems in other ways and their cries were submerged in public silence. Nevertheless, a new direction for the corruption of equal distribution in the healthcare system has been created.

Physician-Patient Relationship (Ph-PR)

Moral problems in Ph-PR have very specific historical grounds in Post-Communist Russia. There is a strong tradition of transparency of all types of social life to State control. There was no place for privacy in any kind of professional activity including medical practice. Even the Russian Orthodox Church for a long time was only a department of government in the Czarist state. Peter I abolished the sacrament of confession in the beginning of the 18th century. Bolsheviks radically strengthened State control and made it more universal. In this political system, the social role of the physician was reduced to that of passive screw in the mechanism of state government. In the Soviet Medical Oath, the superior responsibility of the physician is to "my people and the Soviet government" and he (or she) solemnly swears "to work in a good conscience wherever it is required by society" (that means by State or Party). This "medical screw" has a very low social value. Today the salary of a physician is approximately ¾ that of a charwoman in the Moscow Metro and ⅕ that of a Moscow bus driver. Now we can see a strong wave of strikes organized by medical professional unions to change the existing order of things. Not only do economic problems provoke these strikes, but there is a clearly articulated will to obtain more social value. Therefore, the starting point for moral debates on Ph-PR is not only the vulnerability of patients but also that of physicians. It is impossible to speak about privacy or confidentiality until healthcare providers are sovereign social actors. Physician autonomy and self-determination are necessary preconditions for possible trust on the side of the patient. One episode that took place in a laboratory of anonymous HIV testing gives a good example. This was a telephone conversation with client:

Hello, is this the anonymous diagnostic laboratory?

Yes, sir.

May I come today for testing?

You are welcome.

And have I to bring a passport with me?

. . .?!

This strange question is a result of long social training, and it will be a long time before people believe that physicians have a right not to inform State authorities against their clients and that there is strong legal protection for such rights. But such belief can be based only on respect for the power and authority of the law. In Russia, there have never been strong legal traditions. Russian people are trained to protect their interests not through hearings in courts but by looking for restoration of justice through the mercy of those who govern. Soviet patients used to send letters with complaints (actions) against physicians to the Healthcare Minister or the General Secretary of the Communist Party. It will take a long time to turn the vertical relationship of servile "brotherness" of the patients and physicians under supervision of State authority into a horizontal relationship of civil "otherness" under protection of the law.

The problem of distrust in the Ph-PR common to Western countries and Russia will be solved in different ways. In Russia it is necessary not to redistribute decision-making power between patients and doctors but to recreate power in both parties and to initiate movement toward each other on the grounds of mutual respect.

Psychiatry and Behavior Control

The problem of repressive psychiatry in the Soviet Union had a very narrow political interpretation. The struggle against involuntary mental hospitalization was a part of dissident activity. The main interest was focused on collaboration of psychiatric authorities with the KGB and absence of legal protection against such abuse of human rights. In 1988, the new legal regulation for psychiatric service was adopted by the Supreme Soviet of the USSR. The purpose of the law was to increase the autonomy of psychiatric patients and to give effective protection to their human rights. Criminal penalties were provided for malevolent involuntary mental hospitalization of evidently normal people. Mentally ill patients received the right for lawyer assistance and defense of their interests in court. However, independent organizations of psychiatrists have criticized this law because it leaves room for old-fashioned repressive interpretations. A new bill of special regulation for psychiatric service is now being discussed in Commissions of the Russian Supreme Soviet.

Other debates include the problem of experiments in the field of behavioral control practiced by the KGB and the use of soldiers and prisoners as subjects in experimentation. An independent investigation, organized by the media, is being carried out.

In contrast to Western countries, there have been no ethical questions raised about the potential harms of uncontrolled psychiatry and behavioral control. Consequently, a wide variety of "therapies" have proliferated outside any controls—legal, educational, or financial. A major problem now is to address this lack of constraints and establish necessary social policies and professional guidelines.

Abortion

For a long time, one absolute value—the idea of Communism—gave exact values to all matters and problems in our lives. What was good for the construction of Communism was the absolute Good. The problem of abortion was not excluded. In 1920, the USSR was one of the first countries to legalize abortion. During the period of industrialization, acute lack of labor resources motivated State policy in this field. Party leaders wanted to quickly increase the number of workers by involving women in industrial production, and abortion became one way of liberating women from their traditional family dependency.

In 1936, prohibition of abortion was supposed to help improve the demographic situation, which deteriorated during the period of collectivization of agriculture and the Great terror. Another part of this policy was restriction on the production of contraceptives. In spite of the legalization of abortion during the Khrushchev government (in 1955), the state policy in this field did not change. This policy resulted in a permanent shortage of contraceptives, an increased number of abortions, and an official and rigorously promoted attitude toward women who made such family-limiting decisions as semicriminals or moral deviants. This attitude was expressed in strict limitation of anesthesia. Pain was justified as a sort of social penalty. But it was not harmful to kill a fetus; it was harmful to damage State labor resources.

Current public debate concerning abortion practices reveals the usual opposition of interests between rights of a woman for self-determination and rights of a fetus for life. The dominant feature of this debate in Russia is the appeal to recognize women who decide to have an abortion as normal patients and to treat them with mercy and compassion. The rights of a fetus to life are advocated in an old-fashioned manner by religious organizations.

Teaching Medical Ethics

The program of studies in ethics for students of medical schools was formulated and implemented long before "perestroika" started. It does not require special theoretical studies, and elements of the theory of medical ethics are incorporated into courses of philosophy, history of medicine, and "introduction into the profession. " In general, this theory of medical ethics is heavily overloaded with communist ideology. It stresses duties of healthcare providers to the State, government, Party, and Soviet people. As is pointed out in a popular dictionary of ethics, "Man becomes a moral person when having comprehended the content and meaning of his acts, he voluntarily submits himself to moral require-ments of society." If someone did not voluntarily submit himself to "moral requirements of society, " which were exclusively articulated by the Party, then that person could be submitted involuntarily by the KGB or by psychiatrists. The problems of practical application of ethical principles are supposed to be discussed during the teaching of therapy, surgery, and other medical subjects.

Of course, in the modern situation it is impossible to follow the old-fash-ioned program literally. The majority of teachers make changes by replacing communist ideology with the ideology of "new thinking." "New thinking" emphasizes the priority of universal human values over the values of class, nation, profession, and other groups . Yet most partisans of "new thinking" remain deaf to the rights of the individual against the interests of society.

In 1991, the first course of lectures on bioethics was formulated and imple-mented at Moscow State University at the Department of Philosophy (with about 20 students). The course requires 1 year of theoretical studies and contains all topics usually found in programs of bioethics in the United States. In 1991, the first semiannual course of lectures on the philosophy of healthcare and bioethics was implemented at the Department of Psychology of MSU for a group of clinical psychologists. The main focus of teaching was on the issues of physician-patient relationships and death and dying. In 1991, a course on bioethics was started in Samara Medical School. The specific features of bioethical courses at MSU are connected with the traditions of Russian and European philosophy.

In the Institute of Philosophy and the Center for Human Studies of the Russian Academy of Sciences, there are now several postgraduate students who are specializing in bioethics.

Bioethics and the Media

Bioethical problems are getting more and more attention in Russian newspa-pers and magazines. Among the items most often discussed are organ donation and transplantation, euthanasia, allocation of resources and access to health-care services, experiments on human subjects, and tendencies in AIDS and

HIV infection (this infection in Russia is developed commonly due to the malpractice of medical personnel).

The only journal that attempts to discuss bioethical issues in a regular manner is the bimonthly *Chelovek (The Human Being)*. This journal began publication in 1990 and has included articles by E. Pellegrino on medical ethics in the USA and by B. Yudin about discussions on euthanasia in the Russian media (No. 2, 1990). An extensive report about discussions on prospects of bioethics in Russia ("Round-Table") was published in two issues (No. 6, 1990 and No. 1, 1991), and a round-table discussion on social and ethical problems of transplantology was published in No. 4, 1991. The journal has also published articles concerning ethical problems of biomedical research, including those arising from the Human Genome Project.

In general, the media, the public, and the politicians in Russia do not yet understand that the field of bioethics is very important in the realm of human rights.

Bioethics as a Social Institution

Bioethics as a social institution includes five distinct yet interrelated domains of activity: 1) grass-roots and media activity to help shape and reshape health-care policy; 2) bioethical structures such as ethics committees in hospitals, research institutes, and elsewhere; 3) law making in the field of biomedicine; 4) bioethical education; and 5) bioethics as a multidisciplinary area of scientific research.

The current situation in Russia as it pertains to each of these domains can be summarized as follows.

1. Growing concern about the present and future of the healthcare system is evident in Russian society. This concern is expressed in the media, yet it remains diffuse, and different topics (such as transplantation, euthanasia, abortion, etc.) are not understood as components of the whole. As a result, most such discussions end without definite results.

2. Recently, some leading centers of biomedical research have tried to establish bioethics committees. A new Russian National Committee on bioethics under the aegis of the Russian Academy of Sciences has been formed. The first step of the Committee was the organization of the Commission on protection of animals as subjects of scientific experimentation. Another bioethical institution, The Center of Biomedical Ethics and Law, was organized in Moscow in 1990. It conducts regular interdisciplinary debates on urgent problems of Russian medicine. A proposal to establish an all-Russian Committee on biomedical research will be submitted to the President of Russia and thereby will not be controlled by medical or academic authorities. Ethical assessment and regulation will be among the principal goals of this Committee.

3. In Russian society, much work must be done in the fields of medical law and judicial regulation of healthcare practice and biomedical research. The

current situation in this field is disastrous. Many people were compelled to speak about the necessity for law-making activities, for example, about the need for new legislation after facts about commercial use of organs and tissues from cadavers became public. Implementation of a healthcare insurance program makes the need for legal reforms more noticeable, and lawyers are showing some interest in medical specialization.

In November 1991, the Declaration of Rights and Liberties of Citizens was adopted by the Russian Supreme Soviet (parliament). It establishes the principle of voluntary consent regarding participation in scientific or medical experiments (article No. 8) and the right of every citizen to qualified medical aid in the state healthcare system. Non-state forms of healthcare services were also legalized. A new draft of legislation on "protection of health of citizens of Russian Federation" passed first hearings in the Healthcare Committee of the Supreme Soviet. This law will bring radically new approaches. One of the main ideas of this draft is to transform the whole system of healthcare. The Ministry of Healthcare will be only one of several elements under the control of Society and the State. According to the draft, management of biomedical research, as well as management of medical expertise (including medical statistics), must be implemented by agencies directly subordinated to the Russian president.

Previously, medical and healthcare legislation was mainly declarative and strongly laden with ideology. The new draft, which is much more concrete and definite, stresses rights of patients and their families. It includes six chapters:

I.   General principles
II. Rights of citizens and of different categories of the population to healthcare and medical and social help
III. Protection of rights and legitimate interests of citizens in the sphere of health
IV. System of healthcare of Russian Federation
V.   International cooperation
VI. Activities of professionals (including the rights of physicians and the obligations of physicians)

An important point in relation to this draft is that it must be, after its adoption, a "constitutional law," in that all subsequent legislation in medicine and healthcare will become a "detailization" and extension of it.

4.   The first steps in bioethical education have already been taken in Moscow and Samara.

5.   Fragmentary scientific research work in the field of bioethics has started in the Russian Academy of Sciences. It is possible to find publications on bioethics in medical, biological, judicial, and philosophical journals. Forgotten during the Communist government, the intelligent humanitarian traditions of prerevolutionary Russian medicine become more attractive to modern scholars.

Post Script: Seven Years After

After approximately seven years of reforms that have come since our previous observation, Russian health care is still in the process of transition heavily influenced by the unstable economic and political situation in the country. The vector of the transition is rather unclear. At the moment the system combines in an eclectic manner "for free" and "for profit" programs of provision of medical services. Free provision of medical services that covers in principle all Russian population is achieved through two basic mechanisms—direct financing from the federal and regional budgets in combination with obligatory medical insurance. Obligatory medical insurance, as a federal system, is still in the process of painful development. Both systems in combination could provide ordinary patients access only to a minimal amount of medical services. As it was during the communist administration, special privileges for access to free high quality health care are available for the Russian ruling elite.

"For profit" programs combine direct payment in cash and mechanisms of voluntary medical insurance. The latter have suffered dramatically during the financial crisis in August 1998. "For profit" programs offer high quality and high technology medical services practically in all areas of modern medicine. The existing level of prices is much lower than in the USA and Western Europe, but (in spite of this) not affordable for the majority of the Russian population. Demarcation lines between "for free" and "for profit" programs are not clearly designed in legislation and institutional policies of the Russian Ministry of Health Care. That is why in a lot of cases the mere necessity to pay and the level of payment could be a matter of special negotiations between physicians and patients.

Development of Medical Legislation
and New Features of Physician-Patient Relations (Ph-PR)

During this period several very important steps for legal framing of new patterns of relations among physicians and patients were taken. In 1992 the Russian Parliament had adopted legislation entitled "On Transplantation of Organs and Tissues" that legalized the concept of "brain death" and the "presumed consent" model for harvesting of organs. New legislation on the provision of psychiatric services that gave some guarantees for protection of patients rights and prevention of practices of "repressive psychiatry" existed in the USSR was adopted in the same year. In 1993 the "General Law on Health Care of Russian Federation" was adopted by the Russian Parliament. The law has legalized development of medicine in Russia as a combination of federal, municipal and private medical institutions. It was the first law that guaranteed protection of basic patients rights: informed consent for every medical intervention, protection of privacy and confidentiality, the right to terminate treatment, the right to know one's diagnosis and prognosis, the right to choose a physician and medical institution and some other rights. The law also gave protection to research subjects and framed physician-patient relations in new reproductive technologies. It also has a special article that forbids active euthanasia.

Some important legal norms for development of "for profit" programs in health care were established by the "Federal Law on Protection of Rights of Consumers" (1996). The "Federal Law on Medical Drugs" adopted in 1998 had established research ethics committees in every medical institution participating in clinical testing of new drugs. At the moment it is very difficult to say to what extent such committees exist not only in a "paper form," but in reality too. The law also prescribes organization of an ethics committee for review of programs of clinical testing in a Federal Agency controlling quality of medical drugs.

Several other bills were prepared in the Russian Parliament to modernize this legislation, but none of them was adopted. As examples we could mention bills on protection of patients rights, reproductive rights of citizens, a new medical oath, and a bill with a strange sounding name—"Federal Law On Legal Foundations of Bioethics and Its Guarantees." Legislators defined "bioethics" in this bill as a "set of traditional values in healthcare." The last legislative initiative expresses increasing influence of conservative, traditionally-oriented (including religious) groups aiming to limit abortions, forbid experimentation on aborted fetuses, limit development of new reproductive technologies (e.g. forbidding "surrogate" motherhood), introduce a model of "presumed non-consent" in harvesting of organs for transplantation, and prohibit creation of transgenic organisms that have human genes in their genome. This bill is to some extent a reaction to bills that were proposed and lobbying by some medical "interest groups" wishing to widen liberties of physicians in the provision of new high tech services, for example in the area of reproduction.

Development of new legislation in health care that is more sensitive to the ideas of patients rights and general changes in the mentality and behavioral values of the Russian population influences basic patterns of Ph-PR, making them less paternalistic, more oriented on individual choice, and more tolerant to market-oriented provision of health service. More cases of conflicts among physicians and patients are settled not through complaints to governmental authorities (which was characteristic of the situation in the USSR), but in courts. Most cases are concerned with malpractice, but some (and this group has a tendency to grow) are connected with limitation of patients rights (e.g. treatment without consent).

New legislation and growing experience of Russian biomedical professionals in international scientific collaboration produce some improvement in moral standards of research on human and animal subjects. For example, written consent (not necessarily adequately informed and from this point of view not in the full sense voluntary) is now a usual procedure in recruitment of research subjects. Some research organizations (like Russian Humane Genome

Project) have developed their own moral guidelines for research and application of biomedical knowledge that correspond in most positions to Western standards. The Russian Ministry of Health Care has established its own "Ethics Committee" for review of moral conflicts in medical practice, development of new institutional policies, and improvement of education of medical ethics in medical schools.

An important feature of today in Russia is a growing number of patients groups and organizations that through mechanisms of mutual assistance (in education, provision of information and other ways) are trying to solve health problems in the existing difficult social and economic environment. Correlatively, we could see self-organization of medical professional groups aiming to make better professional and moral standards for the provision of medical services. Organizations of physicians and other medical professionals establish there own ethics committees, develop moral guidelines, etc.

Very important steps (mostly in the area of education) are taken to appropriate the new idea of nursing that has its own independence from physicians in providing health care. New role models for nurses have special importance in the field of provision of health care for patients in terminal conditions in hospices and medical institutions having programs of palliative care.

Development of Bioethical Research and Education

In 1992 Russian National Committee on Bioethics (RNCB) was established inside Russian Academy of Sciences as a nongovernmental and noncommercial research institution that today coordinates most of academic activities in this area.

RNCB (in collaboration with different scientific and medical institutions) has organized several conferences in which philosophers, lawyers, medical doctors and scientists from different regions of Russia participated: "Ethical and Legal Problems of Clinical Testing and Scientific Experimentation on Human and Animal Subjects." (1994), "Death and Dying: Interdisciplinary Interpretation" (1994), "Hospice movement: moral, philosophical and social problems" (1995), "Social Problems of Children's Oncology" (1997), and some others. In 1992 RNCB published a special report entitled "Vaccination and Human Rights" in which practices of involuntary vaccination in Russia were criticized.

Since 1995 RNCB has received grants from the Russian Scientific Program "Human Genome". These grants fund both theoretical (philosophic and moral) and empirical (sociological) studies. Several surveys of the Russian population were performed to reveal attitudes towards different polices of genetic betterment (including eugenic). For example, it was found that one-third of the Russian population is ready to support eugenic policies such as involuntary sterilization of "subnormal" persons (alcoholics, drug abusers, homosexuals etc.) and involuntary abortion of fetuses with genetic "defects."

A growing amount of research in bioethics is now being performed in universities and departments of philosophy of medical schools in Moscow,

Krasnoyarsk, St. Petersburg, Saratov and Volgograd. These research projects cover most fields of modern bioethics with the exclusion of the problem of justice in health care.

Academic journal "Cheloveck" (Human being) publishes many of the bioethical papers in Russia. It had presented debates on euthanasia, definition of death, ethics of scientific research, ethics of modern genetics and so forth. Other academic and medical journals also welcome papers in bioethics. Before 1991 (the time of our first review) there were no books in Russian that could systematically present basic problems of bioethics for scholars and for the public. During the last few years several books were published in the field: A. N. Bartko, E.P Mykhaylova "Biomedical Ethics (theory, principles, problems)" part 1, 1995; part 2 1996; "Biomedical Ethics", editor V.I. Pockrovsky, 1997; "Beginnings of Bioethics", editor A.N. Orlov, 1997; "Introduction to Bioethics", editor B.G. Yudin, 1998; "Bioethics: Principles, Rules and Problems", editor B.G. Yudin, 1998.

Teaching of bioethics is presented in a large number of medical schools around Russia and in some departments of philosophy in universities. Still we could say that the system of bioethical education is only in the process of development.

Literature (for more information)

Tichtchenko, Pavel "Corruption: the Russian experience" in *Bulletin of Medical Ethics*, number 121, September 1966, pp.13–18.

Tichtchenko, Pavel "The Individual and Healthcare in the New Russia" in *Cambridge Quarterly of Healthcare Ethics*, vol 4, number 1, winter 1995, pp.75–79.

Tichtchenko, Pavel; Yudin, Boris, "The Moral Status of Fetuses in Russia" in *Cambridge Quarterly of Healthcare Ethics*, vol 6, number 1, winter 1997, pp. 31–38.

ISLAM

Islamic Code of Medical Professional Ethics

Abdul Rahman, C. Amine, and Ahmed Elkadi

──────────────── INTRODUCTION TO READING ────────────────

Islam offers still another alternative to Hippocratic medical ethics or the liberal ethics of Western political philosophy. The style of contemporary Muslim writings on medical ethics is quite different from the secular medical ethical literature of either the East or West. It is much more explicitly religious in tone, much more so even than the medical ethical writings of most contemporary religious commentators on medical ethical issues. It works very closely with the Quranic texts that it considers relevant to medical decision making. In doing so it makes clear how different the moral reasoning is of one in the Muslim tradition from secular and Judeo-Christian medical ethical discussions. The following text is representative. It was originally written for an international conference on Islamic Medicine in Kuwait in 1981. It concludes with a reprinting of the oath of the Islamic Medical Association of the USA and Canada.

Medicine was defined by Muslim physicians such as Al-Razi (841–926 AD) and Ibn Sina (Avicenna, 980–1036 AD) as the art concerned with the preservation of good health, combating of diseases and restoration of health to the sick. For several centuries, the world has witnessed and benefited from the great advances made by Muslim physicians in the area of health sciences. These advances were not just based on technical skill or intellectual superiority. They were equally well founded on a clear understanding of the role of the Muslim physician as derived from Islamic teachings and philosophy. For thousands of years, ethics have been recognized as an essential requirement in the making of a physician. Although the ancient codes of ethics[1,2] have to some extent stressed this requirement, they were still deficient and contained grave errors.[3] Contemporary codes of ethics tend to be more liberal and less restrictive. The Quranic ethics, on the other hand, stand out as a perfect model for all mankind, all professions and all time.

The medical ethical requirements proposed in this paper are primarily based on Quranic ethics. They include guidelines for the physician's behavior and attitude, both at the personal and professional levels. The same standard of moral and ethical values should guide the physician in his private life and while conducting his professional business as well. A person who lacks moral values in private life cannot be trusted in professional activities, even with the highest professional and technical qualifications. It is impossible for a person to have two different ethical standards. Truthful is God the Almighty when He says:

God has not made for any man two hearts in his body.[4]

The following verses from the Quran are most suited as a guide for the personal characteristics of the physician:

Luqman admonished his son: "My son" he said "serve no God besides God for idolatry is an abominable injustice." We have enjoined man to show kindness to his parents, for with much pain does his mother bear him and he is not weaned before he is two years of age. We said: Give thanks to Me and to your parents; to Me shall all things return. But if they press you to serve besides Me what you know nothing of, do not obey them, be kind to them in this world and follow the path of those who submit to Me: to

Me you shall all return and I will declare to you all that you have done. "My son, God will know about all things be they as small as a grain of mustard seed, be they hidden inside a rock or in heaven or on earth, God is wise and all-knowing. My son, establish regular prayer, enjoin what is just and forbid what is wrong; endure with fortitude whatever befalls you, for this is firmness of purpose in the conduct of affairs. Do not treat men with scorn nor walk proudly on the earth; God does not love the arrogant boaster. Rather, let your gait be modest and your voice low; the harshest of voices is the braying of the ass. "[5]

. . . and those who restrain anger and forgive other men, verily God loves those who do good.[6]

God further states:

It was the mercy of God that you have dealt with them gently and if you were severe and harsh-hearted they would have broken away from about you. Therefore, forgive them, pray for their forgiveness and consult them in the conduct of affairs; then, when you have decided to proceed, depend on God for support: verily God loves those who depend on Him.[7]

Based on the above, the Muslim physician must believe in God and in Islamic teachings and practice, both in private and public life. He must be grateful to his parents, teachers and elders. He must be humble, modest, kind, merciful, patient and tolerant. He must follow the path of the righteous and always seek God's support.

The physician equipped with the above-listed virtues is capable of complying with the needed professional requirements. The professional requirement is to acquire and maintain proper knowledge. God makes it clear in the Quran: ". . . Say: Are those equal, those who know and those who do not know?. . ."[8]
God also states:

. . . Verily, those who fear God among His servants are those who have knowledge . . .[9]

Therefore, the believer is encouraged to always seek knowledge.

. . .Say: O my Lord, advance me in knowledge.[10]

The physician must also abide by the legal rule regulating the profession provided they do not violate Islamic teachings. The need to respect law and order is reflected in the following verse:

Oh you who believe: Obey God and obey the Apostle, and those charged with authority among you . . .[11]

Recognizing God as the maker and the owner of both patient and physician, it is only logical that the care provided to his patient must be in accordance with God's guidelines.

A subject of great importance is the subject of life. Life is given by God and cannot be taken away except by Him or with His permission. God says in the Quran:

> It is He who created death and life, that He may try which of you is best in deed . . .[12]

He also says ". . . Nor can they control death nor life nor resurrection."[13] God further states:

> . . . Whoever kills a human being in lieu of another human being nor because of mischief on earth, it is as if he has killed all mankind and whoever saves the life of a human being, it is as if he has saved the life of all mankind. . . .[14]

The physician therefore has no right to terminate any human life under his care. This also applies to the unborn baby since clear evidence indicates that human life starts at the time of conception. Consequently, the physician has no right to terminate the life of the unborn baby unless it constitutes a definite threat to the mother's life.

The physician must realize that God is watching and monitoring every thought and deed. This was clearly indicated in the verses quoted earlier from Sura 31 of the Quran.[5] The same verses also indicate that the parents' demands are not to be obeyed if they are in violation of God's orders, in spite of the fact that parents are considered to be the most important persons to their children after God. Following the same principles, the physician has no right to follow popular demand or his patient's wishes if they are in violation of God's orders.

Based on sound logic and clear Islamic teachings, the physician has no right to recommend or administer any harmful material to his patients. The most concise yet comprehensive guide in this matter is found in the following verse of the Quran:

> . . . and He makes for them good things lawful, and bad things forbidden . . .[15]

This implies that anything forbidden by God must be bad or harmful; anything proven to be bad or harmful must be forbidden.

The humanitarian aspect of the medical profession must never be neglected nor overlooked. The physician must render the needed help regardless of the financial ability or ethnic origin of the patient. A beautiful hint is found in the following Quranic verses:

> And they feed, for the love of God, the indigent, the orphan, and the captive, (saying) 'We feed you for the sake of God alone: no reward do we desire from you, nor thanks.'[16]

When entrusted with the care of a patient, the physician must offer the needed advice with consideration for both the patient's body and mind, always remembering his basic obligation to enjoin what is just and forbid what is wrong.

The physician must protect the patient's confidentiality, reflecting God's description of the believers: "Those who faithfully keep their trusts and their covenants."[17]

The physician must adopt an appropriate manner of communication and be reminded of the ethics of speech referred to in the Quranic verses quoted earlier in this paper.[5] God also describes the good believers in the Quran and says: "For they have been guided to the purest of speeches."[18]

Situations requiring the physician to examine patients of the opposite sex are always a test of his moral character and his strength. A basic instruction is found in the following Quranic verses:

> Say to the believing men that they should lower their gaze and guard their modesty; that will make for greater purity for them, for God is well acquainted with all that they do. And say to the believing women that they should lower their gaze and guard their modesty . . .[19]

God further says: "God does wish to lighten your burden, for man was created weak."[20]

It is, therefore, advisable that the physician examine patients of the opposite sex in the presence of a third person whenever feasible. This will be an added protection for the physician and the patient.

The physician must not criticize another physician in the presence of patients or health personnel, remembering the wise Quranic advice:

> O you who believe, let not some men among you make fun of others; it may be that they are better than them; nor let some women make fun of others; it may be that they are better than them; not defame, nor be sarcastic to each other, nor call each other by offensive nicknames . . .[21]

God further says:

> God does not love that evil be voiced in public speech, except where the person has suffered injustice . . .[22]

The physician must refuse payment for the treatment of another physician or his immediate family. There is no specific instruction regarding this particular matter in the Quran or Islamic tradition. However, reference is made to another situation which may be used in analogy. God says in regarding Zakat money: "Alms are for the poor, the needy and those employed to administer the funds . . ."[23]

Here is a situation where the persons providing a certain service are entitled to the use of the same service at the time of need. Applying the same principle, the physician who provides the health service to others is entitled to the use of the same service at the time of need.

Last, but not least, the physician must always strive to use wisdom in all his decisions and the reward will be great. Truthful is God almighty when He says: ". . . and he to whom wisdom is granted, is granted a great deal of good indeed . . ."[24]

In closing, reference is made to the Oath of the Muslim Physician adopted by the Islamic Medical Association in 1977(25), and which reflects the spirit and philosophy of the Islamic Code of Medical Professional Ethics proposed in this paper.

In summary, the Muslim physician must believe in God and in Islamic teachings and practice in private and public life; be grateful to his parents, teachers, and elders; be humble, modest, kind, merciful, patient and tolerant; follow the path of the righteous; and always seek God's support. The Muslim physician must stay abreast of current medical knowledge, continuously improve his skill, seek help whenever needed and comply with legal requirements governing his profession; realize that God is the maker and owner of his patient's body and mind, and treat him within the framework of God's teachings; realize that life was given to man by God, that human life starts at the time of conception, and that human life cannot be taken away except by God or with His permission; realize that God is watching and monitoring every thought and deed; follow God's guidelines as his only criteria, even if they differ with popular demand or the patient's wishes; not recommend nor administer any harmful material; render needed help regardless of financial ability or ethnic origin of the patient; offer needed advice with consideration for both the patient's body and mind; protect the patient's confidentiality; adopt an appropriate manner of communication; examine a patient of the opposite sex in the presence of a third person whenever feasible; not criticize another physician in the presence of patients or health personnel—refuse payment for treatment of another physician or his immediate family and strive to use wisdom in all his decisions.

The Oath of a Muslim Physician

Praise be to Allah (God), the teacher, the unique, Majesty of the heavens, the Exalted, the Glorious, Glory be to Him the Eternal Being who created the Universe and all creatures within, and the only Being who containeth the infinity and the eternity. We serve no other God besides Thee and regard idiolatry as an abominable injustice.

Give us the strength to be truthful, honest, modest, merciful and objective.

Give us the fortitude to admit our mistakes, to amend our ways, and to forgive the wrongs of others.

Give us the wisdom to comfort and counsel all towards peace and harmony.

Give us the understanding that ours is a profession sacred that deals with your most precious gifts of life and intellect.

Therefore, make us worthy of this favored station with honor, dignity and piety so that we may devote our lives in serving mankind, poor or rich, wise or illiterate, Muslim or non-Muslim, black or white, with patience and tolerance, with virtue and reverence, with knowledge and vigilance, with Thy love in our hearts and compassion for Thy servants, Thy most precious creation.

Hereby we take this oath in Thy name, the Creator of all the Heavens and the earth and follow Thy counsel as Thou have revealed to Prophet Muhammad (*pbuh*).

Whoever killeth a human being, not in lieu of another human being nor because of mischief on earth, it shall be as if he hath killed all mankind. And if he saveth a human life, it shall be as if he hath saved the life of all mankind . . .[25]

—This Oath is adopted by the Islamic Medical Association of USA and Canada.

Notes

1. Oath of Hippocrates
2. Oath of the Hindu Physician
3. "Professional Ethics; Ethics in the Medical Profession," by Ahmed Elkadi, MD. *Journal of the Islamic Medical Association*, (September):pp. 27–30, 1976.
4. Quran: 33/4
5. Quran: 31/13–19
6. Quran: 3/134
7. Quran: 3/159
8. Quran: 39/9
9. Quran: 35/28
10. Quran: 20/114
11. Quran: 4/59
12. Quran: 67/2
13. Quran: 25/3
14. Quran: 5/32
15. Quran: 7/157
16. Quran: 76/8–9
17. Quran: 23/8
18. Quran: 22/24
19. Quran: 24/30–31
20. Quran: 4/28
21. Quran: 49/11
22. Quran: 4/148
23. Quran: 9/60
24. Quran: 2/269
25. "Oath of the Muslim Physician," *Convention Bulletin of Islamic Medical Association*, October 1977.

INDIA AND HINDUISM

Medical Ethics in India

Prakash N. Desai

─────────────── INTRODUCTION TO READING ───────────────

It is impossible to develop an understanding of contemporary Indian medical ethics without taking into account its ancient and diverse cultural history. To delve into this rich heritage is, however, to confront a multiplicity of beliefs of limitless proportion. In the following article, author Prakash Desai acknowledges the problem of heterogeneity but nonetheless constructs a view of Indian medical ethics from broad-based and enduring Hindu principles. Whether through exploring concepts such as *dharma* (moral law) or *karma,* the cosmic law of cause and effect, Desai provides a glimpse of the cultural and religious building blocks from which an Indian medical ethics is derived. In the final stages of his article Desai outlines how, specifically, the ethical problems of medicine can be addressed through ancient text, myth, and history.

Medical ethics in India is embedded in its ancient and diverse medical and cultural traditions. Unlike the West, where technologies of modern medicine have brought to the fore tensions between the values of its traditions and health delivery, medical ethics in India have not yet become an object of explicit concern. The ethical crises in the West have forced a restatement and reconsideration of the religious meaning of life and death, among other things. In contrast, medicine in India is largely indigenous, and as such is more consistent with the classical and/or folk traditions. The majority of Indians are without adequate and decent health services, which in fact may be the real ethical crisis to be confronted in India. Re-articulation of the ethical aims of medicine, including adequate health care for all, is an important priority. The task is complex. This paper proposes to outline the context from within which medical values emerge and ways in which some ethical dilemmas that confront modern medicine in India today may be resolved.

I. Problems of Definition

Before considering Indian medical ethics, several problems have to be encountered. In the first place, it would be less complex to speak about Hindu ethics than Indian ethics. Although the two terms may appear, synonymous, in the area of medicine there are important distinctions. Well-established medical theory and practices that are distinctly Hindu have existed in India for over two thousand years. These include Ayurveda, and somewhat subsidiary to it, Siddha. For the study of Indian medical ethics, this system of medicine has to be the object of our study. However, the so-called Western or modern medicine[1] that came to India with the Europeans, and later became a dominant medical enterprise, is a major vehicle of health care and with its modern technology raises several ethical dilemmas. Besides these two, the Unani (from Ionian) and Homeopathic systems have a large following in India. Outside of these organized schools of medical theory, there are widespread folk traditions patronized mainly in rural India.

A second problem facing the medical ethicist is the discrepancy between theory and practice. This is a more general problem. In India there has always been a variable and flexible code of ethics for human conduct subject to local interpretation. Changing according to regional disparities and particular folk traditions, always-so-slightly different set of priorities emerges. The rules of human actions and transactions apply more to overt social behavior and less to inner states of mind. This is an issue of sufficient psychological significance to require more elaborate discussion later.

Another problem is that India is not exclusively Hindu. Besides the religious and ethnic minorities that account for almost fifteen percent of the population, there are nearly as many at the periphery of the Hindu fold. This includes the so-called untouchables, whose religious and social practices are at great variance with the classical tradition, and half as many tribals, who are clearly outside the Hindu system of beliefs. Even if we put aside the non-Hindu traditions of India for the sake of the present discussion, the Hindu tradition itself is not a homogeneous system. In the Hindu tradition there is no central organizing structure of authority and arbitration. Without a universally-accepted book or scripture or priestly hierarchy, there are no abiding points of reference. There is no authority that can proclaim a particular code of conduct for all Hindus, much less see to its enforcement. Over the centuries, so many sufficiently different paths to self-realization as well as God-realization have arisen that a common definition of laws of human conduct can hardly be agreed upon.

II. Use of History

Though the diversity and diffusion in Indian society make the formulation of moral imperatives that are binding for all difficult, the historical orientation of the people manifests itself in great respect, and concern for continuity. This concern might easily be regarded as a vital feature of the traditions. *Parampara*, meaning tradition handed down from generation to generation, acts as a force in shaping the behaviors and attitudes of the masses. What has been a particular family's or group's history is often cited as a rationale for human conduct.

Itihas, "it happened thus," is the meaning of history. Taking the example of one's forefathers as a basis for action is of great psychological significance. Ashis Nandy (1980, pp. 4–5) has discussed three strands of Indian history. The *charons*, or minstrels, were wandering individuals or groups who sang of past events and heroic acts of men "giving meaning to the present by projecting its rough realities into a mythologized past." He wrote that "while providing a capsuled world-image and organized ethical criteria to the laity, they built a defensive shield which consolidated the culture through constant affirmation and renewal of its psychophilosophical base." A second strand was personified by those who constructed formal genealogies and thus advanced the significance of generational continuity. The third institution was that of court historians.

Apart from using history in this fashion, making the past and present continuous with each other, there is also a preoccupation with the past. Historical antecedents and precedents are offered as justification for or against actions and attitudes. "Those who forget their past are apt to repeat it" is not an apt idiom for Indians. Their ethos demands that they remember their past and insists that they repeat it. They glow with pride that theirs is an ancient civilization; they speak of their ancestors with a sense of immediacy. The lineage (*gotra*) by which they identify themselves carries with it moral imperatives, specifying some actions and forbidding others. The preservation of the tradition is ensured by the knowledge of the actions of the mythologized heroes, lending authenticity to a living tradition. Thus, for Indians, the history is lived-in. Actions are inspired by the accounts of heroes of the past.

The most ancient Hindu scriptures are the Vedic literature, regarded as revealed, or heard (*shruti*), and the later epics and *puranas* (meaning belonging to the past) which are in the consciousness of everyday life (collectively *smriti*, remembered). It has even been suggested that what is now regarded as Hinduism properly starts with these texts, and the earlier Vedic literature provides a philosophical background to the tradition (Eliade 1987). More than the theoretical and abstract aspect of the religious tradition, beliefs and practices have greater command on the minds of people. Generational tradition stretching back to its legendary heroes holds greater sway over the laity, and those whose task it is to interpret the scriptural edicts must accommodate the changing and yet continuous nature of the tradition.

III. The Aims of Dharma

Another important source of regulation of human affairs is the literature of the *dharmasastra*[2], the law books. Collectively the texts provide organization for personal and social life. The duties and obligations of the householder and the aims of a moral life which connect the individual with the cosmos and the worshipper with the sacred are the two principle purposes of Hindu life embodied in these texts. Inherent in these standards of conduct are the ideals of generational continuity.

The composition of the law books, which began in the pre-Christian era, continued for centuries. This large body of literature when taken together appears to be unnecessarily repetitive, but when cast in the context of the rapidly-expanding territorial contours of Hindu society and the passage of time, the literature represents a unique adaptation of a particular area in a particular era. I would also suggest that the aspect of *dharmasastra* giving uniformity and coherence to Hindu social life was a challenge that was thrown up by an essentially inward-looking, intensely psychological and in the end individualistic pursuit of self-realization advanced by the Upanishadic doctrines. The concept of *dharma* was a return to the earlier Rigvedic ideal of *rta*, order (from *Rig*, cognate with the English rule).

Rta, or order, was an essential need articulated by the Vedic poets. Celestial events like the alternation of day and night and the cycle of seasons were seen as governed by a cosmic law. "Order and truth were born from heat as it hazed up" (*Rig Veda*) 10.190); in this way the philosopher poets visualized an organic connection between the two. The sacrificial ritual connected with early Vedic practices was aimed at the restoration of order. Even today in India, when the rains fail to come for a long time, especially when the monsoon fails in successive years, similar sacrificial rituals are commissioned. The principle of cosmic order was later interiorized to become *dharma*, the ordainer of action and thought.

Dharma (a word derived from the verb *dhru*, meaning to hold, to contain, to maintain or sustain) is that which sustains and holds a people together individually and collectively. It is the law of morality or ethics, performance of which is an obligation and through which one attains well-being both here and now, and later after death. The implications of a life informed by *dharma* are all-pervasive and all-inclusive. It leaves no sector or stage of life without norms and expectations for moral life, and loss of *dharma* leads to fragmentation and chaos. As an organizational principle it has two central ideals: (1) the stratification of people and their social lives into classes or varna, and (2) an ordered transition from one stage of life to another, the *ashramas*. The four classes of social organization and the four stages of life came to entail in each instance a set of obligations and actions. The modern caste system is more a proliferation and cross-multiplication of the original four classes, and the word *jati* (subcaste), like genera, retains some of the original meaning.

The most important of them for our purposes is the notion of *gunas* or strands. These are qualities or properties that inhere in human beings, derived from the substance of one's lineage, thus one's jati, and ultimately the *varna* (Marriott and Inden, 1976). The *Bhagavad Gita*, the celestial song of the Supreme, is a dialogue on the battlefield to urge a prince (belonging to the warrior class) to act according to his *dharma*, and is perhaps the most explicit statement about the connection between *dharma* and *guna*. The dialogue asserts the primacy of one's obligations, and propounds action according to these obligations as the paramount ethical aim of life. It states, "It is more salutary to carry out your own Law poorly than another's Law well; it is better to die in your own Law than to prosper in another's" (*Bhagavada Gita* 25(3).35).

The law of life stages determines sets of actions. From the stage of apprenticeship to that of a householder, a forest-dweller, and finally a renouncer, a person's passage through life calls for actions appropriate to each stage.[3]

The emphasis so far in the realization of ethical aims of life is predominantly on the regulation of behavior. Impulses that tend to result in disruption of the social order have to be under control, social transactions have to be governed by established order, structural principles of hierarchy and boundaries have to be respected. The disjunctions between internal states of feeling and thought and required social conduct have to be set aside. Performance according to *dharma* may then bring about a split between the internal state and the actions of an actor. Often retaining the consciousness of this incongruence, the actor feels no remorse or guilt about intentions, as long as the action is able to keep the intentions from the public knowledge. The emphasis on behavior may thus shift the mechanism of regulation from an internal personal source to the external public force of one's group, family, lineage, or caste (Desai, 1982).

Transactions have moral implications and psychological meaning. The dynamics of intimacy of orbits and a split between public and private selves are related to each other and to the problem of ethics.

A stratified, hierarchical society puts people into different psychological orbits, and the levels of intimacy shared varies according to the place in the larger social order of people in transaction. The laws governing human relationships are not standard for any two persons. Assignment of worth is determined by the psychological significance attached to the levels of need and intimacy according to personal, familial, and caste considerations. These may be compared to the heavenly bodies, their orbits, and the gravitational forces they exert on each other.

Similarly, we can also imagine orbits within a person amounting to a public and private persona. The division between the two is not fixed and changes according to levels of intimacy. But an emphasis on obligations tends to focus on behaviors rather than intentions in Hindu personality. This tendency to split as it were two levels of consciousness is also determined by many other forces in Hindu childhood, a discussion of which is beyond the scope of this paper. Often the split permits actions to be at odds with intentions, behavior at variance with inner states. Distinctions between a private and a public self emerge, allowing different behaviors according to different situations or audiences. Where consistency is not a virtue, the discrepancy does not necessarily lead to inner dissonance. Repentance, penance or shame may follow wrongful acts but not guilt, a word for which there is no equivalent term or concept in Indian languages.

IV. Aims of Medicine

The corpus of Hindu literature pertaining to health and medicine is Ayurveda, by its name the knowledge of long life. *Ayus* or life is the continuance of consciousness, animation and the sustenance of the body (Carakasamhita,

1.30.22, hereafter Car.). Earlier in the *Atharvaveda*, priestly craft included prescriptions for various botanical preparations, donations, propitiatory rites, observance of rules of daily living, fasting, expiation, etc. for the alleviation of pain and cure of disease. According to Winternitz, "In the Vedic texts we find the beginning of a science of anatomy, of an embryology, and of a hygiene. In the *Satapatha Brahmana* (X and XII) and in the *Atharvaveda* (X.2) we find an accurate enumeration of the bones of the human skeleton." (1967, p. 626). The Ayurvedic construction of the human body and the nature of the self were both continuous and consistent with Hindu religious literature. Ayurveda is a prime example of how the secular and the spiritual are overlapping and indivisible domains in Hindu thought.

The *Carakasamhita*, the primary and oldest-known medical text, opens with a scene of an assembly of sages. They had assembled as a sort of a blue-ribbon panel at a retreat in the Himalayas, because the populace was inflicted with diseases which interfered with the observances of religious obligations (Car.I-6.7). Desiring a disease-free state, a source of "virtue, wealth and gratification," (Car.I-1 5) they sought divine guidance. The healthy human body is essential to the realization of life's tasks, including the ethical. Health-seeking was a religious obligation. Ayurveda was created before the creation of the world, so that the potential for protection of health and removal of disease were built into the act of creation. Ethical laws were natural laws, and the Ayurvedic world-view was a part of the Hindu conception of humanity and its place in the universe.

This orientation to health and illness has endured over centuries and continues to inform the expectation of patients and the practice of physicians. Allopathic practitioners are forced in their attitude, if not in theory, to acknowledge their patients' health idioms. The language of hot and cold, light and heavy, wet and dry, permeates the discourse of patients and physicians of all schools, for such properties are common to diets, drugs, disease, and temperamental dispositions. Food and diet with their potential for altering body chemistry, are a constant part of Ayurvedic prescriptions, and there is hardly a patient who does not ask his Allopathic doctor for a regimen of diet to match the disease or the drug.

In India, in the midst of a variety of medical traditions, patients rarely patronize only one tradition, shopping as it were for one that is most congenial to their particular, often chronic, disorder. This 'pick and choose' attitude is not only consistent with the Hindu orientation to life (in which there are few absolutes), but also prevents too obvious a fracture between a patient's tradition-informed help-seeking behaviors and a physician's response to them.

V. Ayurvedic Assumptions

1. The Body

The human body is constructed out of the same substances that constitute the universe. The five created elements are the *mahabhutas: akasha* (often translated as space or void), wind, fire, water and earth. Each is a precursor of a specific body part. Space contains the spoken word and gives rise to the sense of hearing. Wind becomes the tactile organs, touch itself, and is responsible for internal and external movements. Fire is the sense of sight, the eyes, and the form. It inheres in emotion and lustre, alacrity and bravery, and "cooks" the food, transforming it into other substances. Water becomes taste and the gustatory sense organs, and is the source of the fluids in the body, including semen. Earth, the fifth element, is responsible for smell and olfactory sense organs (*Susrutasamhita*III 1.16.20 hereafter Su.).

Food when digested becomes *rasa*, the body sap, and is present in all body parts. As the etymology suggests, *rasa* means 'constantly in motion' (Su.I.14.9). *Rasa* is sequentially transformed into blood, flesh, fat, bone, marrow, and finally semen. These seven are collectively called *dhatus* (from the verb *dhru*, same as that for *dharma*), which hold the body together. The Upanishads had declared that the body is a product of *anna*, food, and the Ayurvedic texts echo the same assertion. In a 1981 translation of the *Bhavaprakash* into Gujarati, Vaidya Prabhashankar Nanbhatt Gadhadavala introduces the text with a commentary, in which he states that nothing other than food and drink enters the body, and thus they are the most important causes of diseases, as well as being medicines (p. 10). With the body and the universe sharing the same elemental constitution, all substances have potential for being medicinal. Thus human beings and nature are harmonious and behave according to the same laws. After all, the entire creation was a product of the body parts of the cosmic giant Purusha (see the 'Purusasukta Hymn' of the *Rigveda*, X.90).

2. The Self

Borrowing from the Samkhya school of philosophy, reality is divided into an eternal, undecaying, conscious *purusha*, and a created and thus decay-prone multiform materiality, *prakriti*. Ayurveda completed the material person by adding to it a force of consciousness. The Upanishads had declared prana or breath to be the property of life, an idea that evolved into notions of consciousness and self (*atman*). It cannot be overemphasized that the inquiry into the nature of the self had been a principal pursuit from the very beginning of the Vedic civilization (Collins and Desai, 1986) and Ayurveda, much like the earlier literature, shows a similar fascination. It conceives of the self as bipartite, a transcendental *atman* and a phenomenal *ahamkara*. The latter is material in origin and equivalent to pride, a false and narcissistic sense of self. *Carakasamhita* and *Susrutasamhita* vacillate in their notion of a self that is transcendental and one that is a property of being alive (Car.IV.1. 70–74 and Su.IV.11). Although the predominant view in the Ayurvedic literature follows a notion of the propertyless *atman* as the life principle, in the later texts self and life are understood as coupled (*jivatma*) and are used interchangeably with the properties of breathing and consciousness and various aspects of thought. *Prana* is the breath from which the idea of the self (*atman*) evolved, and it departs with death.

At the very beginning, in the *Rig Veda* and the Upanishads, *prana* is the breath associated with life, the absence of which is death. *Prani* means a living creature, and *prana* is the life force. The definition of death is respiratory failure, although later on there are indications of the heart and the brain as seats of the *prana*. Folklore allows for "the disappearance of the *prana* into the cranium," as in suspended animation or in certain yogic achievements, and a person may be mistakenly taken for dead, hinting at an idea of brain death.

Breath is understood as pervading the whole body and presages the Ayurvedic humoral theory, in which the wind is a principal *dosha*. When the narcissistic component of the self, particularly the consciousness of being a person, becomes an object of explicit reflection, *prana* is understood as that consciousness. *Prana* is associated with four states of consciousness: waking, dreaming, dreamless sleep, and beyond. The dreaming self, which comprehends object-less images and travels far and wide without limits of time and space, led to speculation about an object-less self. Thus arose the ideas of true (*atman*) and false (*ahamkara*) selves, both interior, but *ahamkara* was superficial, while the *atman* was deeper.

Prana thus becomes the essence of both individual and universal selves. A detailed discussion of this development is to be found in my forthcoming book *Health/Medicine in the Hindu Tradition*.

3. Conception

The questions of when and how life begins are matters of great concern to Ayurveda. It is suggested in the *Carakasamhita* that an embryo is formed with the union of mother, the father, the life principle, appropriateness, nourishment, and the principle of consciousness (Car.IV.3). It is argued that none of these principles by themselves is capable of producing an embryo. If the mother and father are the only factors in the production of an embryo, why would anybody be childless? The life principle, the *atman* or the self, could not reproduce itself, for then it no longer could be considered to be without beginning and end. The argument ends with an assertion that the union of all the variables is essential in reproduction. According to this argument, the beginning of life is the moment of conception. The principle of life is not extrinsic to the semen and the uterine "blood." An analogy of a magnifying lens and the rays of the sun, in neither of which fire is present but with their union becomes manifest, is used to illustrate this assertion. (*Bhavaprakash* 1.2. 32–33 and *Astangahryidaya* II. 1–3).

An elaborate discussion on fetal and congenital abnormalities follows. Defective male or female seeds, unnatural coitus or weakness in any humors (*dosha*) can lead to miscarriage, still-birth, multiple pregnancy, and a variety of birth defects. Psychological circumstances during the pregnancy can affect the characteristics of the unborn child, and infertility may occur in healthy and fertile parents if all the conditions do not come together appropriately. Determination of gender is explained by the preponderance of the male or female seed (Car.III.3). These views are current in India today, and childless couples eat foods regarded as capable of increasing generative substances, pregnant women are protected from psychological strife, and postpartum care of the mother and the baby follow the ancient prescriptions.

4. Gunas

We have already seen that the *gunas* (strands or qualities) are the bases of *dharma*. This theory of intrinsic properties of substances (including persons) may be regarded as the strongest influence of the Samkhya philosophy on Ayurvedic theories, and in turn became the biological or natural theory of ethics. In all matters there are three properties—*sattva*, *rajas*, and *tamas*—meaning goodness, vitality, and inertia respectively. In an undifferentiated state of matter, the three are in an equilibrium, and changes in their balance produce differentiation and give rise to multiform materiality. The three have physical (light, heavy, cool, hot, dull, active, etc.), psychological (calm, serene, passionate, lethargic, stupid, etc.), and ethical (pure, virtuous, compassionate, violent, dark, obscuring, etc.) dimensions according to their context. They have a reciprocal relationship with activities; for example, a person with *rajas* predominant will be active, hot, and passionate, and *rajas* will be promoted in a person by activities like love, battle, and pleasure-seeking.

Among the body substances semen, blood, and fat epitomize the three *gunas*. Through activities like meditation and contemplation, one moves from inertia to serenity, from an undesirable to a desirable state. In everyday usage, *guna* means virtue, and also quality or property. Psychological personality types are described in terms of the *guna* distribution, with explicit ethical expectations. It is clear from the medical texts that these types are not immutable and appropriate intervention (dietary regimen, activities, attitudes, relationships, etc.) can alter the *guna* equilibrium, often essential in curing physical and mental diseases. The moral implications are also obvious. We may regard the potential in every transaction, and in every substance to bring about an alteration in a person's constitution or nature (Marriott, 1976, 1980). This is akin to the *karma* theory in which every action has consequences.

VI. Ethical Aims of Ayurveda

Karma, meaning action, a source of ethical commands, is a law of causality: every action has consequences. *Dharma* assigns actions and *karma* holds a person to them. Morality inherent in every human action has a potential for immediate or later reward or punishment; by this logic life events imply antecedent actions, and where the future consequences serve as commands, past actions are explanations. Thus *karma* may be viewed as having three temporal dimensions. One cannot alter that which is already done, but the present and future represent opportunities for modifying one's fate. The laws of *karma* do not allow arithmetical cancellation of good against bad, since every action has its consequences, and the fruits of both have to be borne. Essential to the theory of rebirth, *karma* does involve predeterminism, but contrary to popular belief predeterminism and fatalism are not the only implications of the laws of *karma*.

In everyday life, actions having consequences are not uppermost in Hindu consciousness. A Hindu does not approach tasks at hand with an idea of helplessness before fate. The karmic laws are invoked generally when unforeseen and undesirable developments like grave illnesses, misfortunes, or accidents occur. When life unfolds in an unexpected and unwanted way, the person tends to find solace in determinants of the past, rather than some inadequacy in effort or deficiency in skill. Even in instances of grave illnesses the response is not fatalistic, but should the treatment prove ineffective there is the escape hatch (Weiss, 1980) of the unknown wheel of *karma*.

Ayurveda interprets *karma* as causal in accidents and diseases, but assigns a vital role to effort, both personal and medical. The "Why me?" question of a patient may best be answered in terms of bad actions of the past, but a patient's fate is not always sealed. Proper care, diagnosis, and treatment will alter the disease. The *Carakasamhita* lays great stress on right conduct, physical and psychological, and considers right conduct to be the best guarantee against ill health. Illnesses produced by disturbances in internal equilibrium are also due to errors in wise and prudent behavior. The texts emphasize moderation as a key to well being.

In the medical texts, action springs from three main desires: The desire for self-preservation, the desire for acquiring the means for a comfortable life, and the desire for a happy state in future existence (Dasgupta, 1975). Attention is constantly riveted to the problems of this life, and the rules of righteous conduct involve more medical than moral principles. Adequate, regular nutritive diet, appropriate proportions of activity, rest and sleep, moderation in sexual behavior, avoidance of excessive greed, anger, sorrow, etc., form the cornerstone of a good and healthy life. Dasgupta explains this orientation by contrasting the two: "Right conduct is not conduct in accordance with the injunctions of the Vedas, or conduct which leads ultimately to the cessation of all sorrows through cessation of all desires, or through right knowledge and the extinction of false knowledge, but is that which leads to the fulfillment of the three ultimate desires. The cause of sins is not transgression of the injunctions of the scriptures, but errors of right judgment or of right thinking" (1975, p. 405). For the medical texts, the medical versus moral dichotomy is spurious, a body and mind in constant interaction with the environment and prone to change with every transaction represent the laws of nature, the ultimate medical morality.

A notable exception to such an interpretation of the ethical aims of life is the explanation offered for epidemics. Epidemics result from collective misdeeds, when a whole community is involved in evil action: it is a lapse of *dharma* on a mass scale. The actions spoken of here are clearly related to scriptural injunctions, and the leaders of the community (the king or the priest) are held particularly responsible for leading people astray. Here the composers of the texts follow the same logic as that of the common person: that unexpected, unusual, or seemingly causally-unrelated events are attributed to the workings of *karma*. Those who are unaffected during epidemics are said to have accumulated good deeds and are therefore protected. In treating people who are afflicted during an epidemic, stress is laid on the virtues of truthfulness, charity, worship, observance of celibacy, and discourse upon scriptures (Car.III-12–20).

VII. The Physician in Ayurveda

If there is anything the compilers of Ayurveda texts rail against, it is quackery. Time and again warnings are issued and the dangers of being treated by a quack are enumerated. The medical texts evince a keen interest in competence, knowledge, skills, and attitude. Learning is highly valued, and a valid inference can be made that rival schools or perhaps lineages must have been involved in public discussion and debate about diagnoses and therapeutics. Teachers are advised to choose their students carefully and students instructed in their choice of mentors. Empathy, listening, patience, generosity, and devotion are the non-cognitive virtues extolled in a physician.

Unfortunately, as Chattopadhyaya (1977) has demonstrated, the physician in ancient India was regarded with highly-charged mixed feelings. Esteem and disdain, trust and suspicion, applause and derision went together. He argues that in ancient India the needs of the hierarchical order mitigated against a separate and independent status for physicians. Brahminical ideology could not permit the evolution of a science that would challenge the assumptions of Hindu metaphysics. The priestly order required that the interpretations of religious laws governing relationships not be contradicted by a materialist science. His explanations about the ambivalence towards physicians are not without merit, but it is difficult to visualize a complete dichotomy between the medical and priestly enterprises.

It is more likely that the classes must have overlapped and physicians must have shared the ideals and prohibitions of the hierarchical order. The place of palpation as an investigative tool is a case in point. Although palpation is an aspect of physical examination, it never becomes the instrument it could have been. The taboos against touching seem to have played a role, and even if fear of contamination is accounted for, the indigenous theory of purity and pollution must have played a major role. After all, the physician was inferior because he mingled with all sorts of people of inferior classes (Chattopadhyaya, 1977). In the practice of a contemporary Ayurvedic physician, the only physical contact with a patient is when the pulse is taken. And the radial pulse and its circulatory significance became a part of Hindu medicine through Unani medicine after the Arabic discoveries. When observation takes priority over theory, existing orthodoxy stands challenged. Science makes commoners out of the privileged. Guarding the secrets of the trade became so ingrained that until recently the practice of medicine had remained familial; medical knowledge and skills passed down from father to son, or to close relatives.

Over time, the doctor-patient relationships have become familiar and intimate. It is as if the family physician has been drawn into an intimate orbit, made into an honorary family member. The physician becomes a counselor and advisor, and a mutuality develops in which the doctor-patient relationship goes far beyond the consulting room. On the other hand, the "dispensary" or the "clinic" is located on main streets open to public view, conveying not only easy access but also a form of advertising. History-taking and most physical examinations take place with other waiting patients sitting around, with little concern for confidentiality in matters of ordinary physical illness. Discussion or examination relating to sexual problems is an exception. Except for modern "private" hospitals, the open wards in public hospitals are no different in this matter. A more detailed examination, not a part of the routine of a general practitioner or an Ayurvedic *vaidya* (doctor), occurs in privacy.

In the Ayurvedic world-view, in which the human being is continuous with the environment, medicinal preparations for internal use pose special problems. A *vaidya* uses natural, usually vegetable products, whereas an Allopathic physician uses "synthetic" preparations which are regarded as very heavy and hot, difficult to assimilate and prone to have side effects. They not only attack the diseased parts of the body, but also the healthy ones. Surgery, unlike internal medicine, does not have the same implications, with a rich ancient tradition of surgical medicine and a body-consciousness that is more physiological than anatomical. Prosthetic devices have been part of medicine and mythology, and organ transplants have been received well wherever available. The psychological and social implications of the match between the donor and recipient in cases of organ transplant need further investigation.

VIII. The Problems of Ethics

Questions about medical ethics in India interact with local custom and tradition in everyday practice. Unusual occurrences may be resolved by a reference to mythology or folklore. This is not to suggest that Indian medicine does not address the problems of ethics. They are intertwined in medical texts, and mythical figures are seen as models of exemplary ethical behavior. Ethical solutions may be inferred and derived from scriptural texts. This is particularly so in the context of modern and recent medical technologies, with which medicine in India had no prior contact.

In the broadest outline, we may conceive of the ethical problems of modern medicine in relation to questions of life and death, of coming into the world and leaving it. Conception, pregnancy, and parenting are involved in the ethics of coming into the world and the ethics of preservation or prolongation of life involve leaving it.

1. Conception

Generational continuity has motivated Indians, ancient and modern, to pray for progeny. Having sons is a way of paying one's debts to the ancestors, an important religious obligation. The importance of father-son unity has been a well established cultural leitmotif from the times of the Vedas and Upanishads (Collins and Desai, 1986).

The great epic *Mahabharata* is a repository of many stories and is rich in details about birth and death, the two endpoints of life. Its ethical norms about begetting sons are indeed very liberal. Having sons is sufficiently important that the laws allow for many possibilities: "Offspring indeed is in the worlds a firm foundation informed by the Law" (1(7)111). The *Mahabharata* goes on to say, "In the eyes of the Law there are these six sons who are the blood and heirs, and these six are neither heirs nor the blood . . . the son fathered by oneself, the son presented, the son purchased, the son born by one's widow, the son born by one's wife before her marriage, and the son born by a loose woman; the others are the son gifted, the son bartered, the son by artifice, the son who comes by himself, the son who comes with marriage, the son of unknown seed, and the son fathered on a lowly womb" (1(7)111). The ancients in their passion for classification are all-inclusive, and advise that one should try and obtain sons in those ways first mentioned above.

The birth of the heirs to the Kuru kingdom, Dhritarastra and Pandu, follow a classic pattern. The young son of the king was not able to produce offspring and died childless, and the lineage was threatened with extinction. In such a moment of distress a different law must apply (*apaddharma*). The mother of the dead king had a son born to her before her marriage. That son, by law, was called upon to impregnate the dead king's wives. Thus were born Dhritarastra and Pandu. This kind of sexual union for purposes of procreation is called *niyoga*, and customs like this are prevalent in India today (Karve, 1962). These mythologies can serve as the basis for ethical acceptability of semen donation, provided the recipient and donor are appropriately matched according to family and caste rules.

Kunti, the wife of Pandu (who is cursed and unable to have children), has been granted a boon, and so invokes the gods beside whom she "lays" to have four sons (the first was born out of wedlock premaritally). But the story about the sons of Dhritarastra is particularly interesting. We may regard this legend almost as a science fiction story, for the embryonic development occurs in pots, test-tubes as it were.

Gandhari, the wife of the blind king Dhritarastra, had been granted a boon by sage Vyasa and had asked for a hundred sons. She conceived, but for two years failed to give birth to the fetus. "And when she felt the hardness of her own belly she began to worry . . . (and) fainting with pain, aborted her belly with hard effort. A mass of flesh came forth, like a dense ball of clotted blood. Vyasa, "best of the mumblers of spells" reappeared, and to fulfill the boon he had granted Gandhari asked to "have at once a hundred *pots set up and filled with ghee*" (emphasis mine), and he sprinkled this ball with cold water. "When the ball was doused it fell apart into a hundred pieces, each an embryo the size of a thumb joint; a full one hundred and one duly developed . . . He put them in pots and had them watched in well-guarded places," and in time one hundred sons and a daughter were born (1(7)107). A myth like this may be advanced as an ethical acceptability of test-tube babies. Similarly, a case can be made for ovum donation and implantation of a fertilized ovum. The desire for offspring is the strongest desire of all, and the fertility was sought through a variety of means long before modern technology.

If we include all the laws that govern cohabitation as a prelude to conception, the scope of our inquiry becomes too broad. Without an injunction against polygamy or out-of-wedlock relationships for the purpose of "begetting sons," the questions raised by modern technology were answered in Hindu India in the context of human sexual relationships. I myself have encountered in a clinical situation a couple's attempt to have a child by the wife sleeping with the husband's friend.

Like most other societies, I must add, tradition sets different standards of sexual conduct for men and women. Hindu texts on love and desire (such as the *Kamasutra*) discuss freely the conduct of sexual behavior for the man-about-town (*nagarika*), including with prostitutes and the wives of other men. Fullest sexual expression is celebrated, but in practice more for men than women, although the *Kamasutra* also included women taking lovers. Marriage, though, is a different matter. Prolongation of one's blood-line is an important ethical aim of life, but in matters of marriage the choice of a partner requires deliberation and observance of one's caste rules, which are not uniform across India or castes. In any event, infertility is a major source of stress, especially for women who bear the brunt of social stigma and psychological strife.

In India semen is highly valued, and the loss of semen is fraught with anxiety. There is fear of "excessive intercourse." "Unnatural losses" (a violation of natural law) accompany fears and feelings of enfeeblement (Carstairs, 1956), physical and intellectual. Gender-specific role and trait differentiation is far less acute in India than in the West. Although socially stigmatized, homosexuality is fraught with fewer psychological complications and subject only to ethical constraints. Institutionalized homosexuality is also to be found, and such groups are associated with particular forms of worship (Carstairs, 1956). Celibacy is a high virtue, and in some esoteric practices (such as *tantra*) elaborate means are sought to avoid loss, and enhance containment, of semen. Mythology is also replete with examples of great sages and yogis whose preservation of semen through celibacy led to an excellent store of semen, giving them radiant energy and superhuman powers.

2. Pregnancy and Abortion

In light of the foregoing discussion, it is apparent that pregnancy would be an occasion of great joy, and, once pregnant, a woman is afforded special physical and psychological care. Preservation of pregnancy and the growth and development of the fetus become a priority for the whole family. It is needless to emphasize that the same degree of emotional investment does not follow when a woman has already had several male and female children. In the context of modern technology, the ethical problem to be confronted is that of surrogacy. Laws of distress take over when a couple is childless, or without a son. We have already witnessed a variety of ways and means to have a son, predating technology. There is one special situation that I would like to illustrate with the help of a myth. This involves the transfer or transplant of an embryo. One can presume a set of permutations that would be ethically permissible from the following, the story of the birth of the god Krishna:

King Kamsa was warned that the eighth child of his sister Devaki and Vasudeva would slay him. The king had his sister and her husband imprisoned and killed the first six of their children. The seventh was saved by a unique strategy, an intervention on part of a goddess. The embryo was removed from the womb of Devaki and implanted in the womb of Rohini, the other wife of Vasudeva. The eighth one, Krishna himself, was saved by an exchange with another newly-born who was in turn killed by the evil king. This is an important part of the legend of Krishna, and appears in various *puranas.*

A similar account surrounds the birth of the last liberated sage (*tirthankara*), Mahavira, in the Jain religion of India. He descended from his divine place as an embryo in the womb of a poor brahmin woman. Dissatisfied with the family into which the *tirthankara* would be born, Indra transferred the embryo into the womb of a Ksatriya woman, exchanging it for the one that was in the womb of the Ksatriya woman.[4] We must rely on accounts like this to construct a case to advise us in the present.

Abortion on the other hand is a more complicated matter. We are confronted here with an issue of a gap between theory and practice. It cannot be overemphasized that rules of conduct derive their legitimacy from and are enforced through the institutions of family and caste, and not organized religion. In commenting on Hindu attitudes, Chandrasekhar (1974, p. 44) states, " But as in all codes of ethics, there is in the Hindu view an admirable and practical dichotomy of the ideal and the permissible. The ideal code of behavior was for the dedicated 'righteous' or saintly minority and the permissible way was for the work-a-day million." Concerning abortion to end a pregnancy that brings dishonor to the person and the family, early texts consider it a sin, equal to the killing of a learned person. Induced abortion, called *bhruna-hatya*, the killing of a fetus, is a word also used for the murder of a brahmin. The practice was condemned in the *Atharvaveda* as well as in the later *smriti* literature. In the *Yagnavalkya* Smriti (AD 400), "the undoubted degradation of women is caused by sexual intercourse with the lowly-born, causing abortion (in oneself) and causing injury to the husband." The same *smriti* considers induced abortion as grounds for abandoning one's wife. (Chandrasekar, 1974, p. 44).

Medical texts like the *Susrutasamhita* describe ways of destroying a fetus in cases of obstructed labor or fetal death. The *Susrutasamhita* also makes exception in cases of danger to maternal life (Su.IV. 1 5.6). Acharya Lolimbaraj, a 17th century Ayurvedic physician, advises that "If the root of the herb *Indrayam* is kept in the vagina, menstrual discharge begins. It is a useful remedy for pregnant women in poor health, widows and women of liberal morals" (Chandrasekhar, 1974, p. 45).

Abortion has been legalized in India since 1972. It appears that the act was created without much religious controversy and does not account for any significant drop in birth rates since its implementation. Some would argue that the problem of population growth is the most serious health problem in the region and can be effectively tackled by education of women, greater access to better health care especially for infants, and a general improvement in standards of living. Both male and female sterilization have been widely practiced in India for over three decades, and the addition of abortion as a means of family planning has not made a significant difference in population control. The major beneficiaries of legalized abortion are women who conceive out-of-wedlock, for whom the pregnancy is a matter of social stigma.

3. Sex Selection

One technological advance that already has and will continue to have a significant impact on health behavior is amniocentesis. In a culture where sons are overwhelmingly favored, the availability of this method of sex-determination is bound to cause a stir. Neglect of female babies and female infanticide in India is neither new nor a negligible problem (Miller, 1981). The news magazine *India Today* (6/15/86) reports in a cover story that in one district of South India, "80% of the female babies born every year have been poisoned to death in the last decade."

Amniocentesis, although not widely or cheaply available yet, shifts the action from the post-natal to the pre-natal period. In a recent talk Sudha Shukla, a crusader for women's rights, bemoaned the lack of responsiveness of doctors and legislators to the women's call (Shukla, 1987). Legalized abortion and gender preferences combine to put female fetuses at great risk. According to Ms. Shukla, the movement against the practice, like other reform movements in India, runs against the social grain and suffers from not being able to draw upon traditional authority, be it medical or religious.

IX. Death and Dying

If the ethical problems encountered around the issues at birth are confounding, those at the other end of life are relatively simple. Not that death does not produce anxieties in the dying and sorrow and loss in the surviving, but the religion itself has long ago found a way of coping with death by the denial of it. In the Hindu consciousness, death is not the opposite of life—it is the opposite of birth. The two events simply mark a passage. What is seriously mourned is an untimely death, because otherwise in time everyone must go, when the old body machine is worn out and when one has paid out the accumulated debts of *karma*. But all this is in a context. Age, sex, marital status, place in the hierarchy, suddenness and the quality of life are natural determinants of response to death. Pain and suffering are not natural conditions, and apart from the fact that sophisticated technologies to prolong life do not as yet exist in India, death is a relief from the actual physical suffering that reduces that quality of life. The overarching philosophical attitude about the passage through life often serves to console the dying and the mourning. Once again an after-the-fact helplessness, produced by death or impending death due to a fatal illness, is coped with by the thought of an eternal *atman* or rebirth.

Not too long ago I was grieving over a personal loss and observed these two distinct but related attitudes. Letters and telegrams that came in from farflung relatives made a special note of the undecaying character of the *atman*, the self of the deceased, and, included quotations from the scriptures. A seven-year-old grand-daughter of the deceased remained somewhat unaffected for the first few days. Then on the occasion of the gathering of the clan as part of the mourning ritual, the young girl suddenly realized the implications. For the next few days she carried around on her person a drawing she made of her grandfather, and asked questions both at home and school about the fate of those who die. Then, a week or so later her grief was resolved. She came home from school one day and announced to the entire family that her grandfather will soon be reborn, and someone, one of her cousins or aunts, will be pregnant with a male baby and that would be her grandfather. In a flash I, too, realized that in her child-like simplicity she had captured the age-old Hindu idea of rebirth—that death was denied.

In this discussion I am deliberate in my emphasis not only on the dying but also on the surviving. In the Hindu ethos, death is a concern not only for the dying, but also for those close to them. Understanding people are ever-so-conscious of this dimension, and carefully conceal or reveal the facts about the condition of a seriously-ill person. There is no pretense about concealing the facts from the dying, and the physician's task is to nurture the will to live in the dying. The will may be sapped by a physician's declaration of helplessness. A physician usually informs the family by a not-so-cryptic message about the need to call to the bedside "all those who need to be present." The impending death is not explicitly pronounced because words have power, the naming of death may invite death quickly. Carstairs relates an incident in which, unaware of the taboo against explicit articulation of the dire prognosis, his counsel to the family of a dying patient invited gentle censure (Carstairs, 1955).

It is difficult to imagine a controversy either between the ethicist and the physician or between the family and the physician on an issue like the DO NOT RESUSCITATE orders. A person should generally be allowed to die peacefully, for artificially or mechanically-sustained life is of little value. In any case, most people prefer to and do die in their own beds. I am reminded of my naivete during my internship when I was working at a small-town hospital. A young boy, acutely ill, was brought by the parents. He was diagnosed as having an intestinal obstruction (intussusception) and had to be operated at once. The father refused to give consent, averring that he wanted his son to die in his hands and at home. I tagged along with the departing family, and pleaded with him to give the boy a chance to avert what was otherwise certain death. My success in bringing the boy to the operating table was short-lived. He died on the table. And I had to announce the death to the family. The sad and accusing eyes of the father still stare at me.

Notes

1. The system is called Allopathy in India. Dunn has suggested the term 'Cosmopolitan' (Dunn, 1977).

2. Kane's *History of Dharmasastra* is the most comprehensive work on all the texts, and remains the best available source for an in-depth understanding of the *dharmasastra* literature.

3. Acquiring knowledge, especially of *dharma* through the study of scriptures, remaining celibate, and serving one's teacher are the principal dictates of the first stage. Getting married, having children, tending to livelihood, and participating in the general social life in the second stage and disengagement from active social life and reflecting in the solitude of a forest are the aims of the third stage. The *sannyasin* or renouncer sheds his previous identity including his sacred thread, is free from all social context, and spends the last years of life in meditation and penance seeking liberation.

4. Both cited in *The Mythology of All Races* (1964).

Primary References

Astangahridaya. Gujarati translation by Vijayshankar Munshi, Sastu Sahitya Vardhak Karyalaya, Ahmedabad, 1983.

The Bhagavadgita in the Mahabharata. Translated by J. A. B. Van Buitenen, University of Chicago Press, Chicago, 1981.

Bhavaprakash. Gujarati translation by Girijashankar Shastri, Sastu Sahitya Vardhak Karyalaya, Ahmedabad, 1981.

Carakasamhita. Translated by Priyavat Sharma, Chaukhambha Orientalia, Varanasi, 1981.

Mahabharata. Translated by J. A. B. Van Buitenen, University of Chicago Press, Chicago, 1973.

Rig Veda. Translated by Wendy O'Flaherty, Penguin Books, New York, 1981.

Susrutasamhita. Gujarati translation by Kalidas Shastri. Sastu Sahitya Vardhak Karyalaya, Ahmedabad, 1974.

Secondary References

Carstairs, M.: 1955, 'Medicine and faith in rural Rajasthan, in P. Benjamin (ed.), *Health, Culture and Community*, Russell Sage Foundation, New York.

Carstairs, M.: 1956, '*Hinjra and jiryan:* Two derivatives of Hindu attitude to sexuality', *British Journal of Medical Psychology* 29, 128–138.

Chandrasekhar, S.: 1974, *Abortion in a Crowded World: The Problem of Abortion with Special Reference to India*, Allen and Unwin, London.

Chattopadhyaya, D.: 1977, *Science and Society in Ancient India*. Research India Publications, Calcutta.

Collins, A. and Desai, P.: 1986, 'Selfhood in context: Some Indian solutions', in M. White and S. Pollak (eds.), *Cultural Transition*. Routledge and Kegan Paul, Boston.

Dasgupta, S.: 1975, *A History of India Philosophy*, Vol. II. Motilal Banarsidass, Delhi.

Desai, P.: 1982, 'Learning psychotherapy: A cultural perspective', *Journal of Operational Psychiatry* 13 (2), 82–87.

Desai, P.: forthcoming, *Health/Medicine in the Hindu Tradition*.

Dunn, F.: 1977, 'Traditional Asian medicine and cosmopolitan medicine as adaptive systems', in C. Leslie (ed,), *Asian Medical Systems*. University of California Press, Berkeley.

Eliade, M.: 1987, 'Indian religions: An overview', in Mircea Eliade (ed.), *Encyclopedia of Religions*, Vol.7. MacMillan and Co. New York.

Kane, P.: 1974, *History of Dharmasastra*. 5 Vols. Bhandarkar Oriental Research Institute, Poona.

Karve, I.: 1962, 'The Indian social organization: an anthropological study', in Desai et al. (eds.), *The Cultural Heritage of India*, Vol. II. Ramakrishna.

Mission, Calcutta.

Keith, A. Berriedale, ed.: 1964, *The Mythology of All Races*, Vol. VI., Cooper Square, New York.

Marriott, M.: 1976, 'Hindu transactions: diversity without dualism', in B. Kapferer (ed.), *Transactions and Meaning: Directions in Anthropology and Exchange and Symbolic Behaviors* Institute for the Study of Human Issues, Philadelphia.

Marriott, M.: 1980, 'The Open Hindu person and interpersonal fluidity', Unpublished manuscript.

Marriott, M., and Inden, R.: 1976, 'Toward an ethnosociology of south Asian caste system', in K. David (ed.), *The New Wind: Changing Identities in South Asia*, Aldine Publishing Co. Chicago.

Mahabharata. Translated by J. A. B. Von Buitenen, University of Chicago Press, Chicago, 1973.

Miller, B.: 1981, *The Endangered Sex: Neglect of Female Children in Rural North India*, Cornell University Press, Ithaca.

Nandy, A.: 1980, *Alternative Sciences*, Allied Publishers Private Limited, New Delhi.

Raghavan, V., and Danderkar, R. N.: 1958, 'Hinduism', in T. Bany et al. (eds.), *Sources of Indian Tradition*, Columbia University Press, New York.

Shukla, S.: 1987, 'Amniocentesis and the women's movement in India', lecture sponsored by India Alert, Chicago, Illinois, July.

Venkatramani, S. H.: 1986, 'Female infanticide: born to die', in *India Today*. New Delhi, June 15 (International Edition).

Weiss, M.: 1980, '*Caraka Samhita* on the doctrine of *Karma*', in W. O'Flaherty (ed.), *Karma and Rebirth in Classical Indian Traditions*. University of California Press, Berkeley.

Winternitz, M.: 1967, *History of Indian Literature*. Translated by Subhadra Jha, Vol. III Motilal Banarsidass, Delhi.

Oath of Initiation

From the Caraka Samhita

──────────── INTRODUCTION TO READING ────────────

The ancient oath from the Caraka Samhita of which Prakash Desai spoke deserves closer examination. The translation presented here is by A. Menon and H. F. Haberman. It reveals some uniquely Hindu elements such as the obligation to remain celibate, eat no meat, and carry no arms. Characteristic of Hindu thought, there is an explicit prohibition on causing another's death. There are some passages remarkably similar to Hippocratic commitments (the commitment to be devoted entirely to being helpful to the patient), but there are also some dramatic contrasts.

Note especially the requirements that "No persons who are hated by the king or who are haters of the king or who are hated by the public or who are haters of the public shall receive treatment." An understanding of the Hindu doctrine of karma, of rebirth in a position based on the way one has led his previous life, may be necessary to understand the moral meaning of such a sentence.

---

1.   The teacher then should instruct the disciple in the presence of the sacred fire, Brahmanas [Brahmins] and physicians.

2.   [saying] "Thou shalt lead the life of a celibate, grow thy hair and beard, speak only the truth, eat no meat, eat only pure articles of food, be free from envy and carry no arms.

3.   There shall be nothing that thou should not do at my behest except hating the king, causing another's death, or committing an act of great unrighteousness or acts leading to calamity.

4.   Thou shalt dedicate thyself to me and regard me as thy chief. Thou shalt be subject to me and conduct thyself for ever for my welfare and pleasure. Thou shalt serve and dwell with me like a son or a slave or a supplicant. Thou shalt behave and act without arrogance, with care and attention and with undistracted mind, humility, constant reflection and ungrudging obedience. Acting either at my behest or otherwise, though shalt conduct thyself for the achievement of thy teacher's purposes alone, to the best of thy abilities.

5.   If thou desirest success, wealth and fame as a physician and heaven after death, thou shalt pray for the welfare of all creatures beginning with the cows and Brahmanas.

6.   Day and night, however thou mayest be engaged, thou shalt endeavor for the relief of patients with all thy heart and soul. Thou shalt not desert or injure thy patient for the sake of thy life or thy living. Thou shalt not commit adultery even in thought. Even so, thou shalt not covet others' possessions. Thou shalt be modest in thy affirm and appearance. Thou shouldst not be a drunkard or a sinful man nor shouldst thou associate with the abettors of crimes. Thou shouldst speak words that are gentle, pure and righteous, pleasing, worthy, true, wholesome, and moderate. Thy behavior must be in consideration of time and place and heedful of past experience. Thou shalt act always with a view to the acquisition of knowledge and fullness of equipment.

7.   No persons, who are hated by the king or who are haters of the king or who are hated by the public or who are haters of the public, shall receive treatment. Similarly, those who are extremely abnormal, wicked, and of miserable character and conduct, those who have not vindicated their honor, those who are on the point of death, and similarly women who are unattended by their husbands or guardians shall not receive treatment.

8.   No offering of presents by a woman without the behest of her husband or guardian shall be accepted by thee. While entering the patient's

house, thou shalt be accompanied by a man who is known to the patient and who has his permission to enter; and thou shalt be well-clad, bent of head, self-possessed, and conduct thyself only after repeated consideration. Thou shalt thus properly make thy entry. Having entered, thy speech, mind, intellect and senses shall be entirely devoted to no other thought than that of being helpful to the patient and of things concerning only him. The peculiar customs of the patient's household shall not be made public. Even knowing that the patient's span of life has come to its close, it shall not be mentioned by thee there, where if so done, it would cause shock to the patient or to others. Though possessed of knowledge one should not boast very much of one's knowledge. Most people are offended by the boastfulness of even those who are otherwise good and authoritative.

9. There is no limit at all to the Science of Life, Medicine. So thou shouldst apply thyself to it with diligence. This is how thou shouldst act. Also thou shouldst learn the skill of practice from another without carping. The entire world is the teacher to the intelligent and the foe to the unintelligent. Hence, knowing this well, thou shouldst listen and act according to the words of instruction of even an unfriendly person, when his words are worthy and of a kind as to bring to you fame, long life, strength and prosperity."

10. Thereafter the teacher should say this—"Thou shouldst conduct thyself properly with the gods, sacred fire, Brahmanas, the guru, the aged, the scholars and the preceptors. If thou has conducted thyself well with them, the precious stones, the grains and the gods become well disposed towards thee." To the teacher that has spoken thus, the disciple should say, "Amen."

JAPAN AND BUDDHISM

The 17 Rules of Enjuin
(For Disciples in Our School)

——————INTRODUCTION TO READING——————

Traditional Japanese medical ethics draws both on Buddhist thought and indigenous Shinto tradition. One example comes from the sixteenth century when an approach to disease commonly known as the *Ri-shu* school was widely practiced. A code known as the Seventeen Rules of Enjuin was drawn up by practitioners of this medical art. Note that similar to the Hippocratic Oath, there is a notion that medical knowledge can be very dangerous. It is disseminated only to members of the school and to no others. These rules even go so far as to require that if a practitioner dies or ceases to practice, he must return his books to the school so that they will not fall into the hands of untrained persons. The view of knowledge, quite consistent with the Hippocratic tradition, stands in dramatic contrast with the ethics of Protestantism, which places great emphasis on entrusting the texts to the lay person, and with secular liberalism, which insists that lay persons should be reasonably informed about the nature of treatments and the consequences thereof.

---

1. Each person should follow the path designated by Heaven (Buddha, the Gods).
2. You should always be kind to people. You should always be devoting and loving.
3. The teaching of Medicine should be restricted to selected persons.
4. You should not tell others what you are taught, regarding treatments without permission.
5. You should not establish association with doctors who do not belong to this school.
6. All the successors and descendants of the disciples of this school shall follow the teachers' ways.
7. If any disciples cease the practice of Medicine, or, if successors are not found at the death of the disciple, all the medical books of this school should be returned to the SCHOOL OF ENJUIN.
8. You should not kill living creatures, nor should you admire hunting or fishing.
9. In our school, teaching about poisons is prohibited, nor should you receive instructions about poisons from other physicians. Moreover, you should not give abortives to the people.
10. You should rescue even such patients as you dislike or hate. You should do virtuous acts, but in such a way that they do not become known to people. To do good deeds secretly is a mark of virtue.
11. You should not exhibit avarice and you must not strain to become famous. You should not rebuke or reprove a patient, even if he does not present you with money or goods in gratitude.
12. You should be delighted if, after treating a patient without success, the patients receives medicine from another physician, and is cured.
13. You should not speak ill of other physicians.
14. You should not tell what you have learned from the time you enter a woman's room, and, moreover, you should not have obscene or immoral feelings when examining a woman.
15. Proper or not, you should not tell others what you have learned in lectures, or what you have learned about prescribing medicine.

16. You should not like undue extravagance. If you like such living, your avarice will increase, and you will lose the ability to be kind to others.
17. If you do not keep the rules and regulations of this school, then you will be cancelled as a disciple. In more severe cases, the punishment will be greater.[1]

Note

1. William O. Reinhardt provided this translation.

Buddhism, Zen, and Bioethics

Kathleen Nolan

―――――――――――――INTRODUCTION TO READING―――――――――――

In the following selection, Kathleen Nolan, an American physician who has served on the staff of the Hastings Center and studied at the Zen Mountain Monastery, Mt. Tremper, New York, takes a sophisticated look at the complex relationship between Buddhism and bioethics.

First, Nolan starts with what is perhaps the most important issue in constructing a view of any Buddhist ethics—whether it is at all plausible to speak of a Buddhist ethics in the first place. She recognizes from the outset that Buddhist principles, particularly that of "Itsunyata"or emptiness, makes it difficult to speak of an absolute system of beliefs. She goes on to argue, however, that the primacy of moral conduct is indeed inherent to Buddhist thought.

Nolan also clearly recognizes that the diversity of Buddhist thought makes it difficult to make categorical statements about a Buddhist bioethics. In accordance with this recognition, Nolan consistently presents a variety of different Buddhist viewpoints throughout the article.

Finally, Nolan does an excellent job of bridging past with present, allowing the reader to understand the significance of Buddhism in contemporary terms with explicit reference to long-standing tradition.

Things are not what they seem.
Nor are they otherwise.
—*Traditional Buddhist Saying*

Because of Buddhism's central focus on transcendental enlightenment, it is sometimes portrayed as a religion that is antithetical, or at least indifferent, to worldly concerns, including ethics. Buddhist scholars and teachers sometimes contribute to such misconceptions, especially in relation to the branch of Buddhism known as Zen (Chinese, *Ch'an*; Indian, *dhyana*), which was introduced to Americans by Zen master D.T. Suzuki in the early part of the twentieth century as an amoral (i.e., non-moral) discipline. These misconceptions are no doubt exaggerated by attempts to articulate the differences between Buddhism and other religions, which often emphasize Buddhists' reliance on direct personal experience, rather than rules or argumentation, as the touchstone of religious and ethical truth. From this avowedly mystical perspective, inquiry into standards of ethical conduct may appear to be unnecessary, and an arbitrary character may appear to be engendered in morality itself.

This is an erroneous conclusion, as modern Buddhist teachers and scholars have begun to recognize ([65];[30];[50];[54];[99]). Early Buddhist texts clearly stress the primacy of ethics, placing morality first among the three central doctrines of the Buddha's teachings—sila (morality), *samadhi* (concentration), and *prajna* (wisdom) ([83], p. 57). Morality is primary, not only because of the dangers of practicing concentration without a thorough moral grounding, but also because the Buddha's Middle Way, or Noble Eightfold Path, was formulated as a "a radical critique of wishful thinking and the myriad tactics of escapism" prevalent in his day, and, indeed, in our own ([29], p. 7). Despite its mystical character, Buddhism is thus an extremely practical religion, a religion of the present life and of the present moment [75]. In fact, enlightenment itself can be understood as wisdom (awakening to the true nature of reality) expressed in the activity of compassion. Moral conduct thus forms the foundation for all spiritual attainment ([78], p. 46), and enlightenment without morality is not true enlightenment ([65], p. 133).

However, many Buddhist teachers have expressed considerable reluctance towards the formulation of analytical systems in which ethics becomes an object. of inquiry independent of enlightenment itself ([32];[57]). As Zen master Soyen Shaku once put it,"Buddhism has nothing to do with utilitarianism or intuitionism or hedonism or what not" ([85], p. 71). This avoidance of systematic analysis bears further exploration, not only because it is potentially quite frustrating to non-Buddhist scholars, but also because it offers important insights into Buddhist moral teachings.

Emptiness, Ethics, and Enlightenment

One of the major themes of early Buddhist scripture was the avoidance of religious controversy and ideological debate [16]. The historical Buddha urged his followers not to become attached even to his own teachings and to avoid denigrating the views of others. Stressing the importance of each person's individual spiritual inquiry, he urged: "Do not accept anything because of report, tradition, hearsay, the handing on in the sacred texts, or as a result of logic or inference, through indulgent tolerance of views, appearance of likelihood, or as paying respect to a teacher" ([83], p. 43).

Consistent with such teachings, the Buddha himself often side-stepped contentious religious questions, either responding indirectly or reinterpreting the question in terms of internal attitudes and virtues[16]. Noting a similar tendency in the thirteenth century Zen mystic Dogen Zenji and other Buddhist teachers, Thomas Kasulis therefore argues that Buddhism establishes a virtue ethics, with a central focus on the moral person, rather than the moral act [50].

This is not an unreasonable interpretation. Buddhist texts do stress the importance of moral virtues ("perfections"), including generosity, tolerance, truthfulness, and vigor [100];[83]. Moreover, many Buddhists accept both the Noble Eightfold Path and the basic Buddhist precepts (see below) as simple, straightforward, practical guides to leading a virtuous life.

On the other hand, it might equally well be argued that reliance on the precepts gives Buddhism a strongly deontological flavor [14]. Alternatively, Buddhism could be understood in consequentialist terms, given its emphasis on *karma* (volitional actions, whether good or evil) and the importance of accepting responsibility for our actions [23]. Buddhism could also be understood as offering a narrative ethics, with its teachings couched primarily in stories, such as those found in the sutras and in Zen's famous *koans* (apparently paradoxical utterances used in meditation to cut through tangles of discursive thought and thus allow transcendental insight) [59]. Or again, based on its teachings regarding the co-origination and interpenetration of all beings, Buddhism could be portrayed as one of the earliest examples of an ethics of relationships ([42];[56].

To force Buddhist ethics into these—or other—categories, however, is to risk missing the point of the Buddha's exhortations regarding authority, even (or perhaps, especially) the authority of intellectual constructs. Categories like these manifest an inherent tendency toward dichotomization and self reification; they can therefore separate morality into observer and observed and falsely imply that definition and description completely capture the "essence" of moral experience. By employing teaching methods that avoid this sort of hypostatization, Buddhism emphasizes its grounding in the formlessness or emptiness of all existence (*sunyata*).

Emptiness—the absence of an independent and abiding essence—is perhaps the most problematic concept in Buddhism; yet, it is often used as a synonym for enlightenment, and it may be said to be the "fundamental realization from which ethics and other human virtues originate" [86]; see also [42] and [56]. Frequently misunderstood as a state of blankness or vacuity [67], emptiness in a Buddhist context instead refers to an experience of reality that is direct and immediate, "empty of concepts, and therefore vivid and dynamic" ([29], p. 81).

This seemingly paradoxical "fullness" of emptiness forms the basis for Buddhist teachings regarding the unity and interrelatedness of all being: form is no other than emptiness, emptiness no other than form. Oneness and differentiation exist simultaneously and interpenetrate perfectly in a co-dependence that is "dynamic and multiple rather than static and single" ([56], p. 248). Such wholeness is conceptually unfathomable, but it finds modern metaphors in such phenomena as holograms (in which every piece of these special laser photographs is reflected and contained by every earlier piece) and quantum physic's theory of nonlocal interaction (in which subatomic particles light years "apart" communicate instantaneously as part of a coordinated and indivisible universe) [95].

Anticipating these modern discoveries by nearly 2,500 years, early Mahayana Buddhists described reality in terms of the "Diamond Net of Indra," in which every particle of the universe contains and reflects all others, and in which nothing is static or fixed [19]. For Buddhists, morality is action in accord with this reality compassion, based on a realization of emptiness, or "no-self." Again, this is not nihilistic, nor should it be understood as simple altruism; to act compassionately is to be in harmony with all beings. Compassionate activity flows naturally from the experience of enlightenment and constitutes the life of a Buddha [65].

Despite the unfamiliar terminology, this philosophical description of Buddhist ethics—in which concentration, wisdom, and morality are inextricably linked, and all are intrinsically empty, without an abiding essence—is neither totally foreign to Western thought [51] nor inherently amoral ([65], p. 144;[18], pp. 5–6). Translated into Western philosophical terms (and with a grateful nod to Heraclitus), we might say that epistemology, ontology, and ethics are inextricably linked, and that all are in flux in a state of becoming rather than being. Noted biologist and philosopher Hans Jonas has recently made precisely such an argument, devoting special attention to the importance of this formulation for resolving the "is/ought" dichotomy that haunts most Western ethical systems [43].

The Buddhist Precepts

Elaborating on Buddhist ethics intellectually cannot substitute for actually manifesting compassionate activity. There is an often told story of a thirteenth century Chinese poet-statesman who asked the most renowned Buddhist monk of his time to instruct him in the essentials of Buddhist doctrine. The monk agreed and replied by reciting a version of the Three Pure Precepts: "Do no evil, do good, and purify your heart." The Chinese poet was indignant, declaring that he was interested in the highest and most fundamental teachings, not something known to every small child. The monk observed, "Known to every child but even a silvery-haired man fails to put it into practice." Abashed, the poet returned home to meditate ([85], pp. 69–70).

Indeed, simplicity is among the highest Buddhist virtues, especially in the area of morality. The correct "answer" to a moral question is generally viewed as less important than what the issue can teach the individuals involved about the nature of reality. There are no ethical dogmas and no central authority or governing body to "represent" or "speak for" Buddhism. Even the so-called Buddhist precepts (see Table 1) are generally considered guides to enlightened behavior rather than externally imposed rules of conduct.

However, the interpretation and use of the precepts serves to distinguish between the various schools of Buddhism [8]. The Theravada school (predominant in Thailand, Cambodia, Laos, and Vietnam) generally takes a more literalistic and prescriptive stance than do other schools, such as the Mahayana, out of which Zen arises, and the Vajrayana, as typified by some forms of Tantric and Tibetan Buddhism. For these latter schools, the vow to end the suffering of all beings takes precedence over any dogmatic adherence to rules ([31];[8]), and the precepts must function in accord with particular circumstances ([65], pp. 140–141;[11], p. 202;[1]).

Table 1
BASIC BUDDHIST PRECEPTS
(Mahayana Tradition)

The Three Refuges
    I take refuge in the Buddha
    I take refuge in the Dharma
    I take refuge in the Sangha

The Three Pure Precepts
    Not doing evil
    Doing good
    Actualizing good for others

The Ten Grave Precepts
1. Affirm life; do not kill
2. Be giving; do not steal
3. Honor the body; do not misuse sexuality
4. Manifest truth; do not lie
5. Proceed clearly; do not cloud the mind
6. See the perfection; do not speak of others' errors and faults
7. Realize self and other as one; do not elevate the self and blame others
8. Give generously; do not be withholding
9. Actualize harmony; do not be angry
10. Experience the intimacy of things; do not defile the Three Treasures (i.e., the Buddha, Dharma, and the Sangha)

—(After Loori, Eight Gates)

The differences among the various schools of Buddhism can become quite pronounced when the precepts are called into service to deal with modern ethical and bioethical dilemmas. Buddhist morality also presents itself differently in different cultures, adapting itself to the vessel that contains it [92]. Moreover, many Buddhist authors offer their views without identifying themselves as coming from a specific culture or school of Buddhism, creating confusion about what "Buddhism" actually has to say about a given topic [44].

Within the context of the tradition, the absence of such labels and distinctions does not seem to present a major problem, perhaps because it is understood that individual Buddhists speak only from their own experience. An appreciation for diversity also follows naturally from Buddhist ontology, as well as from the historical Buddha's emphasis on tolerance and respect for the views of others. Nonetheless, as Buddhists from various schools and cultures enter the dialogues of modern bioethics, it may be useful to note the different contexts from which certain positions are or might be articulated.

I. Reproductive Technology

> *Open your hand, it becomes a cloud; turn it over, rain.*
> —*Zen saying*

Several recent books and articles have addressed issues of sexuality and reproduction from an avowedly Buddhist perspective. Four topics raised in these materials are germane to bioethics: non-coital reproduction; sexuality (including homosexuality); contraception; and abortion.

Non-Coital Reproduction

Very little has yet been written by Buddhists about the "technological" (i.e., non-coital) aspects of reproductive technologies, perhaps because Buddhists have traditionally considered all aspects of nature open to analysis, understanding, and compassionate use; in Buddhism there is nothing "mystically sacrosanct" ([33], p. 55). Buddhist monks, for example, have participated in extensive neurophysiological studies of their practice of meditation, and the Dalai Lama once remarked that if studies in neuroscience or other disciplines revealed errors in Buddhist conceptions about the nature of mind, he would gladly correct the Buddhist teachings ([33], p. 117).

Most Buddhists would presumably extend a similar attitude toward noncoital reproduction. As summarized by Shoyo Taniguchi:

> As long as technology brings benefits to the couple who wishes to have a child, and as long as it does not bring pain or suffering to any parties involved, Buddhism would find no conflict in applying and using modern biotechnology. This is a basic Buddhist standpoint ([94], p. 661).

Avoiding pain and suffering, however, is not always easily accomplished. Early Buddhist texts stress the importance of maintaining the solidarity of families and lay out duties of children to their parents and parents to their children ([83], pp. 117–119). These are primarily social duties, arising from the interconnections of the family. Children, for example, were said to owe an unconditional obligation to their mothers in particular, because of the generosity and compassion manifested in accepting the risks of pregnancy and delivery ([25], p. 71). Thus, in considering the harms that might result from such tech-

niques as donor insemination and surrogate motherhood, it would seem necessary to take into account not only physical risks but also any confusion or pain
resulting from disruption of family relationships experienced by the donors,
recipients, or resulting offspring ([76];[7]).

Buddhist teachers, especially those in the Zen tradition, might also be
expected to use questions about the use of non-coital reproductive techniques
as an occasion to probe basic issues such as the nature of sexual impulses, the
origins of procreative desires, the workings of karma, and the meaning of
compassion. As discussed in the sections that follow, these issues have recently
been explored in some detail.

Sexuality

Presentations of Buddhist attitudes toward sexuality can range from the puritanical and ascetic to the promiscuous and unrestrained [90]. The puritanical
perspective views sexual drives as ensnaring passions, a source of grief and
bondage, and a hindrance to enlightenment. On this view, sexual passion is "a
negative force stirring up an unending flow of wants and needs" ([90], p. 22), a
state of desire that should be suppressed or controlled in the pursuit of non-
attachment. Early Buddhist monastics struggled to follow the Buddha's example of celibacy and frequently meditated on the loathsomeness of the body in
an attempt to free themselves from its enticements.

Some Buddhists express the other extreme, using Tantric disciplines to
redirect and transform sexual desires as an aid to enlightenment. Tantra has
been commended as an approach based upon "the affirmation of life in all its
forms and the validity of the phenomenal world; the innate purity of natural
conditions; . . . the body as a microcosm of the universe; and the necessity of
realizing the truth in this present mode of existence" ([90], p. 60). Sadly,
genuine Tantra has frequently been confused with and sullied by untrained and
self-serving attempts to master its profound mysteries.

Mahayana Buddhism steers a middle way between these two extremes,
recognizing that human sexual urges can lead to deluded, self-centered actions,
yet appreciating that these same drives can form the basis for life-giving and
life-affirming intimacy ([2], pp. 37–48;[65], p. 139). Zen, in particular, has been
characterized as "Tantra purified of excess" ([90], p. 85). As expressed by Zen
teacher Robert Aitken Roshi:

> The sexual drive is part of the human path of self-realization. With our
> modern, relatively permissive sexual mores, we have increased opportunity
> to explore our human nature through sexual relationships. At the same
> time, or course, there is more opportunity for self-centered people to use
> sex as a means for personal power. The path you choose rises from your
> fundamental purpose. Why are you here? ([2] p. 41).

Celibacy formed a central part of the monastic tradition in China and
southeast Asia, but Japanese Buddhism embraced a married priesthood, and
members of the lay Buddhist community have always been expected to attain

enlightenment "within the context of ordinary existence (which, of course, includes the sexual dimension)" ([90]; p. 50). Although celibacy is still an option, many American Buddhist communities have followed the Japanese example, accepting responsible sexual activity in both the lay and monastic communities.

The path of sexual responsibility presumably offers itself to all who seek to realize and manifest Buddha nature ([2], pp. 37–48). However, in the early days of Buddhism, homosexual activity was officially condemned by both the puritan and the Tantric traditions ([90], pp. 139–140, and homosexuals were denied ordination, apparently because it was believed they could not or would not control their sexual behavior [101]. Yet the extent to which special disapprobation fell on homosexual as opposed to heterosexual drives and activities is not clear [101]. For example, the monastic rules for celibate monks (*Vinaya*) proscribe homosexual activity as a breach of the monastic vow, but such activities do not seem to have been singled out as especially evil or immoral: ". . . if a monk's penis enters any orifice of a human being (female, male, hermaphrodite, or eunuch), a nonhuman (demon or ghost), or an animal, even if the penetration is only the length of a sesame seed, it is grounds for expulsion (from the Order of Celibates)" ([90], p. 33).

Nor is it clear how much, if any, condemnation continues at present time. Asked for his opinion on the morality of homosexual activity, the Dalai Lama reportedly replied, "Sex is sex". Similarly, Aitken Roshi observes that Buddha nature is neither heterosexual nor homosexual, yet, at the same time, it is both heterosexual and homosexual ([2], p. 42). Thus, although Buddhist scholar and translator John Stevens suggests that acceptance of homosexuality remains controversial ([2], pp. 139–140), modern Buddhist sexual ethics seems to emphasize the integrity rather than the form of sexual activities, placing a central focus on avoiding sex that is self-serving or disregarding of others ([65], p. 139;[2], pp. 37–48;[90], pp. 140–141).

Contraception

One of the potential harms associated with sexual activity is the conception of an unwanted child. Early Tibetan Buddhists had knowledge of both temporary and permanent contraceptives, but apparently discouraged contraception as a possible interference in the workings of karma ([26] (cited in [90]). On the other hand, the necessity for birth control was always tacitly acknowledged, and various methods of contraception were regularly employed: "abstention from sex (the rhythm method), control of the male's ejaculation, and from the time of the Buddha, birth control pills" ([2], p. 139).

Some of the concerns about the use of contraceptives may have related to matters of safety. While providing abortifacients to pregnant women was forbidden under the *Vinaya* (see below), preparing fertility or contraceptive potions was apparently punished only if the woman who used the preparation died ([2], p. 35 (citing [38]). Although the early Buddhists opposed the taking of life, including prenatal life, marriage and reproduction held no privileged place within the tradition; in fact, these were generally considered secular rather than religious concerns, and there was "a decisive turning away from the [religious] sanctioning of fertility" ([58], p. 21).

These attitudes followed Buddhism as it moved into Southeast Asia, China, and Japan, and gradually evolved into a justification of contraception, so long as it was not used to promote a promiscuous life-style but rather as an aid to family planning and as a means to prevent personal, economic, or social suffering ([58], p. 116). As articulated by Shoyo Taniguchi, a modern Buddhist who writes primarily from a Theravada perspective, prevention of an unwanted pregnancy is justified because "Buddhism does not teach procreation as the essential purpose of marriage" ([94], p. 64). Indeed, intentional contraception may be seen as a form of skillful action:

> . . . Here we can make use of the Buddhist theory of Cause and Effect or of Dependent Co-Arising (aticcasamuppada). The principle of this doctrine is given in a short formula of four lines: "When this is, that is. This arising, that arises. When this is not, that is not. This ceasing, that ceases." Simply put, it means that when the causes and conditions co-exist, there is always its effect. If the causes and conditions do not exist, there is no effect.

> From this teaching, it is possible to draw the following conclusion: If one does not want to have a certain effect conditioned by certain causes, one should prevent the necessary conditions from falling together ([94], p. 64).

Modern Zen teacher John Daido Loori offers a different analysis. He focuses his inquiry on the nature of responsible and compassionate sexuality, using the third precept ("Honor the body; do not misuse sexuality") to thrust the question of what constitutes a violation back on the individuals involved ([65], p. 139). Similarly, Robert Aitken Roshi raises questions about personal vulnerability and our acceptance of cultural attitudes toward sexuality. Speaking of the risks inherent in sexual union, he implies that relying solely on contraceptives for protection is insufficient:

> . . . In my view we must acknowledge that sex and fertility cannot be dissociated, whatever mechanical means we may use as birth control. Unwanted pregnancy is a painful reminder of biologically determined nature at work in our bodies; karma that cannot be evaded. . . . ([2], p.45).

Thus, in keeping with his translation of the third precept as "no boorish sex" ([2], p. 37), Aitken Roshi identifies the most important safeguard for sexual activity to be selfless commitment—the cultivation of a life of true intimacy with another, in harmony with others.

II. Abortion

An old Buddhist story tells of two disciples who were having an argument and sought out their teacher to resolve the matter. The first argued that wholehearted effort and strict discipline is necessary to abandon old habits and awaken to the spiritual life. "You're right", said the master. But the second disciple immediately objected, arguing that the true spiritual path is one of surrender, of letting go, and therefore cannot be obtained by effort. "You're right", said the master. A third disciple, overhearing this, remarked, "But they can't both be right, Master". To which the master replied with a smile, "And you're right, too".

This is what is most poignant about the highly charged and contentious character of the modern abortion debate: that almost every argument—pro and con—seems to emerge from the wellsprings of human sensitivity and compassion. Then, too, very few people realize how much consensus there is about some of the most fundamental issues; for example, over 70% of the U.S. population (in repeated polls over the last two decades) believe that having an abortion involves taking a human life, *and* that abortion should remain a legal option for women who feel they need it.

If Buddhism has something to contribute to the abortion debate, perhaps it is as a voice for this silenced majority, creating a space for honest inquiry into the roots of ambivalence, a place where truth can be spoken without being viewed as a betrayal of either the pro-life or the pro-choice platform. This is certainly the message of Helen Tworkov, editor of *Tricyle*, the nation's leading Buddhist periodical, in her article "Anti-abortion/Pro-choice: Taking Both Sides" [97]. As Tworkov observes, "Everything important about life is important about abortion . . ." ([97], p. 61), and ". . . dharma teachings can be used to validate either pro-choice or anti-abortion politics" ([97], p. 67). She continues:

> For this very reason, abortion places American Buddhists at the crossroads of Western and Eastern perception of the individual, society, and what liberation is all about. Anyone considering abortion from Buddhist teachings—and not from political peer pressure—is thrown back again and again on interpretation and view, on self-analysis and ambiguity. This is Buddhism at its most instructive, demanding an authentic confrontation with oneself ([97], p. 67).

Authentic confrontation begins with the realization that some Buddhists, especially those within the Theravada and Pure Land traditions, view the Buddha's teachings as much less ambiguous and open to interpretation than Tworkov suggests ([94];[32]; [55]). For example, in summarizing Buddhist attitudes toward sexual ethics, John Stevens has noted that, until recent times, the Buddhist position against abortion was quite clear-cut ([90], pp. 138–139). Early Buddhist embryology was quite sophisticated, and participating in abortion was considered a violation of the first precept ("Affirm life; do not kill"), as well as the destruction of a potential Buddha ([26] (cited in 90]). Under the *Vinaya* providing an abortifacient to a pregnant woman was clearly considered murder ([90], p. 139). More recently, Shoyo Taniguchi has given careful attention to other, "particularly Buddhistic," reasons (such as the accumulation of negative karma) for discouraging abortion as an unskillful and harmful response to an unwanted pregnancy ([94], p. 62).

Yet one of Tworkov's main points is that few Buddhists—including those who are pro-choice—would dispute these facts. As she observes:

Among my friends, one consistent difference keeps emerging: non-Buddhists argue, in sweeping socio-economic and historic terms, for pro-choice as the touchstone of women's lives. But when it comes to whether or not the fetus qualifies as life, convincing dialectics often collapse into sighs and hesitation. On the other hand, Buddhist practitioners seem to accept that abortion at any stage, unequivocally, means the taking of life ([97], p. 63).

Given that abortion means the taking of life, the central question for Buddhists, especially for those within the Mahayana and Vajrayana traditions, is "What is the most compassionate action?" For the pregnant woman herself, this means honest and intimate consideration of whether a decision to prevent birth can be made, "on balance with other elements of suffering" ([2], p. 22). To violate the first precept in this setting is no small matter, but to fail to violate it when compassion demands it also generates its own karma ([49], p. 228;[82], p. 376). One becomes heir to whatever one does ([94], p. 62).

Some Buddhists view abortion as a "necessary sorrow" ([57], p. 532), since the practice of compassion is not a practice of perfection, at least as perfection is usually understood:

. . . We take vows to be where the suffering is. In terms of abortion, this means staying open to the suffering of a woman faced with an unwanted pregnancy, to her lover who may or may not want the child, to the suffering of an aborted fetus, to the suffering of an unwanted baby ([97], p. 68).

As Aitken Roshi says, "Once the decision [to abort] is made, there is no blame, but rather acknowledgment that sadness pervades the whole universe . . ." ([2], p. 22).

Because Buddhist priests have, at least in recent years, expressed sympathy for parents who have chosen to abort, performing funeral services and other memorial rituals for aborted fetuses, Buddhism has been viewed as relatively "soft" on abortion [57]. However, as William LaFleur has argued, the very presence of such rituals may reinforce a sense of intimacy with the fetus and thus serve to prevent people from becoming inured to abortion ([57];[58], pp. 204–206). The mizuko kuyo rituals of Japanese Buddhists seem designed to express both gratitude and apology to the aborted fetus (as well as Shintoistic notions of purification and appeasement), thereby establishing a continuing relationship with the parents and relieving their burden of guilt ([57];[58];[88]).

In reinterpreting these rituals for Westerners, Aitken Roshi emphasizes the importance of maintaining compassion for all those involved and of saying farewell to this incomplete but individual and human "child unborn" ([2], pp. 21–22, pp. 175–176). At the same time, he remains always the Zen teacher, using the occasion to raise questions about these profound mysteries, life and death—the passage of waves "on the great ocean of true nature, which is not born and does not pass away" ([2], p. 175).

III. Termination of Treatment

When it comes—just so!
When it goes—just so!
Both coming and going occur each day.
The words I am speaking now—just so!
—*Death poem of Zen Priest Musho Josho, 1306*

Because Buddhism offers a discipline for experiencing the joys and sorrows of life fully and unconditionally, it teaches the possibility of dying simply, clearly, and compassionately. Realizing that life and death are not two separate realities, Buddhists engage the practice of dealing with death in all its manifestations. Some Buddhists, especially those in the Tibetan tradition, "emphasize the potential transformative dimensions of the process of dying, experienced through dedicating one's suffering to the benefit of others and dying without fear, without confusion, and without regret [82]. Others focus on its naturalness ([10;36]), or even deal with it playfully, as something like an art form ([37;48]).

Buddhism is a life-affirming religion precisely because it teaches that dying need not be denied, feared, or blithely ignored; instead, as the Dalai Lama observes, living and dying well become one's personal responsibility:

> Naturally, most of us would like to die a peaceful death, but it is also clear that we cannot hope to die peacefully if our lives have been full of violence, or if our minds have mostly been agitated by emotions like anger, attachment, or fear. So if we wish to die well, we must learn how to live well: Hoping for a peaceful death, we must cultivate peace in our mind, and in our way of life (quoted in [82], p. ix).

Cultivating peace requires a willingness to practice non-attachment, to abandon the desire to possess and dominate ([82];[48];[62];[17]). This is the central message of dozens of books, articles, and audio and video recordings that have brought Buddhist (and other Eastern) visions of living and dying to Western audiences over the last decade. A few of these offerings deal directly with decisionmaking about medical treatment, and many offer insights, gleaned from thousands of years of working with "The Great Matter" of life and death, that can spur new thinking about how to resolve termination of treatment dilemmas and improve care for dying patients.

Healing and Dying

Buddhist teachings encourage people who are dying to take responsibility for whatever situation arises. Particularly in the Theravada tradition, this may be expressed as "accepting one's karma", that is, bearing a painful and incurable illness quietly and patiently in order to allow karma to run its course ([80];[61]. However, this does not mean that people should not try to rid themselves of illness and suffering; rather, people who are suffering (and those caring for them) should work with an illness in skillful ways, seeking a deep, wholistic healing which may manifest as recovery from a disease or injury, or as a peaceful and accepted death.

To heal is literally "to make whole," and engaging the process of dying has enormous liberating potential ([13], p. 10;[82];[62]). Meditation teacher and healing minister Stephen Levine, whose work integrates Buddhism with many other religious traditions, reports that he is frequently asked "How do you know when to stop healing and begin to prepare for death?" ([62], p. 203). His response illustrates the importance of practicing non-attachment in relationship to both healing and dying:

> . . . In reality the opening to healing and the preparation for death are the same. When we are differentiating between healing and preparing for death we are forgetting that each are aspects of a single whole. It is all within the attitude with which one comes to life. If we don't use our symptoms as a message of our holding [i.e., attachments], then any attempt at healing which seeks to suppress that teaching slays a much deeper aspect of being. Is the healing that affects only the body in our best interest? On the other hand, if one welcomes death as an escape, that is a rejection of life, and the same imaginary differences between life and death will occur. In either case we never touch the deathless. We never encourage the exploration of undifferentiated being out of which all healing and wisdom arise ([62], p. 203).

Similar sentiments have been expressed by Tibetan meditation master Sogyal Rinpoche:

> . . . now more than ever before we need a fundamental change in our attitude to death and dying.

Happily, attitudes are beginning to change. The hospice movement, for example, is doing marvelous work in giving practical and emotional care. Yet practical and emotional care are not enough; people who are dying need love and care, but they also need something even more profound. They need to discover a real meaning to death, and to life. Without that, how can we give them ultimate comfort? . . . ([82]. p. 10).

Forgoing Treatments: Affirming Life and Accepting Death

Recognizing that the occurrence of illness, injury, and death can provide a profound stimulus for spiritual exploration and awakening, Buddhists from many different backgrounds and cultures have advocated hospice as an appropriate model of care for dying patients ([32];[62];[72];[48];[5];[80];[61]; [10]). In contrast, the positions that have been articulated concerning withholding and withdrawing medical treatment appear to be quite diverse.

For some Buddhists, respecting the first precept ("Affirm life; do not kill") means taking advantage "of whatever means of treatment and recovery are available," because human life affords a rare and irreplaceable opportunity to transcend suffering through enlightenment ([80], p. 310;[10]). Seeking and continuing treatment is therefore imperative because "there is the possibility for every disease to be cured so long as life continues" ([80], p. 310).

From this perspective, a patient who seeks death as a means to avoid a painful or drawn-out dying process short-circuits the potential for healing inherent in the experience of illness and therefore risks engendering negative karma, including what some Buddhists would understand as a painful "rebirth" ([80];[61];[48];[5];[10];[94]). Thus, if the motive is self-destruction, refusal of treatment becomes virtually indistinguishable from suicide, and both are morally unwholesome ([10];[32];[80];[61];[5];[94]). Similarly, surrogate decisions to forgo life-sustaining treatments, if motivated by self-serving aims (e.g., repugnance towards suffering and disability), are problematic because those seeking or causing the patient's death thereby generate harmful karma ([10];[32];[80];[61]).

If, however, a person does not refuse treatment for selfish reasons but instead acts compassionately (e.g., to end extreme suffering, to relieve family or friends of extreme emotional or economic burdens, or to participate more fully in the dying process), the karmic consequences will be quite different ([48], p. 129;[5];[91]). Thus, based on the particular circumstances, and especially on the intent of the decision-maker, it is possible to distinguish decisions to forgo treatment in order to engage dying as a spiritual process from similar decisions in which the intent is to commit suicide ([10];[32];[72], pp. 74–78;[48], pp. 128–134;[5];[34]).

The line between seeking versus accepting death can be quite fine. For example, in one account of the historical Buddha's teachings, several monks are expelled from the Order for encouraging a monk who was greatly distressed by a serious illness not to fear death; the monk subsequently stopped eating and died, and the monks who had offered reassurance were judged guilty of commending suicide (pp. 74–75;[10], p. 209). However, faced on another occasion with a very similar case, the Buddha offered the following commentary:

> 'Do not commit suicide.' . . . If, however, a Bhikkhu [i.e. monk] is very much afflicted with disease and sees the Sangha [i.e. religious community] and other Bhikkhus attending upon him in his sickness put very much to trouble on account of nursing him, he thinks thus, "These people are very much put to trouble on account of me!" He then contemplates upon his life-span and finds that he is not going to live long and so he does not eat, does not clothe himself properly nor does he take any medicine, then it (i.e., suicide) may be excusable (lit. good) ([84] (quoted in [72], p. 75).

Hence, many Buddhists (especially those from the Mahayana or Vajrayana traditions) stress the importance of being willing to forgo medical or surgical interventions, either as an act of compassion or as a means to avoid distractions during the process of spiritual healing ([82];[48];[62];[36]). Tibetan meditation teacher Sogyal Rinpoche, for example, focuses on the importance of fostering peacefulness in a dying person's environment:

When a person is very close to death, I suggest that you request that the hospital staff do not disturb him or her so often, and that they stop taking tests. I'm often asked what is my attitude to death in intensive care units. I have to say that being in an intensive care unit will make a peaceful death very difficult, and hardly allow for spiritual practice at the moment of death. As the person is dying, there is no privacy. They[sic] are hooked up to monitors, and attempts to resuscitate them will be made when they stop breathing or their heart fails. There will be no chance of leaving the body undisturbed for a period of time after death, as the masters advise.

If you can, you should arrange with the doctor to be told when there is no possibility of the person recovering, and then request to have them moved to a private room, if the dying person wishes it, with the monitors disconnected . . .

Try and make certain also that while the person is actually in the final stages of dying, all injections and all invasive procedures of any kind are discontinued. These can cause anger, irritation, and pain, and for the mind of the dying person to be as calm as possible in the moments before death is . . . absolutely crucial ([82], p. 185).

IV. Active Euthanasia

Because of their primary focus on the intent of the decision-maker, most Buddhists writing about death and dying draw very few distinctions between decisions to forgo treatment and voluntary active euthanasia. Those who frown on decisions to forgo treatment insofar as they have any suicidal or death-seeking character generally oppose active euthanasia on the same grounds [32; 10; 80; 61]. Similarly, those who allow an exception for deciding to forgo treatment based on a compassionate intention may allow the same exception for cases of active euthanasia ([72], pp. 80–81;[63];[36]).

Some Buddhists, however, view active euthanasia as more difficult to justify than decisions to forgo treatment ([5];[48], p. 127;[77]). Chinese Buddhists, for example, may incorporate Taoist perspectives in their views on these issues, seeing termination of treatment as a form of "nonaction", in which nature simply takes its course without human intervention [77]. In contrast, active euthanasia, especially for debilitating but not immediately lethal conditions (such as Alzheimer's disease), might be seen as a more egoistic or "unnatural" attempt to avoid suffering ([21], pp. 107–109).

Perhaps more importantly, death via active euthanasia often involves a mode of death that most Buddhists find highly undesirable: the patient is purposely rendered unconscious ([5];[10];[61]). This kind of drug-induced unconsciousness obscures the normal process of dying and thus robs the dying patient of one of life's most potent opportunities for transcending suffering and death in enlightenment ([61];[69]). Here the precept against using drugs to cloud the mind can be invoked to affirm the Buddhist ideal of participating in one's dying, such that "it is the individual who *actively lets go*, and not medication that serves to kill the patient" ([36], p. 133). Since the precepts provide guidance for relieving suffering, some Buddhists have suggested that to grant people "release" through a painless (i.e., unconscious) death may be to confuse comfort with compassion ([98];[32];[48], p. 229). Others have noted that, given the nature of karma, it is simply "pointless to kill oneself—or aid another to do so—in order to escape" ([48], p. 135).

Thus, most Buddhists would view an unconscious death as personally undesirable; nonetheless, a few have argued in support of laws that would protect the individual's sphere of decision-making about these matters, including the choice for voluntary active euthanasia ([72], pp. 80–81;[63]). Such arguments, like those offered by Buddhists in support of legalized abortion, are not based on a desire simply to respect individual autonomy; rather, they support the notion of an ethics based on "mutuality and interdependence", in which individuals in society provide each other with the greatest possible range of opportunity for compassionate action ([72], pp. 74–81). On the other hand, the effects of legalizing active euthanasia might be harmful to some individuals, exacerbating pre-existing tensions about being abandoned or shunned during dying, especially for vulnerable populations such as the disabled and elderly" ([82], pp. 375–76). Moreover, changes in the law may not actually be necessary, since the mandate to compassionate activity is not dependent on legal sanction ([36];[2]), and compassion for the dying can obviously manifest in many ways other than painless killing ([82];[62];[48]).

V. Issues in Providing Comfort Care

Buddhist authors have addressed several issues related to providing comfort care in ways that may be of interest to bioethicists; among them are three that are addressed in particularly distinctive ways: working with pain, abstaining from nourishment, and caring for patients in a persistent "coma", i.e., a persistent vegetative state (PVS).

Working with Pain

Buddhist meditation practices have frequently been offered as a complement (or an alternative) to sedative and analgesic medication regimens for dying patients ([82];[10];[62];[71];[48]). Most of these practices involve exercises such as counting the breath and simple visualizations, which encourage the release of anxiety and self-absorption in order to open to the truth of the present moment. Because they are not intrinsically related to Buddhism as a religious belief system, these and similar meditation practices are potentially available to any suffering patient; they may work particularly well with patients thought to have otherwise untreatable pain ([62], p. 119;[10];[71]).

Several Buddhist authors also emphasize the importance of having health care professionals learn to work with and accept their own pain and fear of dying ([82];[62];[10];[5];[72];[48]). Stephen Levine describes how "resistance and fear, our dread of the unpleasant" can magnify pain for ourselves and those around us: "It is like closing your hand around a burning ember. The tighter you squeeze, the deeper you are seared" ([62], p. 115). He continues:

> Much of our pain is reinforced by those around us who wish us not to be in pain. Indeed, many of those who want to help—doctors, nurses, loved ones, therapists—because of their own fear of pain project resistance with such comments as, "Oh, you poor baby!" Or a wincing around the eyes that reinforces the pain of those they are treating. Those who have little room for their own pain, who find pain in no way acceptable, seldom encourage another to enter directly into their experience, to soften the resistance and holding that so intensifies suffering . . . ([62], p. 118).

Buddhist authors consistently advocate a skillful approach to pain management, encouraging the use of medications (and meditations) in doses titrated to maximize calm and lucidity ([82];[5];[61];[10]; [48]):

> One of the fears that we can most easily dispel is the anxiety we all have about unmitigated pain in the process of dying. I would like to think that everyone in the world could know that this is now unnecessary . . . The Buddhist masters speak of the need to die consciously with as lucid, unblurred, and serene a mental mastery as possible. Keeping pain under control without clouding the dying person's consciousness is the first prerequisite for this, and now it can be done: Everyone should be entitled to that simple help at this most demanding moment of passage ([82], pp. 180–181).

Abstaining from Eating

Buddhist literature, and especially Zen Buddhist literature, contains many stories in which individuals who were very old or ill simply stopped eating and then died. The historical Buddha apparently gave his approval to this process in circumstances where the individual "is not going to live long" and has become a burden to those providing care ([72], p. 75). Voluntary abstention from eating, or "terminal fasting" (Sanskrit, *sallekhana*) was probably a common practice in India at that time; it would normally be accompanied by other spiritual activities such as meditation or the reciting of sutras as a way of entering death calmly and alertly ([22];[12]).

In Buddhism, abstaining from eating, if not motivated by a desire to escape from life, can be accepted either as a form of self-sacrifice (self-immolation) [32], or as a natural response to terminal illness and aging—a "letting go" rather than a death-seeking action ([48], pp. 126–127;[72], p. 77). However, it is critical that the intent not be self-serving. Philip Kapleau Roshi, for example, cites with approval the case of Zen master Yamamoto, who refused to let either his living or his dying be a burden to his community:

> . . . At the time of his death he was the abbot of a large and respected monastery in Japan. Having grown old—he was ninety-six at the time, if I remember correctly—he was almost completely deaf and blind. No longer

able to actively teach his students, he made an announcement that it was time for him to take his leave, and that he would die at the start of the new year. He then stopped eating. The monks in his temple reminded him that the New Year period was the busiest time at the temple, and that for him to die then would be most inconvenient.

"I see", he said, and he resumed eating until the early summer, when he again stopped eating and then one day toppled over and quietly slipped away ([48], p. 126).

These examples are important not only for the light they shed on the debate within bioethics as to whether "starving" invariably causes discomfort in the dying process, but also for the context they provide for respecting oral or written advance directives from Buddhists about forgoing medically supplied nutrition and hydration. Indeed, given the meaning of voluntary abstention from eating within the Buddhist tradition, recent efforts by some state legislatures to restrict competent adults from using their advance directives to refuse medically supplied nutrition and hydration may represent unconstitutional infringements on the free exercise of religion.

Caring for Individuals in a Persistent Vegetative State

Various Buddhist sources relate death to the cessation of consciousness and the termination of natural respiration, although important "internal processes" are said to continue for some time even after death (see below —Definition of Death) ([10], pp. 204–211;[39], pp. 200–202;[82], p. 253;[72], p. 68). However, patients in a persistent vegetative state (PVS), despite their lowered, or withdrawn, state of consciousness, are considered to be alive, manifesting *prana*— "the life force"—through the presence of spontaneous respiration and other brainstem functions ([10], pp. 204–206;[39], p. 211). For some Buddhists, the presence of this interior consciousness calls for continuing a wide range of supporting treatments (including kidney dialysis, blood transfusions, and medically supplied nutrition):

Even though comatose patients are helpless with regard to their physical body, the conscious mind, which has withdrawn within, may still be working to mentally prepare the patients for death. This process of mental cultivation can continue for as long as the patient still has *prana* present in the body . . . [T]herefore, despite the lack of signs of life [sic], the doctor has the responsibility to insure that the patient can continue to cultivate the mind without interrupting the *prana*, and thus avoid jeopardizing the final phase of the dying process ([10], p. 210).

Without specifying the continuation of any particular therapies, others have raised similar concerns, focusing on the potential of Western scientific medicine to take a purely mechanistic view of patients in PVS or dead by brain criteria ([28], p. 24;[81], p. 27;[41], pp. 181–182):

Fearing that . . . [the current death-with-dignity movement] may not make adequate allowance for profound spiritual interchange between family members and the patient, I cannot help entertaining misgivings about[it] . . . Its members insist that human dignity can no longer be maintained once consciousness has been irrecoverably lost. But, even after the level of consciousness has been lowered and life has fallen into a profound coma, interchange remains possible at the deepest levels of the mind. Under such circumstances, whether the patient can pass from life to death with dignity does not depend on connection or disconnection of a respirator or the loss or presence of consciousness. The important issue is whether the . . . person is treated, not as a physical object, but as a Vessel of the Law and regarded by those around him with respectful, compassionate care and treatment ([41], pp. 210–211).

VI. Advance Directives and Surrogate Decisionmaking

Buddhists have endorsed the concept of advance directives, such as living wills and proxy statements, as a means by which individuals can clarify their intentions and communicate them to others ([82], p. 373;[36], pp. 130–140;[48], pp. 303–307;[10], p. 210;[40], p. 212). There is also support, based on such documents, or on traditional customs and cultural expectations, for respecting the wishes and opinions of the incapacitated patient's family and involving them in ongoing decisionmaking ([36];[48], pp. 303–310;[10], pp. 210–211;[40], pp. 212–215;[91], p. 21).

On the other hand, several reports of practices in Japan, China, and Southeast Asia—countries with large Buddhist populations—indicate that principles other than respect for patient autonomy motivate and shape the forms taken by surrogate decisionmaking ([53], pp. 22–23;[40], pp. 213–214; [2], pp. 51–52;[96], p. 25). Physicians from these cultures may consider it unwise or even cruel to provide full details of a patient's condition to loved ones, and would expect to bear more of the burden of decisionmaking than a pure autonomy model would dictate; they would, in turn, be held to very high standards of empathy and compassion in order to justify the family's on- going trust ([40], pp. 210–211;[53], pp. 22–23;[2], pp. 51–52). In addition, some Buddhist authors would restrict surrogates from making certain types of decisions, such as a decision to pursue involuntary euthanasia, on the grounds that no one can decide for another individual that dying will be used as a spiritual practice ([32], pp. 65–66).

Some philosophers have advanced theories about the nature of personal identity that they claim resemble Buddhist teachings ([74], p. 280); these theories have been used to call into question the assumption that the wishes of a person in good health should be respected when that "same" person becomes ill [27], p. 379). While such claims are interesting, and the purported similarities are worthy of further investigation ([39], p. 197, footnote 5), it is worth noting the conflict and confusion that may arise from engaging abstract or conceptual "Buddhist-like" theories of personal identity; these are the kinds of metaphysical debates that the historical Buddha eschewed ([83], pp. 51–52).

VII. Economics and the Distribution of Scarce Resources

While recognizing each person and each person's dying process as precious, Buddhists writing about termination of treatment and care of the dying are also sensitive to the social and economic contexts in which health care is provided ([5], p. 41;[39], p. 211;[79], pp. 244–279). This is in keeping with Buddhist teachings of interdependence, in which all beings are intimately interrelated and mutually dependent, such that the action of any individual affects all others ([19];[72], pp. 73–74).

Still, the focus of Buddhist ethics has traditionally been personal rather than social morality ([83], pp. 135–149;[31], p. 328), and very little has been written about Buddhist perspectives on the social, economic, and political dimensions of health care ethics, despite calls for greater Buddhist involvement in and attention to these issues ([31];[81]). This remains an area for further inquiry, since intriguing insights may emerge from a Buddhist exploration of the ethical interface between individual and social morality ([44];[52], pp. 10–17;[2];[70]; [35];[64];[80], pp. 311–312).

VIII. Organ Donation

> *The Perfection of Giving: When one thinks, "The giving of the gift here gives rise to a great fruit", then give and take is degrading like the profit of commerce.*
> —*Ethics of Tibet, p. 135*

The possibility of removing organs from an individual at the time of death in order to save the life of another (or to substantially ease the burden of a severe illness) raises interesting questions for those concerned with the care of dying patients. Buddhist authors have addressed these questions under two main categories: 1) how can and should one make a determination that death has occurred? and 2) should the dying process of one individual be disturbed in order to benefit another?

Determination of Death

Many schools of Buddhism have elaborate teachings about death and the process of dying, often centered around the concepts of karma and what is commonly called "rebirth" ([78], pp. 32–34;[82];[10];[61];[48], pp. 255–300;[40]). In these teachings, the process of dying is frequently described as occurring in various stages leading up to rebirth, and respectful care of the dying and newly dead is considered essential to help assure that this rebirth will be propitious ([82], pp. 244–298;[40];[48]). These stages may be understood as the progressive dissolution of the physical and mental elements of existence: "each stage of the dissolution has its physical and psychological effect on the dying person, and is reflected by external, physical signs as well as inner experiences" ([82], p. 250).

Traditionally, Buddhists have identified the loss of consciousness and the cessation of spontaneous respiration as the most prominent external signs of death ([10], pp. 204–211;[39], pp. 200–202;[82], p. 253;[72], p. 68), but important internal processes of dissolution are believed to continue for some time after the vital signs are extinguished. A form of "inner respiration" may continue for from roughly twenty minutes ([82], p. 253) to two hours ([40], p. 227) after the cessation of breathing and heartbeat, and the life force may remain present in subtle forms for from several hours ([40], pp. 227–228) to several days ([48], pp. 164–165). Most Buddhists therefore try to avoid moving the body for several hours after death and will generally wait from one to three or more days before proceeding with burial or cremation, in order to insure that the individual's dying process remains undisturbed ([48], pp. 164–165). Chanting and other ceremonial rituals are considered appropriate during this period, and for several weeks after death ([48] p. 176).

Nothing in these traditions would forbid the medical or legal determination of death by whole brain criteria; indeed, it is tempting to correlate descriptions of the dissolution of "inner respiration" and the "departure of the life force" with the loss of brain, and particularly, brainstem function ([39];[40];[41];[l0]). However, it may never be possible to say with absolute certainty exactly when the "integrating power" of the substance of life has been irretrievably lost ([40], p. 222–223). Moreover, despite the absence of an integrative force at the systemic level, some Buddhists would find evidence of the continued presence of life in the continued function of cells and organs, whether in the warmth and heartbeat of brain-dead patients maintained on life support systems or in the growth of hair and fingernails of seemingly lifeless corpses, giving evidence of continued cell division for several days after complete cardiorespiratory collapse ([32], p. 67;[40];[81]).

Thus, while recognizing the need for legally and socially binding determinations of death, Buddhists also call attention to the uncertainty inherent in determining that something that can be called "death" has occurred ([11], pp. 294–299;[48], p. 269). Categories and boundaries are useful, as a practical matter, but within Buddhist teachings, points of so-called transition—such as birth and death—are discussed with great respect for their ultimate intangibility ([78], p. 33). Some traditions, such as Zen, would also direct attention to fundamental religious questions such as "What is the nature of the self?" and "Why does Buddhism teach that 'life is the unborn and death is the unextinguished'?" ([65], p. 122).

Giving and Receiving Organs

Major debates have taken place in Japan over the proposed introduction of brain criteria for the determination of death, especially in the context of retrieving organs for transplantation ([45];[3];[47]). Although much of the opposition to the proposed standards has been attributed to perceived conflicts with Buddhist teachings, many of the issues involved seem to arise from other traditional Japanese values and beliefs. Feldman, for example, attributes the reluctance of some Japanese to donate organs to their "Buddhist ideas about reincarnation" ([28], p. 24), but concerns about survival in the afterlife and bodily reincarnation actually fit more closely with Confucian and Shinto beliefs about the unity of the body and spirit than with Buddhist notions of rebirth ([41], p. 185).

However, Buddhists may indeed be extremely sensitive about the need for organs to be donated freely ([59], p. 351) and for recipients not to accept an organ out of an unseemly grasping for and attachment to life ([28];[32]). Buddhists understand a peaceful death as offering the best opportunity for spiritual awakening ([82], p. 186), and the taking of organs risks disturbing the dying process, possibly causing distraction or even pain: "This is a time of the suffering of pain of sickness and death. At such a time, not even a finger must touch (the body). The touch of a finger will seem like a blow from a great boulder . . ." ([40], p. 229).

To avoid these potential harms requires that the prospective donor make the choice to donate freely and with right intention (i.e.; not for personal gain) ([32]; [82], pp. 376–377; [48], p. 169; [10], pp. 211–212). Tibetan meditation master Sogyal Rinpoche elaborates on this point in his response to a thoughtful series of questions posed by a student:

> Should we donate our organs when we die? What if they have to be removed while the blood is still circulating or before the process of dying is complete? Doesn't this disturb or harm the consciousness at the moment before death?

> Masters whom I have asked this question agree that organ donation is an extremely positive action, since it stems from a genuine compassionate wish to benefit others. So, as long as it is truly the *wish* of the dying person, it will not harm in any way the consciousness that is leaving the body. On the contrary, this final act of generosity accumulates good karma. Another master said that *any* suffering and pain that a person goes through in the process of giving his or her organs, and every moment of distraction, turns into a good karma ([82], p. 376).

Remarkably, this feature of generosity is so central to the Buddhist approach to the morality of organ transplantation that it even takes priority over the question of the determination of death; that is, it has been argued that—given a willing donor—a determination of death prior to organ retrieval is not truly essential ([82], pp. 376–77;[48], p. 169):

> Dilgo Khyentse Rinpoche explained: "If the person is definitely going to die within a few moments, and has expressed the wish to give his organs, and his mind is filled with compassion, it is alright for them to be removed even before the heart stops beating' ([82], pp. 376–377).

On the other hand, some Buddhists feel uncertain about the benefits to be attained by the those who *receive* the organ(s), since they may be acting selfishly

([32], p. 66), by hoping "for the death of another person in order to benefit from their organs" ([28], p. 24) or by striving to avoid death at the cost of pain to another ([40], p. 219;[48], p. 170). Some have also questioned the commercialism and self-interest that may motivate transplantation efforts ([72], pp. 115–120;[48], pp. 169–170). In light of these difficulties, one prominent Buddhist author has called for increased research into the pathology of conditions leading to the need for transplantation and maximum efforts toward developing alternative therapeutic approaches such as the artificial heart ([41], pp. 182–183).

IX. Genetics

> *Nothing is wasted in a splendid reign.*
> *—Zen saying*

Perhaps the earliest mention of Buddhist thought in the bioethics literature appeared in a paper dealing with genetic counseling published in the *Hastings Center Report* in 1971. [60]. At that time, Marc Lappe first introduced the standard of compassion (that is, unselfish action, in a Buddhist sense) as a potential guiding principle for prenatal genetic counseling. Using metaphors from Buddhism and other Eastern religions, Lappe argued that relying on the standard of compassion would avoid the eugenic tendencies associated with the "Western predilection for attempting to create 'ideal situations'" ([60], p. 7). Instead, the goal of genetics from an Eastern perspective would be to minimize the impact of suffering coincident with genetic "defects" ([60], p. 8). This standard, Lappe argued, would not always lead to an easy validation of the practice of aborting fetuses with detectable genetic abnormalities, unless those abnormalities would inevitably lead to great suffering ([60], p. 8).

The attitudes expressed by Buddhists toward disability (whether genetic, congenital, or acquired) vary quite widely. Pinit Ratanakul reports that in Thailand, for example, doctors are reluctant to withhold any available treatment from impaired newborns, since such an action might reflect a repugnance of the patient's pain and suffering rather than true compassion ([81], p. 27). Similarly, the Venerable Mettanando Bhikkhu claims that "More than any other religion in the world Buddhism values life, especially human life, whatever grotesque [sic] form life may assume . . ." ([10], p. 202). He then goes on to explain the basis for this view:

> The probability of being born as a human is so rare, that it has been compared to the probability of a turtle surfacing at random in the wide ocean and accidentally popping its head through the center of the only yoke floating in the ocean. Life is an irreplaceable opportunity to cultivate one's happiness in this lifetime and those to come ([10], pp. 202–203).

In contrast, K.N. Siva Subramanian reports that in Sri Lanka neonatal mortality is generally high, and Buddhists apparently take comfort in the belief that the death of an impaired infant is the result of the workings of karma: "Quality of life rather than sanctity of life is a consideration because of a strong belief in rebirth . . ." ([91], p. 21). In China, too, harsh conditions seem to have led to substantial support among the general public for both active and passive euthanasia of infants with very severe impairments, particularly neurological impairments [77]. Ren-Zong Qiu has argued that impaired infants in China stand in need of protection because of a cultural history of infanticide (of both female infants and "monsters", i.e., infants with severe deformities), an economy that makes raising an impaired newborn an "unbearable burden", and a political atmosphere that encourages parents to withdraw treatment from an impaired child in order to be able to have and raise a healthy one [77]. Another possible explanation of the observed and reported tendency to withdraw support from infants with impairments can be found in Taoist and Confucianist teachings emphasizing the importance of leading a meaningful life, as full members of the human community.

At the same time, both Taoist and Buddhist teachings have been used to uphold the ideals of tolerance and active acceptance of disability. For example, a famous Chinese story recounts how the Taoist sage Yu cheerfully embraced a deforming illness:

> . . . His heart was calm and his manner carefree. He limped to the well, looked at his reflection in the water and said, "My, my! How the Maker of Things is deforming me!" [His friend] Szu asked, "Does this upset you?" "Why should it?" said Yu. "If my left arm becomes a rooster, I will herald the dawn. If my right arm becomes a crossbow, I'll shoot down a bird and roast it. If my buttocks turn into wheels and my spirit into a horse, I'll go for a ride. What need will I have for a carriage? I was born when it was time to be born, and I shall die when it is time to die. If we are in peace with time and follow the order of things, neither sorrow nor joy will move us. The ancients called this 'freedom from bondage.' Those who are entangled with the appearance of things cannot free themselves. But nothing can overcome the order of nature. Why should I be upset?" ([37], p. 69).

Several reports on Japanese views of genetic issues have recently emerged ([7];[9];[68]), but again in this arena, it seems that substantial further work will be necessary in order to parse the impact of Buddhist thought from the influence of Japanese values and beliefs derived from other sources. Moreover, in many areas related to genetic technology, Japanese standards may be tracking Western or international attitudes rather than evolving in accord with any particular Japanese religious or cultural tradition [7].

As noted in relation to new reproductive technologies, Western Buddhists might be expected generally to take a favorable attitude toward genetic interventions, especially those clearly designed to respond compassionately to human suffering. For example, the Dalai Lama was once asked "If, at some future time . . . you could make by genetic engineering, with proteins and amino acids, or by engineering with chips and copper wires, an organism that had all of our good qualities and none of our bad ones, would you do it?" To which the Dalai Lama replied, "If this were possible it would be most welcome. It would save a lot of effort!" ([33], p. 35).

Buddhists for thousands of years have, in fact, chosen to put forth the effort to study and know the self—but primarily in ways other than through the sciences and technology. As Buddhist scholar Robert Thurman observes, this does not represent a failure of will or intellect, but a considered response to the direct realization of the dangers inherent in developing powers to affect the world around us which far outstrip our powers over ourselves ([33], pp. 55–57):

> In ancient India, when the Buddha established the Buddhist educational institutions, reality was approached as both outer environment and inner self, the same as in the West. The inner self, however, was chosen as the more important to understand and the more practical to control and engineer to suit human needs. This was not because of a naive belief in the irreducible human spirit or because of any sort of mysticism. Materialists were already flourishing at that time. The Buddhists themselves used materialistic reductionism in contexts where practical, especially in the development of medicine . . .

Underlying the choice of what aspect of reality, outer or inner, is more important to understand and control, is the complex of views about what reality is, what life within that reality is, what human life in particular is, what its purpose is and what its needs and prospects are. Without knowing the answers to these questions, if we just rush off and analyze aspects of the environment, modify what seems modifiable, and satisfy immediate needs without a long-term perspective, our procedure is not likely to succeed . . . ([33], p. 55).

X. Other Issues

Buddhists have devoted a great deal of attention to some topics that until recently have remained somewhat on the fringe of mainstream bioethics, especially environmental ethics ([4];[6];[15];[17];[19];[20];[24];[35];[44];[46];[70]; [73];[87];[89];[99]) and the care and use of animals by humans ([49];[66];[89]). Unfortunately, discussion of Buddhist approaches to these topics deserves a fuller treatment than the present essay will allow.

New topics also seem likely to emerge as Buddhism finds its footing in the West and begins both to challenge and respond to the myriad biomedical experiences and questions of American practitioners. Indeed, one of the major ways in which Buddhism may contribute to bioethics over the next few years is through expanding the range of topics regularly included in its discourse.

XI. Conclusion

The function of Buddhist ethics is to nourish and heal, manifesting wisdom in compassionate activity. In such activity, self is forgotten and the intimate harmony of the vast and infinitely interconnected universe is revealed. For Buddhists, this is a vital ethical matter—*the* vital ethical matter—because every thought, every word, every action, however small and seemingly insignificant, affects the whole. As Francis Cook says, "It is not just that 'we are all in it' together. We all *are* it, rising or falling as one living body" ([19], p. 229).

A Buddhist ethic is thus an ethic of responsibility, for oneself and for the whole phenomenal universe. Yet this is not simply "doing good", for in compassion "there is no effort involved, no sense of separation, no giver or receiver . . ." ([65] p. 22) This is the realization and actualization of selfless enlightenment:

> *To study the budda-way is to study the self. To study the self is to forget the self. To forget the self is to be actualized by myriad things.*
> —*Dogen Zenji, "Genjokoan" [93]*
> **Zen Mountain Monastery**
> **Mt. Tremper, New York**

Acknowledgments

Partial support for the preparation of this material was provided by the Hastings Center Project on Priorities in the Clinical Application of Human Genome Research, funded by the National Center for Human Genome Research of the National Institutes of Health # R01 HG00418–0.

Special thanks to Marna Howarth and the library staff at the Hastings Center for cheerful and efficient assistance, and to John Daido Loori (Abbot) and his students at Zen Mountain Monastery—for all their teachings. All errors of concept and interpretation are the responsibility of the author.

Bibliography

1. Aitken, R.: 1991, "Interpreting the Precepts", *Buddhist Peace Fellowship Newsletter* (Spring), 23–24.

2. Aitken, R.: 1984, *The Mind of Clover*, North Point Press, San Francisco.

3. Akatsu, H.: 1990, "The Heart, the Gut, and Brain Death in Japan", 20 *Hastings Center Report* 2, 2.

4. Ames, R.T. and Callicott, J.B.: 1989, "Introduction: The Asian Traditions as a Conceptual Resource for Environmental Philosophy", in J.B. Callicott and R.T. Ames (eds.), *Nature in Asian Traditions of Thought: Essays in Environmental Philosophy*, State University of New York Press, Albany.

5. Anderson, P.: 1992, "Good Death: Mercy, Deliverance, and the Nature of Suffering", II *Tricycle* 2, 36–42.

6. Badiner, A.H. (ed.): 1990, *Dharma Gaia: A Harvest of Essays in Buddhism and Ecology*, Parallax Press, Berkeley, California.

7. Bai, K., Shirai, Y., and Ishii, M.: 1987,"In Japan, Consensus Has Limits", 17 *Hastings Center Report* 3 (Supplement), 18S-20S.

8. Barber, A.W.: 1991, in C.W. Fu and S.A. Wawrytko (eds.), *Buddhist Ethics and Modern Society: An International Symposium*, Greenwood Press, New York.

9. Bernard, J., Kajikawa, K., and Fujiki, N.: 1988, *Human Dignity and Medicine*, Excerpta Medica ICS 774.

10. Bhikkhu, V.M.: 1991, "Buddhist Ethics in the Practice of Medicine", in C.W. Fu and S.A. Wawrytko (eds.), *Buddhist Ethics and Modern Society: An International Symposium*, Greenwood Press, New York.

11. Bibel, D.J.: 1992, *Freeing the Goose in the Bottle: Discovering Zen through Science, Understanding Science through Zen*, Elie Metchnikoff Memorial Library, Oakland, California.

12. Bilimoria, P.: 1992, "The Jaina Ethic of Voluntary Death", 6 *Bioethics* 4, 331–355.

13. Birnbaum, R.: 1989, *The Healing Buddha*, Shambhala, Boston, Massachusetts.

14. Boonyoros, R.: 1991, "Buddhist Ethics in Everyday Life in Thailand: A Village Experiment", in C.W. Fu and S.A. Wawrytko (eds.), *Buddhist Ethics and Modern Society: An International Symposium*, Greenwood Press, New York.

15. Callicott, J.B. and Ames, R.T. (eds.): 1989, *Nature in Asian Traditions of Thought*, State University of New York Press, Albany, NY.

16. Chappell, D.W.: 1991, "Buddhist Responses to Religious Pluralism: What are the Ethical Issues?" in C.W. Fu and S.A. Wawrytko (eds.), *Buddhist Ethics and Modern Society: An International Symposium*, Greenwood Press, New York.

17. Chau, S.S. and Kam-Kong, F.: 1990, "Ancient Wisdom and Sustainable Development from a Chinese Perspective", in Engel, J.R. and Engel, J.G. (eds.), *Ethics of Environment and Development: Global Challenge, International Response*, The University of Arizona Press, Tucson.

18. Cook, F.D.: 1978, *How to Raise an Ox*, Center Publications, Los Angeles, California.

19. Cook, F.D.: 1989, "The Jewel Net of Indra", in J.B. Callicott and R.T. Ames (eds.), *Nature in Asian Traditions of Thought*, State University of New York Press, Albany, NY.

20. Crawford, C.: 1991, "The Buddhist Response to Health and Disease in Environmental Perspective", in C.W. Pu and S.A. Wawrytko (eds.), *Buddhist Ethics and Modern Society: An International Symposium*, Greenwood Press, New York.

21. Danto, A.C.: 1987, *Mysticism and Morality*, Columbia University Press, New York.

22. Davis, D.S.: 1990, "Old and Thin", 15 *Second Opinion* (November), 26–32.

23. De Silva, Lily, "The Scope and Contemporary Significance of the Five Precepts", in C.W. Fu and S.A. Wawrytko (eds.), *Buddhist Ethics and Modern Society: An International Symposium*, Greenwood Press, New York.

24. De Silva, P.: 1991, "Environmental Ethics: A Buddhist Perspective", in C.W. Fu and S.A. Wawrytko (eds.), *Buddhist Ethics and Modem Society: An International Symposium*, Greenwood Press, New York.

25. Dharmasiri, G.: 1989, *Fundamentals of Buddhist Ethics*, Golden Leaves Publishing Company, Antioch, CA.

26. Donden, Y.: 1980, "Embryology in Tibetan Medicine", in *Tibetan Medicine, series 1*, Library of Tibetan Works and Archives, Dharamsala, India.

27. Dresser, R.: 1986, "Life, Death, and Incompetent Patients: Conceptual Infirmities and Hidden Values in the Law", 28 Arizona Law Review 3, 373–405.

28. Feldman, E.: 1985, "Medical Ethics the Japanese Way", 15 *Hastings Center Report 5* (October), 21–24.

29. Fields, R: 1992, *How the Swans Caine to the Lake: A Narrative History of Buddhism in America (3rd Edition)*, Shambhala, Boston, Massachusetts.

30. Fu, C.W. and Wawiytko, S.A. (eds.): 1991, *Buddhist Ethics and Modern Society: An International Symposium*, Greenwood Press, New York.

31. Fu, C.W.: 1991, "From Paramartha-satya to Samvrti-satya: An Attempt at Constructive Modernization of (Mahayana) Buddhist Ethics", in C.W. Fu and S.A. Wawrytko (eds.), *Buddhist Ethics and Modern Society: An International Symposium*, Greenwood Press, New York.

32. Fujii, M.: 1991, "Buddhism and Bioethics", Bioethics Yearbook Vol. 1 (Theological Developments in Bioethics: 1988–1990), Kluwer Academic Publishers, Dordrecht, The Netherlands.

33. Goleman, D. and Thurman, R.A.F. (eds.): 1991, *MindScience: An East-West Dialogue*, Wisdom Publications, Boston.

34. Groth-Marnot, G.: 1992, "Buddhism and Mental Health: A Comparative Analysis", in Schumaker, J.F. (ed.), *Religion and Mental Health*, Oxford University Press, New York, 270–280.

35. Heisig, J.W.: 1990:, "Toward a Principle of Sufficiency", 8 *Zen Buddhism Today: Annual Report of the Kyoto Zen Symposium* (October), 152–164.

36. Hill, T.P. and Shirley, D.: 1992, "Death in the Buddhist Tradition", in *A Good Death: Taking More Control at the End of Your Life*, Addison-Wesley Publishing Company, Inc., Reading, Massachusetts.

37. Hoffman, Y. (ed.): 1986, *Japanese Death Poems*, Charles R. Tuttle Co., Inc., Rutland, Vermont.

38. Horner, I.B.: 1982, *Book of The Discipline (6 volumes)*, Pali Text Society, London, England.

39. Ikeda, D.: 1987, "Thoughts on the Problem of Brain Death (1): from the Viewpoint of the Buddhism of Nichiren Daishonin", 26 *The Journal of Oriental Studies* 2: 193–216.

40. Ikeda, D.: 1987, "Thoughts on the Problem of Brain Death (2): from the Viewpoint of the Buddhism of Nichiren Daishonin", 27 *The Journal of Oriental Studies* 1:203–232.

41. Ikeda, D.: 1987, "Thoughts on the Problem of Brain Death (3): from the Viewpoint of the Buddhism of Nichiren Daishonin", 27 *The Journal of Oriental Studies* 2: 151–192.

42. Inada, K.K.: 1991, "Buddhist and Western Ethics: Problematics and Possibilities", in C.W. Fu and S.A. Wawrytko (eds.), *Buddhist Ethics and Modern Society: An International Symposium*, Greenwood Press, New York.

43. Jonas, H.: 1984, *The Imperative of Responsibility: In Search of an Ethics for the Technological Age*, University of Chicago Press, Chicago.

44. Jones, K.: 1990, "Getting Out of Our Own Light", in A.H. Badiner (ed.), *Dharma Gaia: A Harvest of Essays in Buddhism and Ecology*, Parallax Press, Berkeley, California.

45. Kajikawa, K.: 1989, "Japan: A New Field Emerges", 19 Hastings *Center Report* 4 (Supplement), 29S-30S.

46. Kajiyama, Y.: 1990, "Fundamentals of Buddhist Ethics", 8 *Zen Buddhism Today: Annual Report of the Kyoto Zen Symposium* (October), 41–60.

47. Kato, I.: 1988, *Brain Death and Organ Donation*, Japan Medical Association.

48. Kapleau, P.: 1989, *The Wheel of Life and Death*, Anchor Books, New York, New York.

49. Kapleau, P: 1981, *To Cherish All Life: A Buddhist View of Animal Slaughter and Meat Eating*, Zen Center Publications, Los Angeles.

50. Kasulis, T.P.: 1990, "Does East Asian Buddhism Have an Ethical System"? 8 *Zen Buddhism Today: Annual Report of the Kyoto Zen Symposium* (October), 41–60.

51. Kawamura, E.: 1990, "Ethics and Religion —From the Standpoint of Absolute Nothingness", 8 *Zen Buddhism Today: Annual Report of the Kyoto Zen Symposium* (October), 71–85.

52. Keyes, K.: 1987, *The Hundredth Monkey* (2nd edition), Vision Books, Coos Bay, Oregon.

53. Kimura, R.: 1986, "In Japan, Parents Participate but Doctors Decide", 16 *Hastings Center Report* (August), 22–23.

54. Kirita, K.: 1990, "Buddhism and Social Ethics", 8 *Zen Buddhism Today: Annual Report of the Kyoto Zen Symposium* (October), 1–10.

55. Klevnick, L. and Hayes, R.: 1986, "Women & Buddhism: Buddhist Views on Abortion", 6 *Spring Wind —Buddhist Cultural Forum* 1–3 November), 166–172.

56. LaFleur, W.R.: 1978, "Buddhist Emptiness in the Ethics and Aesthetics of Watsuji Tetsuro," 14 *Religious Studies* (June), 237–250.

57. LaFleur, W.R.: 1990, "Contestation and Consensus: The Morality of Abortion in Japan, 40 *Philosophy East and West* 4 (October), 529–542.

58. LaFleur, W.R.: 1992, *Liquid Life: Abortion and Buddhism in Japan*, Princeton University Press, Princeton, NJ.

59. Lancaster, L.R., 1991, "Buddhism and the Contemporary World: The Problem of Social Action in an Urban Environment", in C.W. Fu and S.A. Wawrytko (eds.), *Buddhist Ethics and Modern Society: An International Symposium*, Greenwood Press, New York.

60. Lappe, M.: 1971, "The Genetic Counselor: Responsible to Whom?" 1 *Hastings Center Report* 2 (September), 6–11.

61. Lesco, P.A.: 1986, "Euthanasia: A Buddhist Perspective", 25 *Journal of Religion and Health* 1 (Spring), 51–57.

62. Levine, S.: 1982, *Who Dies?* Anchor Books, New York, New York.

63. Levine, 5.: 1992, "No Second-Guessing: An Interview with Stephen Levine", II *Tricycle* 2, 48–50.

64. Lindbeck, V.: 1984, Thailand: Buddhism Meets the Western Model, 14 *Hastings Center Report* (December), 24–26.

65. Loori, J.D.: 1992, *The Eight Gates of Zen: Spiritual Training at an American Zen Buddhist Monastery*, Dharma Communications, Mt. Tremper, New York.

66. Lorri, J.D.: 1992, "Food: Just the Right Amount", II *Tricycle* 2 (Winter), 78–79.

67. Loy, D.: 1991, "Buddhism and Money: The Repression of Emptiness Today" in C.W. Fu and S.A. Wawrytko (eds.), *Buddhist Ethics and Modern Society: An International Symposium*, Greenwood Press, New York.

68. Macer, D.R.: 1992, *Attitudes to Genetic Engineering: Japanese and International Comparisons*, Eubios Ethics Institute, Christchurch, New Zealand.

69. MacLean, V.: 1992, "Through a Glass, Darkly", II *Tricycle* 2, 51.

70. Macy, I.: 1991, *World as Lover, World as Self*, Parallax Press, Berkeley, California.

71. Miller, O.H.: 1991, "A Sharing of Breaths", *The Quest* (Autumn), 65–69.

72. Nakasone, R.Y.: 1990, *Ethics of Enlightenment: Essays and Sermons in Search of a Buddhist Ethic*, Dharma Cloud Publishers, Fremont, California.

73. Nordstrom, L.: 1990, "Zen, Ontology, and Environmental Ethics", unpublished manuscript.

74. Parfit, D.: 1984, *Reasons and Persons*, Oxford University Press, Oxford.

75. Premasiri, P.D., 1991, "The Relevance of the Noble Eightfold Path to Contemporary Society", in C.W. Fu and S.A. Wawrytko (eds.), *Buddhist Ethics and Modern Society: An International Symposium*, Greenwood Press, New York.

76. Qiu, R.: 1989, "AIDS Confronts the Law in China", 19 *Hastings Center Report* 6, 3–4.

77. Qiu, R.: 1993, "Chinese Medical Ethics and Euthanasia", *Cambridge Quarterly of Healthcare Ethics* (forthcoming).

78. Rahula, W.: 1974 (2nd edition), *What the Buddha Taught*, Grove Press, New York.

79. Ratanakul, P.: 1986, *BioEthics: An Introduction to the Ethics of Medicine and the Life Sciences*, Thammasat University Printing House, Bangkok, Thailand.

80. Ratanakul, P.: 1988, 'Bioethics in Thailand: The Struggle for Buddhist Solutions", *The Journal of Medicine and Philosophy* 13, 301–312.

81. Ratanakul, P.: 1990, "Thailand: Refining Cultural Values", 20 *Hastings Center Report* 2 (March/April), 25–27.

82. Rinpoche, S.: 1992, *The Tibetan Book of Living and Dying*, Harper, San Francisco, San Francisco, California.

83. Saddhatissa, H.: 1987, *Buddhist Ethics: The Path to Nirvana*, Wisdom Publications, London.

84. Sanghabhadra (Bapat, P.V. and Hirakawa A., trans.): 1970, *Samantapasadika: Shan-Chien-P'i-P'o-Sha, A Chinese Version by Sanghabbhadra of Samantapasadika*, Bhandarkar Oriental Research Institute, Poona.

85. Shaku, S. (Suzuki, D.T., trans.): 1987, "Buddhist Ethics", in *Zen for Americans*, Dorset Press, New York (original copyright 1906 by Open Court Publishing Company, Peru, Illinois).

86. Shibayama, Z.: 1974, *Zen Comments on the Mumonkan*, Harper & Row, San Francisco, California.

87. Sivaraksa, S.: 1990, "A Buddhist Perception of a Desirable Society", in Engel, J.R. and Engel, J.G. (eds.), *Ethics of Environment and Development: Global Challenge, International Response*, The University of Arizona Press, Tucson.

88. Smith, B.: 1992, "Buddhism and Abortion in Contemporary Japan: Mizuko Kuyo and the Confrontation with Death", in Cabezon, J.I. (ed.), *Buddhism, Sexuality, and Gender*, State University of New York Press, Albany.

89. Snyder, G.: 1991, "Indra's Net as Our Own", XII *Ten Directions* 1, 7–9.

90. Stevens, 1.: 1990, *Lust for Enlightenment*, Shambhala Publications, Inc., Boston.

91. Subramanian, K.N.S.: 1986: "In India, Nepal, and Sri Lanka, Quality of Life Weighs Heavily", 16 *Hastings Center Report* (August), 20–22.

92. Sze-bong, T.: 1991, "The Conflict Between *Vinaya* and the Chinese Monastic Rule: The Dilemma of Disciplinarian Venerable Hung-i", in C.W. Fu and S.A. Wawrytko (eds.), *Buddhist Ethics and Modern Society: An International Symposium*, Greenwood Press, New York.

93. Tanahashi, K. (ed.): 1985, *Moon in a Dewdrop: Writings of Zen Master Dogen*, Northpoint Press, San Francisco, California.

94. Taniguchi, S.: 1990, "Bio-medical Ethics from a Buddhist Perspective", *Buddhist Digest English Series* 26 (July), 58–70.

95. Talbot, M.: 1991, *The Holographic Universe*, HarperCollins Publishers, New York.

96. Tian-Min X.: 1990, "China: Moral Puzzles", 20 *Hastings Center Report* 2, 24–25.

97. Tworkov, H.: 1992, "Anti-abortion/Pro-choice: Taking Both Sides, I *Tricycle* 3 (Spring), 60–69.

98. Tworkov, H.: 1992, "Tender Mercies' (editorial), II *Tricycle* 2, 4.

99. Ueda, S.: 1990, "The Existence of Man—Life 'One Inch Off the Ground'" 8 *Zen Buddhism Today: Annual Report of the Kyoto Zen Symposium* (October), 165–171.

100. Wayman, A. (trans.): 1991, *Ethics of Tibet: Bodhisattva Section of Tsong-Kha-Pa's Lam Rim Chen Mo*, State University of New York Press, Albany, New York.

101. Zwilling, L.: 1992, "Homosexuality as Seen in Indian Buddhist Texts", in Cabezon, J.I. (ed.), *Buddhism Sexuality, and Gender*, State University of New York Press, Albany.

CONFUCIANISM, TRADITIONAL AND CONTEMPORARY CHINA

Medicine—the Art of Humaneness: On Ethics of Traditional Chinese Medicine[1]

Ren-Zong Qiu

──────────── INTRODUCTION TO READING ────────────

In this article, Ren-Zong Qiu, China's best known and most distinguished bioethicist, argues that traditional Chinese Medicine, cannot be divorced from its Confucian cultural context. Thus, much of the article focuses on outlining basic tenets of Confucian thought. After brief remarks on the history of Chinese medicine, Qiu outlines various dimensions of Confucian thought including the centrality of the concept *Ren. Ren,* or "humaneness," is a Confucian ideal that pervades all human relationships including that of the physician and patient. To practice *Ren* is, essentially, to love one's "fellow man." Qiu discusses the practices of traditional Chinese physicians and their relation to Confucian ideals. In this vein, he describes how Confucian ideals (principally Ren) relate to a physician's attitude towards himself, his patients, and his colleagues. In the last section of the article, Qiu discusses characteristics of traditional Chinese Medicine, where he casts Confucian ideals into a Western philosophical framework, further exploring their intricacies.

This essay will discuss exclusively the ethics of traditional Chinese medicine (TCM). Although traditional medicine with Confucianism[2] as its ideology dominated China up to 1911 when the republic was founded, its ethos remains rooted in the mind of Chinese people both laymen and professionals. I will discuss the ethics of Chinese medicine of the next two periods from 1911 to 1949 and from 1949 to now, especially that with Marxism as its ideology, in another essay.

I. Historical Notes

Chinese medicine has a long history of at least two thousand years, though the first explicit literature on medical ethics did not appear until the seventh century, when a physician named Sun Simiao wrote a famous treatise 'On the Absolute Sincerity of Great Physicians' in his work *The Important Prescriptions Worth a Thousand Pieces of Gold*. In this treatise, which is called the Chinese Hippocratic Oath, he required that a physician develop first the sense of compassion and pity, commit himself to make efforts to save every living creature, treat every patient on equal grounds, and not seek wealth by his expertise.[3]

In the thirteenth century another physician, Zhang Gao, in his *On Medicine* presented twelve anecdotes as examples of retributions for good or bad medical services. Three centuries later, an Imperial court physician, Gong Xin, wrote 'Warnings to Enlightened Physicians' and 'Warnings to Mediocre Physicians' in his *Medical Lessons in Ancient and Modern Times*. He emphasized a physician should have the sense of humaneness and justice in his heart and not to strive for his own profits. His son, also an Imperial court physician, Gong Tingxian, wrote down 'Ten Maxims for Physicians' in his *Back to Life from a Myriad of Sickness*. He reiterated the warnings his father had given and put stress on mastering the principles of Confucianism. In the same vein Chen Shigong wrote his 'Ten Maxims for Physicians' and 'Five Admonitions to Physicians' in his *Orthodoxy in Surgery* in the seventeenth century. He paid more attention to the ethics of relations with colleagues as well as with female patients. In the nineteenth century, Huai Yuan in his 'Warning to Physicians' included in his work *A Thorough Understanding of Medicine in Ancient and Modern Times* required a physician to rouse compassion and pity within himself, to love and respect himself, but to give up hopeless cases.

However, all these maxims, exhortations, admonitions, and warnings are personal advice or suggestions of then famous and prestigious physicians based on their personal experience of practicing medicine, but not professional codes in any sense because there never have been medical professional organizations in traditional China, so they have no binding power on physicians.

II. Confucian Cultural Context

In modern Chinese, the English terms 'ethics' and 'morality' are now usually translated into 'daode' and 'lunli', respectively. But the original meaning of 'daode' in Chinese is 'logos' ('dao' or 'tao') and 'virtue' ('de'), and that of 'lunli' is the principle of interpersonal relations.

Unlike its western counterpart, Chinese philosophy was not differentiated into well-defined sub-disciplines or branches. Strictly speaking, there was no explicitly defined ethics as an independent sub-discipline. Rather, the Chinese philosophy as a whole was an ethics, especially for the Confucian philosophy. The principles of Confucian ethics could and should be applied to politics, military affairs, religions, asthetics, medicine, etc. That is, 'study the whys and wherefores of things, seek knowledge, cultivate one's moral character, manage the family, administer the country, and calm down the land under heaven.' (*The Great Learning*) Confucius has dominated Chinese medicine for almost two thousand years, though not only Confucians, but also Taoists, Buddhists, hermits, herb physicians, and shamans were practicing medicine in traditional China. Confucian medical ethics is the application of Confucian ethic in medicine. So we have to skim through Confucian ethics before we come to discuss the TCM ethics.

Confucianism was of course not the only school of philosophy in traditional China. Apart from it, there were also Yangism, Mohism, Taoism, Nominalism, and Legalism,[4] among others. Because of that, since the early Han Dynasty on, the emperors only respected Confucianism and rejected all others (in most times). However, Confucianism assimilated elements that it deemed useful from other schools of philosophy. Nevertheless, Confucianism became the dominant ideology and penetrated into the mind of Chinese people and conventions of Chinese society as an inseparable component of Chinese culture. The only philosophies that could challenge its dominant position were Taoism and Buddhism, which had a strong influence during some historical periods, but they still could not compete with it.

Confucian ethics is intimately interwoven with its socio-political ideal, which was properly represented in a Confucian classic, *The Book of Rites*, the author of which cited what Confucius had said or what he thought Confucius should have said as follows:

> When the Great Logos (Tao) is brought into practice, everybody under heaven serves the public's interests, chooses those who are virtuous and able to handle official affairs, keeps their word, and performs good neighborliness. They pay respect to others' parents and love others' children as their own and make elders have a good end. The robust play their due role; children grow up well, widowers, widows, orphans, the childless, infirm, and sick are treated well; every man has a nice job; every woman marries a good husband. They do not fear leaving their goods on the street; they need not safeguard them at home. They do not need persons of talent to serve them. They only fear that such persons will not utilize their own abilities. Plots and conspiracies are stopped; schemes, robbery, and thievery do not take place; gates and doors need not be shut. This is the Great Harmony. (*The Application of Rites*)

To achieve this ideal goal—'The Great Harmony World'—the world needs persons who behave virtuously, so-called 'junzi' (a man of noble character or a gentleman) or 'renren zhishi' (a person with humaneness or lofty ideals), whom Confucius characterized as one who 'never seeks life at the expense of humaneness but sacrifices his life for the accomplishment of humaneness.' (*The Analects of Confucius*; English translation, p. 99[5])

'Ren' (humaneness, benevolence, kindheartedness) is the most basic concept in Confucianism. The word 'ren' appears hundreds of times in *The Analects of Confucius*, but is never given a precise definition. A Confucian rival, Mohist, defined 'ren' as 'to love others as love one's own body', and 'a person with humaneness loves himself as well as others not as a means for use, unlike loving a horse' (*The Classics of Mohism*). This definition may agree with its main sense in which Confucius used the term 'ren': 'In answer to Fanchi's questions about humaneness, the master said: "to love one's fellow-men".' (*The Analects of Confucius*, p. 81)

How did Confucius justify 'ren'? To achieve the noble goal of the Great Harmony in which everybody under heaven serves the public's interests, they pay respect to others' parents and love others' children as their own. This requires everybody to have a heart of humaneness—loving others.

The Confucian ideal is embodied in 'li' (rites, etiquettes, conventions[6])—symbols of a socio-political system. 'Ren' (humaneness) and 'li' (rites) seem to be two sides of a coin—internal intentions and external norms. Confucius said: 'Humaneness is to self-control and return to the practice of rites' (*The Analects of Confucius*, p. 76). The constituent parts of humaneness are to 'look at nothing which is contrary to the rites; listen to nothing contrary to them; speak nothing contrary to them; do nothing contrary to them.' (The *Analects of Confucius*, p. 76)

Is there any possibility that a person could practice 'ren' (humaneness)? Yes, there is. Why? Because humaneness is rooted in human being's psychology. Etymologically, 'ren' . . . is derived from person . . . and two . . . means affection or love. The emotion of affection has its origin between parents and children (Cai, 1937, p. 14). Everybody has affection for his or her parents and children. So the concept 'ren' is inseparably linked with another concept 'xiao' (filial piety) which is the starting point of 'ren'. Confucius said:

> Let youth practice filial duty; let it practice fraternal duty; let it earnestly give itself to being reliable; let it feel an affection for all; and then let it be particularly fond of humaneness. (*The Analects of Confucius*, p. 22)

Humaneness is the extension of an affection for parents to others. The principles of humaneness and filial piety have had a strong influence upon Chinese medical ethics. I shall discuss that in the third section.

But there are two problems that remain to be solved: (i) Why does everybody have a similar affection between parents and children and for his fellow-men? Because 'in our nature we approximate one another; habit put us further and further apart.' (*The Analects of Confucius*, p. 109) (ii) Why can man extend his affection for parents or children to others? By the way of analogy. In the negative sense, humaneness means 'do not do to others what you would not desire yourself.' (*The Analects of Confucius*, p. 76) In the positive sense, humaneness means help others to establish themselves and have success as you did for yourself, 'to make analogy of others with oneself is the method of practicing humaneness.' (*The Analects of Confucius*, p. 49)

But it seemed that the solutions of these two problems were not satisfactory. How does one guarantee a person will extend the affection for himself or for his parents and his children to his fellow-men?

Men Ke (Mencius, 390–305 BC) tried to provide this guarantee. He argued with a scholar named Gaozi that human nature is virtuous. Here are his arguments; (i) It is the innate nature of human beings that makes one become a person with humaneness, just like the innate nature of wood makes it to be transformed into a cup or tray; (ii) The nature of human being is toward virtue, just like water flows downward. It flows upward because of external force, not of its nature; (iii) The nature of human being is different from that of dog or ox. The former is virtuous, but the latter not. Men Ke's conclusion is: Everybody has the sense of compassion and pity. The sense of compassion and pity is humaneness. Humaneness is innate in everybody's heart, not something imposed on him from outside. (*Menzi2*)

But how does one explain so much evil or vice in the world? Men Ke explained that the reason is the failure to give full play to human nature because it is stifled by human desires. So to cultivate one's moral character is no more than to scant desire. But where does the desire come from? He gave no answer.

Xun Huang (286–238 BC), a later Confucian, agreed that everybody has approximately the same nature, but the nature of the human being is vicious. Doing good comes by nurture. (*Xunzi*) Why is human nature vicious? Because everybody has his or her interests and desires. So such vices arise as fighting, murder, and riot which should be suppressed by 'li' (etiquette) and 'fa' (laws). Then man could do good, just like a piece of wood was processed and turned into a furniture or a pile of clay into a pottery. But how does one explain so much good done by the noble persons? Xun Huang had to concede that the sages have no desires and vices.

The Confucians in later ages attempted to take a middle road. They argued that human nature could be virtuous but was not always (Dong Zhongshu), or human nature is a mixture of virtue and vice (Yang Xong), or there are three grades in the human nature: the upper is virtuous, the lower is vicious, and the middle can be either (Han Yu) etc. (Cai, 1937, pp. 78–79, 82, 96, 105–106, 128)

However, all sections of the Confucian school agreed that humaneness is a virtue that could emanate from inside oneself to all aspects of life: If you have humaneness in your heart, you practice humaneness ('ren') in the relation with your parents, that is 'xiao' (filial piety), in the relation with your children, that is 'ci' (kindness), in the relation with your friends, that is 'yi' (sincerity) and 'xin' (reliability), in relation with your patients, that is 'ci' (compassion), in the relation with your monarch or superiors, that is 'zhong' (loyalty), in the relation with your inferiors or subjects, that is 'hui' (kindness). You practice humaneness fully, that is 'zhong'. You treat others in the same way in which you do yourself, that is 'shu'. You guide your behavior with humaneness, you follow 'li' (rites). Then you can administer the country and calm down the land under heaven.

III. Medicine Is the Art of Humaneness

This section will discuss the ethics of Confucian medicine, which constitutes the mainstream of TCM. Among the physicians of Confucian medicine, some were professional practitioners, some retired officials or intellectuals failing to pass the Imperial Examination, who took the practice of medicine as charities.

Medicine and Confucianism originated from different sources. The fusion of these two might be related to the fact that emperors in many dynasties encouraged their subjects to worship only Confucianism and to reject other systems. But I think the essential reason is that the theory of Confucianism accorded with the aim of medicine more appropriately than others did. The ethical theory of Yang Zhu's is a kind of egoism. He said 'my life is mine. I want to do nothing to benefit the others under heaven even only pulling out one hair from mine' and 'to do something for others, such as ruling the state, should be a spare time activity after preserving my own life.' (*Menzi*, Lu Buwei, Qiu) This version of egoism is incompatible with the aim of medical activity— saving the life of others or ameliorating the symptoms of others or relieving others from pain or suffering. Taoists held that the human being consists of Yin and Yang just as all other things do in the universe, so he is no more precious than they. It took a relativistic view on life and death—there is no difference between life and death; life is death and vice versa (*Laozi*, *Zhuangzi*). Taoist naturalism and relativism also did not promote the aim of medicine. Buddhists emphasized saving all lives under heaven, but they paid more attention to the next life rather than this one. On the contrary, Confucianism not only treasured human life highly, ('Being predestined to come into being by heaven, the human being is precious because he extraordinarily surpasses all creatures' (see Qiu)), but also heavily stressed 'loving others', 'serving others' and never said a word about the next life.

In Confucian opinion, medicine is nothing but the application of Confucianism in a healing field.

1. Medicine As the Art of Humaneness

Confucians usually said: 'Whoever has no chance to work as a good prime minister, may work as a good physician.' (Unschuld, 1979, p. 98) Both a good prime minister and a physician practice humaneness, though physicians were never in a same status as prime ministers were in the Confucian society.

When Confucians argued the thesis of medicine as the art of humaneness, what they put stress on was that Confucianism and medicine are inseparably, complementary of each other, and that medicine is an essential part of Confucianism. The explicit arguments were given by an imperial physician in Northern Song Dynasty (960–1127) named Zhao Chonggu. As he wrote:

Confucians know 'li' (rites) and 'yi' (justice). Physicians know what are benefits and harms. If you do not cultivate the virtues of 'li' and 'yi', you will be against the teachings of Confucius and Mencius. If you cannot distinguish between benefits and harms, you will damage the lives of people. How can you despise Confucius and practice medicine? How can you separate medicine from Confucius? (Xu Chunfu)

They argued that if you master medical knowledge, you can use it to treat the sickness of your monarch and parents, to practice the principles of 'zhong' (loyalty) and 'xiao' (filial piety), to treat the sickness of your inferiors or children, and to practice the principle of 'ci' (compassion or kindness). (Zhang Zhongjin, Cheng Guopeng) In Chinese history great efforts were made to incorporate medical training as a necessary part of the general education of a Confucian because Confucians asserted only those who understand the art of medicine can be called children who fulfill their duty toward their parents. And if you do not know medicine at all, you have to rely on incompetent physicians. That means you violate the principles of 'ci' (kindness) and 'xiao' (filial piety), so you have to know medicine as a parent of your children and a child of your parents. (Cheng Guopeng)

The Confucian theory of humaneness and associated principles are a valuable legacy to Chinese physicians. But some principles such as filial piety have been exerting a negative impact upon the development of medicine even today: Anatomy was seriously undeveloped; the voluntary donations of dead bodies for medical education or organs for transplantation are very rare up to now, because 'body, hair and skin are all inherited from parents, and no one is permitted to damage them at all.' (*The Classics on Filial Piety*)

2. The Physician's Responsibility

Confucian physicians characterized in various ways their responsibility as 'to cure the sickness to save the patient'. This coin has two sides. The positive one is to do good:

'Physicians should keep humaneness in their hearts; this is a justified maxim. They should help the people as much as possible and perform far-reaching good deeds.' (Gong Tingxian; Unschuld, p. 71[7])

'The principle of medicine is the principle of humaneness. Its basis is innate compassion, and help is its duty.' (Zhang Ren: 'Preface' to (Wan Chuan); Unschuld, 1979, p. 99)

The negative is to do no harm:

'One cannot destroy life in order to save life.' (Sun Simiao)

'It is impossible for a man not to fall ill, and it is impermissible for a physician not to treat patient.' (Zhao Lian)

They further argued that this responsibility is a very weighty one, because the fate of patient's life or death lies in his hands. If a physician treats patients carelessly or does not use medicine skillfully, he will kill even more people. (Song Ci; Shen Jin'ao)

Why? Because physicians have powerful knowledge in their hands. Gao Mei in his 'Preface' to *Medical Cases: A Guide to Diagnosis* (Ye Gui) made an analogy of using drugs with the use of soldiers: the decision over life or death is made in the short span of time between two breaths. (Ye Gui; Unschuld, 1979, p. 99) In view of many incompetent physicians who failed to cure patients, Xu Yanzuo wrote a special article entitled 'Incompetent physicians kill men' and warned in a somewhat exaggerating tone that men rarely die from disease, frequently they die from drugs, but what he said was really an explicit accusation against iatrogenic disease with a consequentialist flavor. (Xu Yanzuo; Unschuld, 1979, p. 113)

But I want to add two observations: (1) interestingly enough, some physicians claimed to give up hopeless cases. They pointed out that two reasons were responsible for such decisions not being made: (i) emotional ties with relatives played a part; (ii) reluctance to stop lay in the hope of great profit. (Huai Yuan; Unschuld, p. 105) All the same, a non-professional physician tended not to make an active effort to treat the patients whom they thought incurable. (Li Tao)

(2) Some Confucians anticipated the dilemmas now facing medicine, as Gu Yanwu (1613–82) pointed out:

> The physicians of antiquity were able to give life back to men and were capable of killing men. Physicians today are neither capable of keeping men alive, nor are they able to kill men. They are solely capable of reducing man to a state which represents neither life nor death and which finally ends in death. (Shen Jin'ao; Unschuld, pp. 106–7)

Heavy responsibility requires a physician to be a virtuous person. Yang Chuan (265–420) said that 'we only can trust or rely on such physicians who have the heart of humaneness and compassion, are clever and wise, sincere and honest.' (*On Physics*, see Zhou)

How should one cultivate these virtues that are requisites for a physician? In addition to a good family background and rich experiences of practicing medicine as Xu Chunfu (1520–96) said in his 'Famous Physicians' in an exaggerating way: 'Don't take the drug prescribed by a physician to whom medical knowledge has been passed on for less than three generations. You never can become an excellent surgeon unless you have suffered bone fracture nine times' (Liu et al., p. 194). The most important is 'zhengji' (to rectify oneself). An anonymous author argued: 'The "tao" of practicing medicine is that you must rectify yourself before you rectify things. To rectify yourself means to understand principles in order to bring your skill into full play. To rectify things means to treat patient with medication . . . If you have not rectified yourself, how can you rectify things? If you can not rectify things, how can you cure a patient's disease?' (Anomyn)

How does one rectify oneself? Confucian physicians put stress on two essential points: cultivating humaneness and mastering skill. As Shi Zhiyuan wrote:

Medicine consists of humaneness ('ren') and skill ('ji'). 'Some master the skill and are wanting in humaneness. These are the greedy physicians. Others possess humaneness, yet they lack skill. These are the incompetent physicians. Incompetency and greed are apt to harm men.' (Xu Yanzuo; Unschuld, p. 108[8])

It seems that Confucian physicians always put humaneness first. In Gong Tingxian's 'Ten Maxims for Physicians' he listed keeping humaneness in the heart and grasping Confucianism as first and second places, then the mastery of medical knowledge. (Gong Tingxian; Unschuld, pp. 71–2) Chen Shigoing in his 'Ten Maxims for Physicians' emphasized: 'Above all they are to know the principles of Confucianism, only then will they be able to understand the principles of medicine.' (Chen Shigong; Unschuld, p. 78)

In the literature of TCM ethics we can find many writings in which the intentions of preserving human life and helping others without rewards were highly praised, and the intentions of seeking profits or even earning a living were fiercely attacked. When a disciple came to Li Gao (1180–1251) to learn from him, he asked the young man: 'Do you want to learn to be a physician looking for money or a physician propagating the principles?' (Liu et al., 1980, p. 31) A much-told tale is as follows:

A famous physician in the period of the Three Kingdoms was living by Lushan Mountain (now Jiangxi Province). When he cured a seriously ill patient, he asked him to plant five apricot trees. (Mildly ill patients are asked to plant one apricot tree.) After several years, he had a hundred thousand apricot trees that became a green and luxuriant forest. If somebody wanted to get a container of fruit when the apricots were ripe, he only had to bring a container of rice to exchange. Dong used the exchanged rice to assist the poor and help travellers. The beneficiaries amounted to twenty thousand persons every year. This was called: The Spring's Warmth in Apricot Forest. (Zhou)

In Chen Shigong's 'Ten Maxims for Physicians', the seventh Maxim is that physicians should

not take money for drugs from the poor or those in distress, from travelling beggar priests, be they Buddhists or Taoists, nor from messengers of local administrators who come for treatment. It is befitting to provide these people with drugs free of charge, . . . such conduct is applied humaneness. (Chen Shigong; Unschuld, 1979, p. 79)

It was argued that if self-interest is at play, the principle of humaneness is violated.

But it is very difficult to justify demanding physicians to provide free medical services without any rewards. Some Confucians assimilated the Buddhist concept of retribution in contrasting pursuits for fame and profits with unselfish help: Unselfish help to patients would be rewarded later in a physician's life or good luck would befall him or his sons and grandsons; otherwise misfortune would be predestined to him and his offspring.

So Confucians strongly fought against the professionalization of medicine. Zhao Xueming (1719–1805) argued that physicians are expected to help people, but recently many made medicine a profession. They saw in it a better way to make money than any other occupation. (SCTM, p. 225) Finally Confucians made some concession. They no longer attacked the intention of earning a living and recognized two reasons of practicing medicine: to earning a living and to help one's fellow-men. (Xu Yanzuo: Unschuld, 1979, p. 109)

The emphasis on physician's virtue and right motivation might be a means of controlling the use of medical knowledge, especially when professional codes and laws governing medical suits are lacking. But it was not as adequate as the codes and laws without cultivating one's virtue.

3. Physician-Patient Relationship

Many Chinese physicians stressed that a physician should treat patients as equals. In his famous 'On the Absolute Sincerity of Great Physicians' Sun Simiao wrote:

> A Great Physician should not pay attention to status, wealth or age; neither should he question whether the particular person is attractive or unattractive, whether he is an enemy or friend, whether he is a Chinese or a foreigner, or finally, whether he is uneducated or educated. He should meet everyone on equal ground. He should always act as if he were thinking of his close relatives. (Sun Simiao; Unschuld, 1979, p. 30)

It was argued that the reasons why a physician should behave in such way lie in: (i) Both rich and poor are living people; (ii) the effects of drugs are same to both of them. (Gong Tingxian; Unschuld, 1979, pp. 63, 72, 74) Even when physicians are asked to examine prostitutes, they should treat them like the daughters of decent family. (Chen Shigong) An exemplary instance was cited in which a famous physician in the Ming Dynasty (1368–1644), Wan Chuan, cured the four-year-old son of his enemy (Zhou).

But some argued that physicians should pay more attention to the patients who were administrative officials such that they thought it was necessary to mention it in the maxims for physicians. In Chen Shigong's 'Ten Maxims for Physicians' the tenth is 'If a physician receives a call from an administrative official, he has to respond to this promptly and should not be negligent. He has to meet these people with sincere respect . . .' (Chen Shigong; Unschuld, 1979, p. 80) In fact, in such a Confucian bureaucratic society like traditional China, it is very difficult for physicians to treat all patients as equals. Confucians only attacked individual physicians who sought their own profits or acted conscientiously to the rich but carelessly to the poor, but never questioned whether the health care system or allocations of resources as a whole were just.

Physicians should take into account whether the costs of treatment constitute an unbearable burden for patients. Xu Dachun (1693–1772) in his 'On

Ginseng' criticized those physicians who used ginseng to treat patients were both killing the patients and breaking up their families. But why did the patients who had taken ginseng die without repentance? Because they confused expensive drugs with effective ones. Xu further criticized that it was forgivable for a physician to kill a patient with improper use of drugs, but his deeds of killing a patient and breaking up his family were more vicious than what a robber or a thief did. (SCTM, pp. 228–229)

Great attention was paid to physicians' sexual morality. Many emphasized the prohibition on a physician's sexual relation with his patient and to make every effort to prevent it. In Chen Shigong's 'Five Admonitions to Physicians' the second is 'when making a visit to a sick married woman, widow, or a nun the physician has to have a companion. Only then can he enter the room and undertake the examination.' (Chen Shigong; Unschuld, 1979, p. 77) Xu Dachun further maintained that 'everything imaginable has to be done to avoid suspicion.' (Unschuld, 1979, p. 80) Thus a line was tied on the wrist of female patient and the physician diagnosed by feeling her pulse through the line at a distance. It always led to the wrong diagnosis.

Chinese physicians seldom talked about patient autonomy except for powerful patients. A strong paternalism was passed from ancient times to present. In his *A Thorough Understanding of Medicine in Ancient and Modern Times*, Huai Yuan argued for paternalism as follows: 'Medicine is applied humaneness. To see other people suffer rouses compassion and pity within myself. When the ailing themselves cannot make any decisions, I will make them in their place. I always put myself in their place.' (Huai Yuan; Unschuld, 1979, p. 102) But this paternalism disappeared in the case of powerful patients such as kings or ministers. We read some biographies of then famous physicians in the *Historical Records* that those patients always made decisions against their physicians. Chinese physicians also scarcely talked about the protection of patient's privacy except for women patients. Chen Shigong insisted that a physician is never allowed to speak of the care in the boudoirs 'even in the presence of his own wife.' (Chen Shigong; Unschuld, 1979, p. 77)

Interesting enough in TCM ethics, maxims or admonitions were prescribed not only for physicians but also for patients. Gong Xin has written 'Warnings to Enlightened Physicians', 'Warnings to Mediocre Physicians' and 'Warnings to Patients' (Gong Xin; Unschuld, 1979, p. 71–2), and his son Gong Tingxian 'Ten Maxims for Physicians' and 'Ten Maxims for Patients.

4. Physician-Physician Relationship

Trust and harmony are most precious. The principles of handling the relation between colleagues are trust and harmony—the application of humaneness to this aspect, as put in many maxims for physicians. For instance, in Chen Shigong's 'Ten Maxims for Physicians' the third is about the relationship between colleagues:

Colleagues from the vicinity should not be offended thoughtlessly or treated arrogantly. When associating with them one should be friendly and cautious. Older colleagues should be respected, learned ones should be regarded as teachers, conceited ones should be avoided, and to those who are not as advanced as oneself one should offer one's help. In this way slander and hatred are avoided, because trust and harmony are the most precious. (Chen Shigong; Unschuld, 1979, p. 78)

On the other side of the coin, the slandering or even criticizing of colleagues before patients was fiercely attacked as a violation of the principle of humaneness.

There are a number of reasons why a physician should esteem highly trust and harmony between colleagues: (i) the moral reason—physicians should practice consistently the principle of humaneness also in the relation with colleagues; (ii) the epistemological reason—the practice of medicine is fallible, as an ancient physician Chun Yuyi in the early Han Dynasty said: 'It is impossible for a physician infallibly to diagnose the disease and make a decision about life or death' (Si Maqian); (iii) the pathological reason—the failure of the use of earlier drugs is due to an imbalance on special occasion; (iv) the social reason—medicine is an enterprise in which knowledge is handed down by way of master-disciple relationship in a community of colleagues, so colleagues have to protect each other and on no account are they to expose one another.

But Confucian physicians confused these two things: physicians should not slander their colleagues, but they should discuss medical issues with them in a critical way.

However, physicians of TCM tended to be reluctant to communicate with their colleagues and kept secret the prescriptions that they thought to be useful and that usually caused these prescriptions to be lost, though making these prescriptions public was praised as a good conduct in the literature on TCM ethics.

In traditional China there were no medical organizations and professional codes to regulate and control the relations between physicians and patients as well as these between physicians, apart from the maxims, admonitions or warnings set forth by individual physicians. Hence there was no guarantee for all that the prestigious physicians said on medical ethics. The only control or restraints came from the penetrating influence of Confucian ideology.

IV. Characteristics of TCM Ethics

First, in Confucian ethics more attention was paid to virtues that a moral agent should have and how he could have them. The so-called 'xiusheng yangxing'— cultivation of one's moral character—is the starting point of becoming a person with humaneness and achieving his lofty goal. To be a person with humaneness, one should make an effort along two lines: to cultivate one's compassion to others so as to have humaneness in one's heart, and to behave according to rites which embody the principle of humaneness. But it seems that Confucians in various dynasties put more stress on the first, because 'the achieving of humaneness must come from oneself'. (*The Analects of Confucius*, p. 76) The way of cultivating the sense of humaneness is subduing oneself or self-control. Subduing oneself means subduing one's own desire: to give priority to what others like and dislike over what one likes and dislikes. What differentiates a person with humaneness from the one without humaneness is that the latter knows only what he wants but does not know what others want. In subduing oneself in medicine, a physician should help patients without consideration of rewards, not to pursue fame or profits, not exploit patients' trouble to get rich, not depreciate colleagues. How should one subdue oneself in an effective way? It seems that the only way is to study the Confucian classics. This method of cultivating moral character is still practiced in modern China, though the effect is doubtful.

The 'li' seems to be external norms for human conduct, as well as the maxims, admonitions, exhortations, or warnings in medicine. But 'li' was too vague to be a set of normative guidelines for human conduct. My colleague Professor Li Zhehou interpreted 'li' as 'a socio-political system with the characteristics of hierarchy based on the blood relationship of clan' (Li Zhehou, p. 16) That is what the maxims, admonitions, warnings in medicine were. All these were too vague to have the binding force on physicians.

Even so, Confucians put more weight on internal feelings than external restraints, as Confucius himself said: 'The achieving of humaneness depends upon oneself, how can [it depend] upon others!' (*The Analects of Confucius*; English translation, p. 76) 'If one is not humane, what is the use of knowing rites?' (op. cit., p. 129)

The virtue ethics of Confucianism could perhaps be used as an antidote to the shortcomings of modern normative ethics. If a man wants to do anything he eagerly desires, he will make every effort to avoid the restraints of ethical norms, if he has no heart to follow them. But by itself the advice of cultivating moral character is not enough. Perhaps, it is necessary to work along two lines cultivating one's virtue within and restraining one's conduct without. The reason is perhaps that the nature of human beings is both virtuous and vicious at least for most of them. Secondly, Confucian theory of humaneness as well as its medical ethics may be characterized as deontological. 'Humaneness', 'filial piety', 'fraternity', 'sincerity', 'compassion', 'loyalty' etc. seem to be *a priori* imperatives. It is absolute for a person with humaneness to follow these principles in spite of whatever consequences will occur. Confucius said: 'A person with humaneness never seeks life at the expense of humaneness, but sacrifices himself for the accomplishment of humaneness.' (*The Analects of Confucius*, p. 99) On the contrary, Confucians were always disgusted with the concerns of interest: 'The Gentleman is conscious only of justice, the base person only of interest.' (*The Analects of Confucius*, p. 36)

Confucians of later ages further emphasized that all these principles mentioned above are heavenly ones—the principles imposed upon human beings by heaven. Arguing to demarcate between justice and interest, as wrote Dong Zhongshu: 'We are only concerned with justice, we are not concerned with interest; we are only concerned with understanding what are the principles, we are not concerned with how much merit we achieve.' Another

Confucian, Zhu Nanxia, said in a more deontological tone: 'As for sages, they do everything naturally rather than for any purpose. If one does something for a purpose, this purpose is his selfish desire; there is no heavenly principle in it. That is the line demarcating between justice and interest.' (Cai, p. 102)

It was Yang Zhu and Mo Di who first put forward the utilitarian ethics in China. The former may be labeled an egoist utilitarian, the latter an altruist utilitarian. Yang Zhu argued that one must value oneself because 'my life is mine, I benefit from it so much that even the monarch's rank of nobility is no match from my life, the wealth of all over the world cannot be changed for my life, and one day I lose my life, I never get it again' (Lu Buwei). Mo Di argued that what a person with humaneness wants to do is for the purpose of promoting the interests of people under heaven and to rid them from harms, such as war, robbery, killing etc. which originated from not loving each other so as to reach mutual benefits (*Mozi*). The later Mohists defined 'gong' (merits) as 'benefiting people' and 'li' (interests) as 'something which you are pleased to get' (*Mozi*: 'The Classics of Mohism', 'Commentaries of Classics') In modern Chinese the English word 'utility' is translated into 'gongli'.

Both these two utilitarian theories were fiercely attacked by Confucians. Men Ke criticized that Yang Zhu's claim of 'for myself' is without any respect to his monarch and Mo Di's claim of loving each other to reach mutual benefits is without any respect to his father, and it is birds or beasts that are without any respect to monarch and father. (*Menzi*)

In the TCM ethics all the requisites which a physician should meet or all the maxims he should follow are also heavenly principles without regard to which consequences will happen. It was argued that when the care of a patient is not good, one should not blame the physician who followed Confucian principles for the failure.

Now the Confucian dogma 'justice important and utility trivial' was blamed for hindering the development of science-technology and commodity economy and the transition from mediaeval ages to modern ages as well as for impeding the improvement of health care in traditional China.

Thirdly, in TCM ethics analogical reasoning is more often used than its modern Western counterpart.

Confucians held that it is a fact that a human being has the attitude of compassion to others, as Men Ke put: 'Everybody has the sense of compassion and pity'. How can one infer from this that 'a human being ought to love others'? On the basis of the principle 'Tao', which according to Zhu Xi's interpretation, is both the truth of what it is and the norms of what it ought to be. (Qian Mu, p. 91) In their opinion 'tao' in the universe is a model for the order which should exist in a society. As it was written in *The Book of Changes*: 'Heaven is lofty and honourable; earth is low . . . Things low and high appear displayed in a similar position. The noble and mean had their places assigned accordingly.' (p. 377) So with the help of 'tao' we can infer from 'is' in nature to 'ought' in human society: 'is' and 'ought' fuse into one in the concept of 'tao'.

As for the theory of humaneness, the fusion of 'is' and 'ought' in it is based on a psychological doctrine: Everybody has the sense of compassion to others.

I have mentioned above that the method of practicing humaneness is analogy for Confucius: The nature of everybody is similar. Humaneness is to put oneself in the place of other or to treat other people as you would do yourself. There are two points in it: the one is knowing—inferring from what is that I like or dislike to knowing what is that another likes or dislikes. The other is about practicing: 'Do not do to others what you would not desire yourself (*The Analects of Confucius*, p. 76) or 'Help others to get what you have got'.

Is there any necessary connection between knowing and practicing? Men Ke made an attempt to bridge the gap with his psychological theory of 'the nature of human being is virtuous'. It seemed to be unsuccessful.

There seemed to be a kind of deductive reasoning in the relation between the Confucian theory, principles of medical ethics, and conduct of physicians, but without *modus tollens*.

Parents and children, husband and wife, brothers and sisters, friends, monarch and his subjects, physician and patient and so on, all these are various forms of interpersonal relationship. Filial piety ('xiao'), kindness ('ci'), chastity ('jie'), fraternity ('ti'), trust ('xin'), sincerity ('yi'), loyalty ('zhong'), compassion ('ci') etc. are the application of humaneness in respective relations. But these principles centered on humaneness never have been refuted by any unethical conduct because the theory and principles are both ambiguous enough that people do not know which part of the statement system should be refuted. On the occasion of refutation it was usually resolved by revising the theory or adding some auxiliary theory for instance, on the nature of human being. So the Confucian theory as well as ethical principles of TCM have been stable during the long history.

Is it the case that whoever has good intention necessarily will do good? Yes. In Confucians' opinion, there is a necessary connection between good intention and good conduct. If you did not do good, it only proved that your intention was not good, that you had no sense of humaneness, you did not understand the principles of Confucianism, you tried to seek your own fame or profit, you did not work hard to study the Confucian classics, and so on.

These peculiarities of ethical reasoning in TCM are closely interrelated with its virtue theory and deontological theory, and together with them hindered the development of normative ethics and utilitarian theory in Chinese medicine because of their absolute dominance.

Notes

1. The Chinese character 'ren' has been translated into various English words: benevolence, kindheartedness, humanity, but I prefer the word 'humaneness' Professor P. U. Unschuld invented (Unschuld).

2. The founder of Confucianism is Kong Qiu (551–479 BC).

3. Sun Simiao (581–682), a physician who mainly is a Taoist but tainted with Confucianism, Buddhism, and shamanism.

4. The founders of Yangism and Mohism are Yang Zhu (395–335 BC) and Mo Di (480–420 BC) respectively. The founder of Taoism may be Li Ran, his dates of birth and

death are unknown, perhaps at the same time with Confucius. The main proponents of Nominalism are Hui Shi (370–310 BC) and Gongsun Long (320–250 BC). The master of Legalism is Han Fei (280–233 BC).

5. The translation is somewhat different from the English version, the same below.

6. I will choose 'rites' as the English counterpart of 'li' below.

7. In Unschuld's book (1979) is collected the main literature on TCM ethics. It is very helpful for any who are interested in this issue. I made some changes in the citations when I felt it was necessary according to my understanding of the texts.

8. Professor Unschuld might mistake Shi Zhiyuan as Jiang Shi.

References
Primary Sources
The Analects of Confucius, see IP (part 1, vol. 1, pp. 41–66), and the English translation by J. R Ware: 1955, The *Sayings of Confucius*, Mentor Books, New York.

Anomyn, On *Prescriptions of Pediatrics*, see Zhou (1983). *The Book of Changes*, see the English translation by J. Leggs: 1971, Mentor Books, New York.

The Book of Rites, see IP (part 1, vol. 2, pp. 592–611).

Chen, Shigong, *Orthodoxy in Surgery*, vol. 2, printed in the period of Xianfeng's reign, Qing Dynasty.

Cheng, Guopeng, 'Preface' to *Understanding of Medicine by Heart*, see Liu et al., p. 61.

Institute of Philosophy et al. IP: 1973, *Materials of Chinese Philosophy*, part 1: Pre-Qing Dynasty, vol. 1, 2, Zhonghua Books, Beijing.

Gong, Tingxian: *Back to Life From a Myriad of Sickness*, vol. 8, pp. 59–60, printed in the period of Wanli's reign, Ming Dynasty.

Gong, Xin: *Medical Lessons in Ancient and Modern Times*, vol. 8, printed in the period of Kangxi's reign, Qing Dynasty.

Huai, Yuan: *The Thorough Understanding of Medicine in Ancient and Modern Times*, printed in 1936.

Laozi: *The Classics of Tao and Virtue*, see IP (part 1, vol. 1, p. 233–256).

Lu, Buwei: *The Springs and Autumns of Lu's*, see IP (part 1, vol. 1, pp. 108–110).

Menzi, see IP (part 1, vol. 1, 185–230).

Mozi, see IP (part 1, vol. 1, pp. 69–103; vol. 2, pp. 237–361).

Shanghai College of Traditional Medicine SCTM: 1980, *Selection of Ancient Medical Texts*, Shanghai Press of Science and Technology.

Shen, Jin 'ao: *A Book of Respecting Life of Shen's*, Congwen Books, Hubei, printed in the period of Tongzhi's reign, Qing Dynasty, vol. 1, p. 1.

Song, Ci: *Collected Papers on Redressing Grievances*, see Zhou.

Si, Maqian, Historical Records, 'Biography of Canggong', see SCTM (p. 33).

Sun, Simiao: *Important Prescriptions Worth a Thousand Pieces of Gold*, printed in the period of Wanli's reign, Ming Dynasty, vol. 1, pp. 9–11.

Sun, Simiao: *Supplementary Prescriptions Worth a Thousand of Pieces of Gold*, printed in the period of Guangzu's reign, Qing Dynasty, vol. 29, pp. 2–3. Wan, Chuan *Wanmizhai's Book Series of Medicine*, printed in the period of Guangxu's reign, Qing Dynasty.

Xu, Chunfu: *Medical Traditions in Ancient and Modern Times*, printed in the period of Jiajing's reign, Ming Dynasty.

Xu, Yanzuo: *Concise Words on the Essence of Medicine*, printed in the period of Guangxu's reign, Qing Dynasty.

Xunzi: see IP (part 1, vol. 2, pp. 373–473).

Ye, Gui: *Medical Cases—Guide to Diagnosis*, printed in the period of Daoguang's Reign, Qing Dynasty, Suzhou.

Zhang, Gao: On *Medicine*, printed in 1933, Nanking: Library of Chinese Study, vol. 10, pp. 31– 39.

Zhang, Zhongjing: 'Preface', to On *Fever*, see Liu et al., pp. 61–70.
Zhao, Lian: *An Important Supplement to the Introduction to Medicine*, printed in the period of Guangxu's reign, Qing Dynasty.
Zhuangzi, see IP (part 1, vol. 2, pp. 259–303).

Secondary Sources
Cai, Yuanpi: 1937, *A History of Chinese Ethics*, The Commercial Press, Shanghai. Li, Tao: 1930, 'Ethics of Chinese medicine', *Chinese Medical Journal* 16, 239–242.
Li, Zhehou: 1985, *On the History of Ancient Chinese Ideas*, The People's Press, Beijing.
Liu, Zhengmin et al.: 1980, *The Foundation of Ancient Chinese Medical Texts*, The Press of Health, Beijing.
Qian, Mu: 1962, *Commentaries to the Four Books*, The Press of Chinese Cultures, Taipei.
Qiu, Ren-Zong: 1985, 'The intersection of human values and public policy—a Chinese view', in Z. Bankowski and J. Bryant (eds.), *Health Policy, Ethics, and Human Values*, CIOMS, Switzerland.
Unschuld, P. U.: 1979, *Medical Ethics in Imperial China—A Study in Historical Anthropology*, University of California Press, Berkeley.
Zhou, Yimou (ed.): 1983, *Chinese Physicians on Medical Morality*, Human Press of Science and Technology, Changsha.

Sun Szu-miao and the Origins of the Debate on Medical Ethics in China, From *Medical Ethics in Imperial China*

Paul Unschuld

──────────── INTRODUCTION TO READING ────────────

Ancient China had a long history of scholarship in medicine including medical ethics. The most thorough study of this literature available in English comes from the German historian, Paul Unschuld whose book, *Medical Ethics in Imperial China,* contains extensive translations of the most important texts. In the following excerpts from his volume (reprinted here with some footnotes omitted), he describes the earliest available literature focusing on the writing of Sun Szu-miao [spelled Sun Simiao in the previous selection by Ren-Zong Qiu], a seventh century, CE, physician reflecting Taoist and Buddhist influences who began what Unschuld describes as a long process of differentiating professional medical ethics in China from the underlying Confucian world view. Unschuld sees this as part of a process of gaining for physicians control over "secondary resources of medicine," i.e., the material and non-material rewards of the practice. These excerpts contain the full text of a particularly significant portion of Sun Szu-miao's writing, here called "On the Absolute Sincerity of Great Physicians."

Unschuld then goes on to present a Confucian response from an eighth century physician, Lu Chih. Appealing to the classical Confucian virtues, humaneness and compassion, Lu Chih reflects the traditional attitude that medicine should be the domain of everyone in the population, not just "mere" professionals. The classical Confucian view was that every family should have someone who could practice medicine out of a sense of familial loyalty, not just for money.

With the exception of several short quotations from earlier times the texts to be discussed in this study date from the seventh century AD up to the end of the nineteenth century. Following the explanations given above, one might assume that the debate over ethics in Chinese medicine coincided with the broadly conceived program for the training of medical doctors in the Chinese Middle Ages. Such an assumption would be quite risky; its sole justification may be the fact that we have no knowledge of an earlier Chinese source going beyond mere suggestions of ethics or discussing the ethics of the physicians at length.

The sources used here are taken from medical literature. . . . In part we are dealing with individual sections from medical literature, which were devoted to questions of medical ethics. Although some of these statements are repetitive, I have translated every section on ethics which I could locate. I present them unabridged, in order to make this primary source material accessible to the widest possible audience. The goal is to create a basis for further discussion centering on the theme of ethics in medicine. In addition to these individual sections I have examined a considerable number of prefaces to medical literature for their relevant statements. In these cases I have had to make a selection from this prolific material. It is important to emphasize that the authors cited below took a definite stand in favor of medicine, either by editing medical literature itself or simply by composing prefaces to it. Thus they represent an aggregate who wish to influence the pattern of resource distribution to their private advantage or in the direction of the interest of the social group with whom they share a comprehensive paradigm. There are no "impartially objective" statements. Every participant may be identified with the interests of one of the groups involved.

The texts speak mostly for themselves. Wherever material was available, it seemed appropriate to provide the social background of the specific authors and to point out the central features of their formulated ethics.

Sun Szu-miao (AD 581?–682) appears to be the first Chinese author to have devoted a separate section of a paradigmatic nature to questions of medical ethics. In the official history of the T'ang dynasty his biography describes him as an extraordinarily talented man, who devoted himself to the teachings of the *I-ching*, of Lao-tzu and of the *yin-yang* philosophers, and also took an interest in the magical calculation of numbers. Besides other smaller works, he compiled the lengthy *Pei-chi ch'ien-chin yao-fang* (generally known as *Ch'ien-chin fang*) and, three decades later, a supplementary work, the *Ch'ien-*

chin I-fang. Both works have been often reprinted and still constitute an important source for the practices of traditional Chinese physicians.

Where or how Sun Szu-miao received his medical training is not known to us. It is, however, highly unlikely that he was in contact with one of the medical schools established after AD 629. Usually referred to as a Taoist, he seems to have been equally influenced by a considerable amount of Buddhist thought. He already possessed a strong reputation during his lifetime, based on his education and his achievements as a physician. This resulted in several appointments to positions at the court, none of which he ever accepted.

At the beginning of his voluminous work, *Ch'ien-chin fang*, Sun Szu-miao devoted a separate section "to the absolute sincerity of Great Physicians" ("*Lun ta-I ching-ch'eng*"). It is important to call attention to several points which he touches upon in this section. In the first place, he gives a general frame of reference to "his" medicine. He does not provide many details concerning the concepts he thought a "Great Physician" should follow. Yet from the few terms he mentions it appears that he advocated the medicine of systematic correspondence only. This medicine was a syncretic conceptual system based on the theories of the Five Phases (*wu-hsing*) and *yin-yang*, as well as on a mode of treatment derived from the concepts of magical correspondence. Furthermore, its contents and its terminology were influenced by the concepts of demonic medicine. Sun Szu-miao could have chosen pure demonic medicine (of which he was a strong supporter elsewhere, as can be seen from his introductory remarks to his Classic of Spells [*Chin-ching*]) or he could have chosen pragmatic, symptom-oriented pharmacotherapy, or even the above mentioned "religious" medicine of some Taoist sects, as a theoretical basis for his and his colleagues' healing practice. This is especially so because demonic medicine and pragmatic pharmacotherapy may have constituted the most prevalent paradigms of medical practice among the populace of his time (and throughout all subsequent centuries until the end of the Confucian era). We do not know the reasons for Sun Szu-miao's decision to point out only the medicine of systematic correspondence as the basis of a Great Physician's practice. It should be mentioned again though, that this system's underlying paradigm reflected the social concepts inherent in Confucian ideology. In contrast, demonic medicine and symptom-oriented, pragmatic pharmacotherapy flatly contradicted several claims and assumptions of Confucianism. Demonic medicine is based on a world view of "all against all," where one's own morality is neither an assurance of a healthy life as an individual nor a guarantee of a harmonious existence in society. Pragmatic pharmacotherapy is equally amoral, in that it rests on an assumption that illness can be prevented or cured by the intake of certain substances and that, therefore, no specific moral lifestyle is necessary for maintaining or regaining health. Confucianism, however, closely ties together maintenance of social order and of individual health; its social ideology starts from the notion that a certain lifestyle along fixed moral rules will contribute to both social harmony and personal well-being. To be sure, the medicine of systematic correspondence as it has come down to us in its earliest texts, compiled between the second century BC and the eighth century AD (most notably the Yellow Emperor's Inner Classic [*Huang-ti nei-ching*]), also contains various allusions to Taoist concepts. Yet these are marginal and do not overshadow the basic parallels that exist between this healing system and Confucian ideas of a desirable social structure.

Next to presenting "his" theoretical framework, Sun Szu-miao pointed out the necessity of a thorough education and rigorous conscientiousness. He may have done so in reference to the establishment of the first medical schools for Confucian scholar physicians during his lifetime, an innovation which may have been regarded by freely practicing physicians as jeopardizing their image.

Then follow explanations both on the basis of values, such as "compassion" (*tz'u*) and "humanity" (*jen*), and on the basis of maxims, such as "to aid every life and every man" or "one, cannot destroy life, in order to save life," which are taken from the Confucian and Buddhist comprehensive paradigms.

Sun Szu-miao seems to have understood that when visiting the sick the psychological aspects of the relationship between physician and patient must be taken into account. In order to gain trust, and thus unhindered access to "secondary" resources of medicine (that is, material and non-material rewards), the physician has to appear affectively neutral. The first signs of a group consciousness appear in Sun Szu-miao's explanations, when he criticizes the habit of belittling other physicians for the sake of one's own advantage. This shortsighted conduct is a decided disadvantage for a group in the process of obtaining professionalization and yet, according to all reports, it was displayed by the majority of practitioners at that time and later. In our own past, outstanding leaders of various professions have noticed this tendency; they therefore organized smaller elite groups within their larger group of professionals. These select groups were open only to candidates who had given evidence of high quality service. At the same time these core groups gave the impression of unity to the outside and avoided any critique of one another in front of non-members of the group. This was done in order to gain a much higher potential of trust and to obtain those resources which were not accessible to persons merely interested in individual profit.

The demarcation of a core group against the less exemplary mass is articulated in Sun Szu-miao by his choice of the term *ta-i* (closely related to *t'ai-i*, "court physicians") and his reference to the inefficiency of all the other physicians. For this reason he was not concerned with all the physicians, but only with those who stood out as "Great Physicians." To organize this elite group would have been a logical step, and in the West it was carried out, though considerably later. Yet in the Confucian society this did not happen.

In the end Sun Szu-miao deals with the problem of rewards. Greed was evidently one of the most serious grounds for the suspicion in which the public held the practices of physicians. Prince Huan of Ch'i made statements to this effect. If the public is to be persuaded that at least the "Great Physician" is not out for the material goods of his patients, one has to point out another system of reward, and make it sound credible that this compensates for the renuncia-tion of the goods of those patients whom one wants to treat.

Sun Szu-miao referred back to a statement by the founder of Taoism, Lao-tzu (604–? BC), in order to depict an incentive for rewards which was to render material desires unnecessary. In claiming that good deeds would be rendered by one's fellow-men while bad deeds would be requited by spirits, he was not far from an emphasis contained in the Confucian comprehensive paradigm, namely the stress on a this-worldly "reward" by fame which will be retained in later generations. Also he came close to the Buddhist idea which respectively foresees reward or retribution by supernatural powers in either the present life or a later life, if not even in another world.

To sum up we can say that the explanations formulated in this manner were based on values and concepts immanent in the three comprehensive para-digms influencing Chinese society during the time of Sun Szu-miao with almost similar strength. In addition they were oriented toward the gain of trust and provided a protective function. This protective function is the essential trait of a formulated ethics. In order to draw a profile of himself and his "better" colleagues, Sun Szu-miao could, at least theoretically, have put the excellence of his product in the foreground. Yet for a brilliant thinker of the stature of a Sun Szu-miao, what was at stake was the transformation of the outcome evaluation of his activity into a process evaluation, in order to surmount the status of a craftsman. Here are his own words:

On the Absolute Sincerity of Great Physicians

The saying goes back to Chang Chan [fourth century]: The difficult parts and the fine points in the [medical] classics and the literature on the prescriptions date back to the distant past.

Nowadays we have diseases which take a similar course with [different patients], yet from the outside they appear to be different; and there are others, which take a different course with [different persons], yet from the outside they appear to be similar. For this reason it will never suffice to examine exclusively with ears and eyes the symptoms of excess [*shih*] or deficiency [*hsü*] in the five granaries [*wu- tsang*] and the six palaces [*liu-fu*] as well as the flow [*t'ung*] or the blocking [*sai*] of the blood [*hsüeh*] and the pulses [*mai*], and the constructive [*jung*] and protective [*wei*] influences. In the first place one has to examine the symptoms of an illness which can be felt in the pulses to determine the specific ailment. Only someone who gives his undivided mental attention can begin to elaborate on these symptoms. This undivided attention must be given even to the last details which are related to the irregularities in the depth and the mark-ing of the various kinds of pulsations [*ts'un, k'ou, kuan, ch'ih*], which condition the variations in the position of the acupuncture points [*shu-hsüeh*], and which are responsible for the deviations in the thickness and strength of flesh and bones. Today, however, the prevailing effort is to grasp the most subtle details with the crudest and most superficial thought. This is truly dangerous!

If there is an excess and we still increase it, if there exists a deficiency and even more is taken away, if a congestion prevails and is further intensified, if there is a flow and still more is drained, if there is chill and further cooling is applied, and if in the case of heat an increase of temperature is brought about, then the specific illness has to deteriorate exceedingly. Where there is still hope for life I then see the approach of death!

It has indeed never happened that spirits distributed [the understanding] for the difficult aspects and the details which are necessary for physicians, people versed in the prescriptions, soothsayers and magicians. But how else can a person gain access to these secrets? At all times fools could be found who studied the prescriptions for three years and then they simply maintained that there was no disease in the world which could not be cured. Thereafter they treated diseases for three years and reached the conclusion that there was no useful prescription in the world. Thence ensues that it is absolutely necessary for the student to master the foundations of medicine in its most general significance, and to work energetically and unceasingly. He is not to gossip, but has to devote his words exclusively to the medical teachings. Only then will he avoid errors.

Whenever a Great Physician [ta-i] treats diseases, he has to be mentally calm and his disposition firm. He should not give way to wishes and desires, but has to develop first of all a marked attitude of compassion. He should commit himself firmly to the willingness to take the effort to save every living creature.

If someone seeks help because of illness or on the ground of another difficulty, [a Great Physician] should not pay attention to status, wealth or age, neither should he question whether the particular person is attractive or unattractive, whether he is an enemy or a friend, whether he is Chinese or a foreigner, or finally, whether he is uneducated or educated. He should meet everyone on equal ground; he should always act as if he were thinking of himself. He should not desire anything and should ignore all consequences; he is not to ponder over his own fortune or misfortune and thus preserve life and have compassion for it. He should look upon those who have come to grief as if he himself had been struck, and he should sympathize with them deep in his mind. Neither dangerous mountain passes nor the time of day, neither weather conditions nor hunger, thirst nor fatigue should keep him from helping wholeheartedly. Whoever acts in this manner is a Great Physician for the living. Whoever acts contrary to these demands is a great thief for those who still have their spirits!

From early times famous persons frequently used certain living creatures for the treatment of diseases, in order to thus help others in situations of need. To be sure, it is said: "Little esteem for the beast and high esteem for man," but when love of life is concerned, man and animal are equal. If one's cattle are mistreated, no use can be expected from it; object and sentiments suffer equally. How much more applicable is this to man!

Whoever destroys life in order to save life places life at an even greater distance. This is my good reason for the fact that I do not suggest the use of any living creature as medicament in the present collection of prescriptions. This does not concern the gadflies and the leeches. They have already perished when they reach the market, and it is therefore permissible to use them. As to the hen's eggs, we have to say the following. Before their content has been hatched out, they can be used in very urgent cases. Otherwise one should not burden oneself with this. To avoid their use is a sign of great wisdom, but this will never be attained.

Whoever suffers from abominable things, such as ulcers or diarrhea, will be looked upon with contempt by people. Yet even in such cases, this is my view, an attitude of compassion, of sympathy and of care should develop; by no means should there arise an attitude of rejection [in regard to the afflicted person].

Therefore a Great Physician should possess a clear mind, in order to look at himself; he should make a dignified appearance, neither luminous nor somber. It is his duty to reduce diseases and to diagnose sufferings and for this purpose to examine carefully the external indications and the symptoms appearing in the pulse [of patients]. He has to include thereby all the details and should not overlook anything. In the decision over the subsequent treatment with acupuncture or with medicaments nothing should occur that is contrary to regulations. The saying goes: "In case of a disease one has to help quickly," yet it is nevertheless indispensable to acquaint oneself fully with the particular situation so that there remain no doubts. It is important that the examination be carried out with perseverance. Wherever someone's life is at stake, one should neither act hastily nor rely on one's own superiority and ability, and least of all keep one's own reputation in mind. This would not correspond to the demands of humaneness!

And then in visiting the sick, wherever beautiful silks and fabrics fill the eye, the physician is not allowed to look out for them either to the left or to the right. Where the sounds of string instruments and instruments of bamboo fill the ear, he should not evoke the impression that he delights in them. Where delicious food is offered in stunning succession, he is to eat as if he experienced no taste. And, finally, where liquors are placed one next to the other, he will look at them as if they did not exist. Such manners have their origin in the assumption that if one single guest is not contented, the whole party cannot be merry. A patient's aches and pains release one from this obligation less than ever! However, if a physician is tranquil and engrossed in merry thoughts, in addition to being conceited and complacent, this is shameful for any human frame of mind. Such conduct is not suitable to man and conceals the true meaning of medicine.

According to the regulations of medicine it is not permissible to be talkative and make provocative speeches, to make fun of others and raise one's voice, to decide over right and wrong, and to discuss other people and their business. Finally, it is inappropriate to emphasize one's reputation, to belittle the rest of the physicians and to praise only one's own virtue. Indeed, in actual life someone who has accidentally healed a disease, then stalks around with his head raised, shows conceit and announces that no one in the entire world could measure up to him. In this respect all physicians are evidently incurable.

Lao-tzu has said: When the conduct of men visibly reveals virtue, the humans themselves will reward it. If, however, men commit their virtues secretly, the spirits will reward them. When the conduct of men visibly reveals misdeeds, the humans themselves will take retribution. If, however, men commit their misdeeds secretly, the spirits will take retribution. When comparing these alternatives and the respective rewards which will be given in the time after this life and still during this life, how could one ever make a wrong decision?

Consequently physicians should not rely on their own excellence, neither should they strive with their whole heart for material goods. On the contrary, they should develop an attitude of goodwill. If they move on the right path concealed [from the eyes of their contemporaries], they will receive great happiness as a reward without asking for it. The wealth of others should not be the reason to prescribe precious and expensive drugs, and thus make the access to help more difficult and underscore one's own merits and abilities. Such conduct has to be regarded as contrary to the teaching of magnanimity [*chung-shu*]. The object is help. Therefore I enter into all the problems in such detail here. Whoever studies medicine should not consider [these problems] insignificant![21]

Thirty years after Sun Szu-miao had composed this section in the *Ch'ien-chin fang*, he wrote the similarly voluminous work *Ch'ien-chin i-fang*. The 29th and 30th chapters were devoted to the practices of magic and the so-called techniques of interdiction. At the opening of the 29th chapter, Sun Szu-miao cited a brief ethics by the respective practitioners, evidently from an older shamanistic work. When and in what context it was compiled originally is not known. At the time he wrote his first book, Sun Szu-miao possibly already knew of this text and was influenced by it. The older text lacks the paradigmatic feature of Sun Szu-miao's own explanations of the ethics of physicians. In addition it does not emphasize elite groups and other aspects which were introduced by Sun Szu-miao. The unknown author addressed his colleagues rather than the public; as the following rendition of the text discloses, the author devoted himself largely to the need of his group for protection from their contemporaries and from the spirits.

Five Exhortations

First: not to kill; second: not to steal; third: not to live immorally; fourth: not to engage in perfidious talk; fifth: not to drink wine, nor to be envious.

Ten Types of Good Conduct

First: to assist those who are in need and difficulties; second: to bury dead men and perished birds and animals which are found on the way; third: to respect demons and celestial beings; fourth: not to kill, nor injure anyone, and to develop a compassionate attitude; fifth: not to envy the rich and despise the poor; sixth: to preserve a temperate disposition; seventh: not to set value on the expensive and scorn the cheap; eighth: not to drink wine, nor eat meat or pungent foods; ninth: not to indulge in music or women; tenth: to keep one's disposition and character well-balanced, not to lapse alternately into a bad mood and then again into a good mood.

Eight Taboos

First: to look at dead bodies; second: to look at blood from an execution; third: to look at processes of birth; fourth: to look at the six types of domestic animals when they give birth; fifth: to look at children in mourning and at people shedding tears; sixth: to embrace small children; seventh: to sleep with women; eighth: to speak with strangers about the practices.

Four Restrictions

First: It will not do to wear soiled, contaminated clothing. Communication with the spirits would thereby be prevented.

Second: It will not do to curse maliciously and to utter insults.

Third: It will not do to discuss fraudulent teachings with other people and to call on the saints in this connection.

Fourth: It will not do to drink wine, to eat meat, to kill or injure someone and not to live true to the right principles.

Then it says: It will not do to recite texts of interdiction at contaminated places.

Then it says: It will not do to perform interdictions with persons who do not believe in them.

Then: It will not do to impart the procedures of interdiction to outsiders.

Then: It will not do to hold texts of interdiction with impure hands.

Then: It will not do to make noise and to lark about with outsiders.

Then: It will not do to speak slightingly of the gods.

Then: It will not do to beat any of the six kinds of domestic animals or men in anger, neither will it do to ride in carts or on horses.

Whoever transgresses against three maxims out of the sum of those cited here will not succeed in the practices of interdiction. Whoever is able to avoid offences will bring on great success with his interdictions.[22]

A Confucian Response

Approximately one-hundred and fifty years after Sun Szu-miao had developed his own instructions for medical ethics and had put them down in the *Ch'ien-chin fang*, Lu Chih (AD 754–805) expressed the view of a Confucian scholar in regard to both medicine as such and the group who practiced medicine independently as a means to earn money. Already in his young days Lu Chih had successfully passed the examinations for the career of civil servant, and graduated at the age of eighteen to a *chin-shih*. After some time spent in less important administrative positions, he finally received a key position in the Han-lin academy and became an intimate friend and adviser of the emperor. His political writings are known to posterity. Lu Chih can thus be considered a representative of the ruling class of his time. His views on medicine and its practice therefore carry special weight:

> Medicine is based on practiced humaneness [*jen-shu*]. The sentiments of the physicians are focused on living men; hence it is said: "Medicine is practiced humaneness." When someone suffers from a disease and seeks a cure, this is no less important than if someone facing death by fire or by drowning calls for help. Physicians are advised to practice humaneness and compassion. Without dwelling on [externals such as] tresses and a cap that fits, they have to hasten to the relief of him [who asks for it]. This is the proper thing to do. Otherwise accidents such as burning or drowning take place. How could a man who is guided by humaneness calmly tolerate such a happening?
>
> Yet in many places there are physicians who make use of the needs of others and who appropriate their goods to themselves in a fraudulent way. This is a case of very diligent partisans of greed. How can this be reconciled with "practiced humaneness"? Very many have adopted this [frame of mind] and their deeds are by no means admirable. Why on earth are they not rewarded for it by misfortune?
>
> Nowadays it can frequently be observed that the descendants of [good] physicians accumulate luxury, live in happiness and in splendor and are elected to the higher ranks. In the last instance this is yet another expression of a reward through heavenly principles. What need is there then to plan only for the profit which arises from an occasion and to then be considered a thief?
>
> The attitude of humaneness and righteousness [i] is in contrast to the magic arts. The latter contradict the heavenly principles which are provided for living creatures. Whoever devotes himself to such [practices] cannot pass for an example.[23]

I wish to comment on several points in this statement. In the first paragraph of this short essay Lu Chih indicates that medicine should be a matter of course for everyone who is endowed with "an attitude of humaneness" as indeed all men are, according to Mencius, who demonstrated this with his example of the well. The logical consequence of this thought is that the "primary" resources of medicine have to be distributed evenly among the population. In the second paragraph Lu Chih then points to those who practice medicine for money-making, and in this context he partially questions Sun Szu-miao's system of rewards. In casting doubt on the certainty that a higher power will impose a punishment on physicians for their fraudulent machinations, he adds again to the distrust which, according to his opinion, should be shown to these practitioners. In the third paragraph he argues accordingly that those who make use of medicine in the sense preferred by him will be richly reimbursed by society, not necessarily in their own but at least in the succeeding generation. In his conclusion he makes a very obvious critique of the Taoists' involvement with alchemy and magic. Sun Szu-miao was in fact numbered among those so involved.

It is remarkable in Lu Chih's statements that he does not show contempt for medicine as a resource, but merely for its practice as a profession. Notwithstanding observations of this nature on the part of a high level representative of the political hierarchy, authors throughout later centuries repeatedly sensed the need to increase the value of medicine in the face of orthodox Confucianism, and expressed this in the prefaces to their medical works. Such efforts were not limited to the group of physicians who remained outside the career of the Confucian examinations and the civil service. Among the Confucian scholars who tried to overcome the ideology of discredit directed at this field of activity were also those who dealt with medicine beyond the "domain of families," either because they had been appointed civil servants or because of their private interest.

Notes

21 Chang Lu. *Ch'ien-chin fang yen-i*

22 Sun Szu-miao, *Ch'ien-chin i-fang*, ch. 29, pp. la–lb.

23 Lu Chih, *Lu Hsüan kung lun*, in Hsü Ch'un-fu, *Ku-chin i-t'ung ta-ch'üan*, ch. 3b, pp. 13a- 13b.

Medical Ethics and Chinese Culture

Ren-Zong Qiu

──────────INTRODUCTION TO READING──────────

In addition to being an authority on traditional Chinese medical ethics, Ren-Zong Qiu is also a leading figure in modern medical ethics in China. In the following selection he summarizes developments in post-revolutionary

China. He divides the article into three sections: the first discusses the development of contemporary Chinese medical ethics, the second is devoted to a comparison with its Western counterparts, and the third discusses these characteristics with relation to Chinese culture. This article covers a wide range of bioethical issues, including euthanasia, reproductive technology, family planning, and the health care system, and does so with reference to contemporary trends, and probing analysis of why those trends exist in China today.

Section three serves to complement previous articles in this chapter on ancient Chinese medical ethics. In this section Qiu briefly examines the role of Buddhism, Confucianism, and Taoism in Chinese culture and its subsequent influence on contemporary medical ethics.

Introduction

This paper consists of three sections. In the first section, I sketch the development of Chinese medical ethics with a focus on the contemporary stage of this development. The second section is devoted to the characteristics of Chinese contemporary medical ethics in comparison with its Western counterpart. In the third section, I attempt to provide an explanation of these characteristics in terms of Chinese culture and to highlight the influence of Chinese culture on medical ethics.

Section One

Chinese medicine has a history of at least two thousand years. The first explicit literature on medical ethics did not appear until the seventh century when a physician named Sun Simiao wrote a famous treatise titled "On the Absolute Sincerity of Great Physicians" in his work *The Important Prescriptions Worth a Thousand Pieces of Gold.*[16] In this treatise, later called the Chinese Hippocratic Oath, Sun Simiao requires the physician to develop first a sense of compassion and piety, and then to make a commitment to try to save every living creature, to treat every patient on equal grounds, and to avoid seeking wealth because of his expertise.

Traditional Chinese medical ethics is the application of Confucianism in the field of medical care. Confucian ethics is a form of virtue ethics with a strong deontological basis. Its focus has been on the virtues that a moral agent should have and the ways they can be acquired. The starting point of this morality is the cultivation of one's character by becoming a person with compassion. All the requisites which a physician should meet, and all the maxims that he or she should follow without regard to consequences, are heavenly principles.

In premodern China, medical ethical issues were addressed only in the preface of medical texts. All maxims, exhortations, admonitions, and warnings were personal advice or suggestions of well-known and prestigious physicians of that time. These guidelines were based on the personal experience of noted physicians, but were not professional codes in any sense. There have never been medical professional organizations in traditional China, so codes would not have any binding power on physicians.[10] Only on January 1, 1937, was "The Creed of Doctors" published by the Chinese Association of Doctors as the motto of modern medical practitioners in China.[18]

In 1949, after the founding of the People's Republic of China, the government cancelled the licensing system. Even though mistaken medical judgments were made after this time, the courts and lawyers were not allowed to become involved. Social control of medical practice relied mainly on regulations of health administrations and ideological education by the Communist Party Committee of Hospitals. Medical personnel were required to read Mao's article titled "In Memory of Comrade Norman Bethune" and to generate criticism and self-criticism according to Mao's teachings before and during the notorious Cultural Revolution.

Medical ethics has become one of the most flourishing disciplines in the People's Republic of China during the last decade. The current stage of Chinese medical ethics began with a conference on the philosophy of medicine which was held in Canton in December of 1979. At the plenary session of this conference a report titled "Philosophical Issues of Medicine in the 1970s" was made, part of which was devoted to medical ethics.[11] After this conference the discussion of medical ethics focussed on two issues: the concept of death and euthanasia, and the delivery of medical care without discrimination.[11] Before the publicity of two legal cases, one on active euthanasia, the other on artificial insemination by donor (AID),[15] the discussion was circumscribed by academic and professional circles. These circles were comprised of physicians, philosophers, and health care administrators who were publishing in specialized journals and attending conferences or colloquia on philosophy of medicine or medical ethics.

After the publicity on the cases, medical ethics drew attention from lawyers, journalists, policymakers, legislators, and the public. For example, after broadcasting divergent opinions about the first legal case on active euthanasia in a dialogue aired on a popular program called "Half Hour at Noon,"[10] Central People's Broadcasting Station received more than a thousand letters from its audience all over China. Of them, 85 percent favored some form of euthanasia, while 15 percent—including a school girl in the fifth grade of a primary school—were against any form of euthanasia. The widow of the late Premier Zhou Enlai, Mrs. Deng Yinchao, took the time to write a letter to the station to support the discussion. She said: "A couple of years ago, I wrote a living will to the effect that when I become terminally ill and medicine is no longer useful, the effort to save my life must not be made."

In January of 1989, another discussion on euthanasia was aired by the Central People's Broadcasting Station on a program called "English Service." The First National Conference on Social, Ethical, and Legal issues relating to euthanasia was held in Shanghai in June of 1988 with an attendance of 112 physicians, medical scientists, nurses, philosophers, lawyers, and health care administrators.

Euthanasia

During this decade, one of the primary medical ethical issues to be addressed is euthanasia. There are two Chinese translations of the English word "euthanasia": *anlesi* which means peaceful and happy dying, and *wutongzhisi* which means painless killing. The first is more widely accepted.

On almost every point there has been dissent among physicians, philosophers, lawyers, and the public. At the Shanghai conference on euthanasia, only one thing was agreed on unanimously by all participants: the suggestion that the criterion for death of the person be brain death. The other suggestion was that society ought to accept the right of a terminally ill patient to choose his or her way of dying and should encourage the practice of writing a living will. These recommendations were accepted by all but two participants.[7]

However, there seems to be common assent that the following four kinds of patients fall within the category of those for whom euthanasia may be considered: the comatose, the terminally ill, seriously defective newborns, and very low birth weight infants. If the criterion of brain death is accepted and the irreversibly comatose can be defined as dead, they should not be excluded from the category.[13]

Can euthanasia be identified as a special modality of death differentiated from natural death, accidental death, suicide, murder, and manslaughter? At the Shanghai conference, some participants characterized it in the following way:

> Under the condition of expressing her or his will orally or written, previously or presently, patients who are terminally ill and not incompetent (may reasonably request euthanasia). If no living will is left, the withholding or withdrawal of useless, painful, or burdensome treatment or active measures to end his or her life painlessly may be taken out of compassion and a desire to be of assistance. (Such an act) is done out of respect for his or her dignity and right to choose a way of dying. If the person is incompetent, these procedures may not be done against his or her will.[7]

It was argued that this characterization can be applied to the seriously defective newborn and very low birth weight infant with some modification. The problem in the case of euthanasia as characterized above is: What is the cause of death? Is it the action of withholding or withdrawing treatment, the action of ending life, or the disease process? Another problem is: How can the motive of this action be classified? Was it done from compassion or from some selfish intention?

Is euthanasia ethically justifiable? Most Chinese ethicists argue that the principles of beneficence, autonomy, and justice can be applied to justify euthanasia in certain circumstances. But behind the agreement there is a discrepancy in the argument. The holistic argument is that which emphasizes the benefit euthanasia may bring to the whole society. The argument from individualism is that we should respect the right of the terminally ill to choose a way of dying that is in his or her best interests. If a terminally ill patient prefers to live as long as possible no matter how painful the life will be, and there is no financial problem to prevent access to the needed medical care, we should respect her or his choice.

There have been cases in which patients committed suicide by hanging themselves, or have cut an artery with a knife, or have jumped from a window after their request to withdraw treatment was refused. Physicians felt themselves to be in an embarrassing dilemma when faced with such cases. Euthanasia can help us to avoid these tragic outcomes. In the case of seriously defective newborns and very low birth weight infants, euthanasia is intended to prevent an existence filled with suffering, at least in the current circumstances of China. It can be seen in letters from radio and television audiences who respond favorably to the idea of euthanasia. One elderly person wrote: "I don't want to die in a painful way." Another person who had the experience of caring for a terminally ill relative wrote: "I have no heart to see my kin dying in such a way."

On the other hand, the main objections brought forth against euthanasia are:

Psychological	When people are close to death, they often have a stronger will to continue life.
Ethical	The heavenly principle of medical ethics prohibits a physician from doing anything which might bring the patient closer to death.
Social	Any form of euthanasia can be misused as a disguise for murder.
Medical	Euthanasia will hinder the development of medicine.

Does euthanasia violate existing Chinese law? Most Chinese lawyers give a positive answer. Euthanasia violates the existing Chinese marital law, criminal law, and civil law. In the official explanation of criminal law, there are two factors which are very important in judging if an action constitutes a murder: one is motive—whether or not the agent intends the death of the innocent victim; the other is effect—whether the action is the cause of the victim's death. In the case of euthanasia, the motive of the agent and the effect of the intervening action are the same as in the case of murder. However, some have suggested that it is possible to change the current explanation by applying the principle of double effect.[7]

Is euthanasia acceptable to the Chinese public? Surveys show that the percentage of respondents favoring active euthanasia as well as passive euthanasia is higher than we expected. In a survey which my colleagues and I made in 1985,[13] four actual cases were described: a newborn with serious heart disease (cardianastorophe, angioplany, hypoplastic left heart, ventricular septal defect, auricular septal defect); a one-month-old female baby with microencephaly; an irreversibly comatose patient; and a dying cancer patient with intractable pain. The percentage favoring euthanasia was 14.7 percent, 62.4 percent, 37.1 percent, and 39.4 percent, respectively. In the first case, 42.9 percent of the respondents favored the parents as final decisionmakers, whereas 33.5 percent favored a committee, and only 17.1 percent thought that the physician should make the decision alone. In the second case, 58.5 percent of the respondents held the view that even though a one-month-old baby is a person, it is permissible to take his or her life if that quality of life is very low. Another survey showed that 37.09 percent of respondents favored euthanasia and 46.02 percent thought that it should be done by specialized workers. In this survey, 54.97 percent thought that the decision should be made by consultation between physician and family, 26.82 percent favored the patient as decisionmaker, and 8.94 percent favored the physician. One interesting finding was that attitudes towards euthanasia reflect professional, educational, and age differences. Respondents who were medical personnel or engaged in other intellectual pursuits, the well-educated, and young people held a more favorable attitude toward euthanasia.[3]

These surveys show that more and more Chinese medical personnel and laypersons take quality of life into account when considering euthanasia. The respondents reflected a balance of different values. Both the principle of respect for the sanctity of life embodied in the practice of making every effort to prolong life no matter what the cost and the paternalism embodied in the practice of decisionmaking by the physician without informed consent seem to be weakened. A story of a peasant who rescued a diseased pig was published on the first page of *People's Daily* and praised as a model of moral action. Another similar story was that of a train which made an unscheduled stop at a station so that an ill passenger could be treated. We can see that a change in the focus of morality has taken place since the Cultural Revolution.

Reproductive Technology

Reproductive technology as it is now practiced or being developed through research in China includes prenatal sex selection, artificial insemination by husband (AIH), artificial insemination by donor (AID), and in vitro fertilization (IVF). AIH seems not to have raised any ethical issues. Procedures such as IVF and organ transplantation, which require advanced technology to implement, are limited by Chinese policy to development in a few centers.

The application and development of reproductive technology benefits infertile couples. Among newly married couples, the rate of infertility is approximately 5 to 10 percent.[20] Where the reproductive technology has not been available, people have resorted to other means such as the practice of a "borrowed wife" to solve their problems. In some villages, infertile couples have agreed to pay a "borrowed wife" and her husband payments of 10,000 yuan (about US $2000) for a girl and 20,000 yuan (about US $4000) for a boy. This practice can be called "surrogate motherhood by natural insemination."

In China, AIH and AID are now widely practiced. Sperm banks have been set up in eleven provinces.[7] In Beijing and Changsha, "test tube babies" have been born after conception by IVF, and people are currently considering surrogate motherhood.

While doctors have been working out the technical problems in reproductive technology, the related social, ethical, and legal issues have gained increasing public interest. After sex identification by amniocentesis, 90 percent of female fetuses were aborted. In 1986, the male to female ratio of infants was 108.4:100. Now it is about 112:100[5] which may be due mainly to what is termed "postnatal selection," that is, female infanticide (a crime under existing laws). Prenatal sex selection is also a factor. The Ministry of Health currently prohibits the practice of prenatal sex selection.[8]

Except in a few centers in larger cities, there has been no regulation of IVF. Those who practice AID do not apply any criteria for selection of either donors or recipients: there are no special procedures required, no application forms which the success of the procedure or the condition of the child could be confirmed, no records, no follow-up studies, and so on. Even private doctors at the community level practice AID using as a donor, perhaps, the shoemaker who happens to live near the gate. Fees are charged, so doctors engaging in this practice receive a considerable amount of money from infertile patients.

The legal status of AID children is not guaranteed. There was a case in Shanghai[8] which illustrated the conflict between traditional values and modern technology. In this case, the AID child was not given legal status and was not accepted by the extended family. This was due to the fact that their traditional values did not allow for one who does not come from the blood lineage of the husband's family to be recognized as part of that family.

Family Planning

Family planning and the policy of "one couple, one child" is the most thorny problem in China. In order to cope with overpopulation, the Chinese must do something to control this difficulty. The goal of the public on this matter is to make sure that the Chinese population does not exceed 1.2 billion by the year 2000. But it is not so easy to achieve such a goal because a slowing of population growth is in conflict with the government's new economic policy, with Chinese traditional values, and with the wishes of a great number of peasants. The results of an unpublished survey made by the Chinese Society for Sociology in 1979 shows that a considerable percentage of city inhabitants (19.44–30.95 percent) and the majority of peasants (51.34–79.53 percent) want to have two or more children. The issues involved are:

1. Is it ethically justifiable for a government to limit the right of its citizens to reproduce? I think that, in principle, I agree with Professor H. Tristram Engelhardt on this question. He argues: "Reproduction, unlike sexual

intercourse, concerns more than the consenting individuals providing gametes. The production of a new person involves not only obligations of parents towards children, but also their duties towards society and others who may become financially obliged to protect and nurture the new individual."[21]

2. Although the limitation may be justifiable in principle, what should be done when the policy runs counter to the wishes of many people? Whenever this occurs, either the use of coercion is necessary to achieve compliance or the policy becomes unenforceable. There is little difficulty in big cities, where most inhabitants favor having one child, but in some rural areas either the rate of growth of population is beyond the limit of the government, or, in certain so-called advanced areas of family planning, there is some form of coercion.

3. How much emphasis should be focussed on abortion? The government claims that the primary emphasis on population control policy is on contraception, not abortion. But in rural areas contraception has been unsuccessful and so the peasants resort to abortion. From 1971 to 1983 the number of abortions totalled 92 million. Since 1983, the figure has not been available.

4. Although, generally speaking abortion is not considered to be an issue in China, what should be done about the risks and problems posed to all concerned? Many women in rural areas have undergone abortion so many times that officials responsible for maternal care worry about their health. In addition, since there is no problem in using the tissues or organs of aborted fetuses for transplantation, abortion may be sought for these purposes. Late abortion is an issue because it may cause adverse effects on the mother's health and because a fetus older than 28 weeks is given the status of human being. The Chinese Ministry of Health promulgated in the 1960s a regulation to prohibit the abortion of a fetus older than 28 weeks. Late abortion not only involves multiparous women, but also involves unmarried girls who are pregnant. Both groups make every effort to hide the truth at the first stage of pregnancy. Now the rate of sexual relations and pregnancy among the unmarried is higher than it was. This increase is due to changes in the sexual behavior patterns of young people. Unfortunately, changes in the ethical environment lags behind this behavioral change. In addition, sex education and contraceptives are not so accessible to young people.[14]

Many Chinese officials and scholars now worry about the fact that the quality of life of the entire population is deteriorating. In many villages, all of the villagers are relatives with the same surname, bringing about for some of them the label "idiot village." In these communities no person can be found intelligent enough to be responsible for the management of the village, so many subsidies are granted by the government every year. The number of handicapped is estimated at about 50 million, but the criteria according to which one can be classified as handicapped are more stringent than those in the United States. Since Mr. Deng Pufang took the position of president of the Chinese Association for the Handicapped, conditions relating to the handicapped have greatly improved. But it still may be a long time before the hand-icapped are integrated into societal life. Social support for their care is mini-mal so the burden has to be imposed upon the family. According to our study, the cost of care for a handicapped child is about 60 percent of a worker's aver-age salary and one parent must resign from his or her job to look after the child at home. Some handicapped children are mistreated and abused. Now they can enter colleges and universities, but they still experience discrimina-tion in the workplace. So the idea of improving the quality of life for the entire population and preventing the birth of handicapped children is in the best interests of society, of the family, and of the handicapped person herself or himself within the current social and economic conditions of China. This way of thinking brought about the draft of the Eugenic Law and the Law of Compulsory Sterilization for the Mentally Retarded in Ganshu and Liaoning Provinces.

Health Care System

The Chinese health care system is a mixture. The public health care program covers roughly 200 million people. Its beneficiaries are mainly workers but also include professionals and employees in state-owned factories and institutes. Although their medical care is free, they must pay the costs of medical care for their children. All Tibetan people, however, have the privilege of free medical care. Some villages have developed cooperative health care programs. Most peasants in rural areas, owners and employees in private enterprises, and the unemployed must pay the costs of medical care by themselves. As a result, in some poor villages, especially in the remote mountainous areas, health care is not accessible. Under the public health care program, the demand for treat-ment always exceeds the supply. High-ranking officials have privileges regard-ing medical care and enjoy special treatment. Ordinary people, if they are to be treated satisfactorily or to be admitted into the hospital in time, have to get in through the back door, so to speak, by means of various channels.[9]

Currently the government is attempting to reform health care by imple-menting the lease-contract-responsibility system which has proven to be very successful in agriculture. Under this program, the more patients a physician treats, the more money he or she can earn. As a result, there is a kind of trust crisis in the fiduciary relationship between physicians and patients. If the physi-cian makes an all-out effort at treatment, the patient or his or her relatives will wonder if the physician only wants to get more money from the treatment. If the physician's treatment is rather conservative, they will wonder if the physician and hospital manager want to save the scarce resources for high ranking officials or other privileged patients. In October of 1989, some economists and ethicists who have been involved in the field of medical care met with health administra-tors and advisors of the Ministry of Health to argue against the implementation of the lease-contract-responsibility system in health care. This meeting was also attended by the Minister of Health, Professor Chen Mingzhang.

Section Two

What are the characteristics of Chinese contemporary medical ethics? It depends on which frame of reference is used. In this section I would like to describe the characteristics of Chinese contemporary medical ethics in reference to its Western counterparts. I would also like to consider modern Chinese ethics as compared with traditional Chinese medical ethics.

Euthanasia

Euthanasia, especially active euthanasia in general and that practiced in the case of seriously defective newborns and low birth weight infants, seems to be getting increased support from professionals as well as the public in China. The percentage of respondents from different social strata who support euthanasia is very high in the surveys made in various locations by different kinds of medical professionals working in varying institutes.[22] Most lawyers maintain the view that euthanasia, especially active euthanasia, violates existing Chinese laws. Most physicians and ethicists, on the other hand, seem not to reject active euthanasia. In journals and newspapers or on the radio, those who have come forward to argue against euthanasia are in the minority. Is it possible that there is a silent majority who are against euthanasia? It seems not to be the case. Although the audience who wrote to the radio station might be the segment of the public who were interested in and sensitive to this issue, in many surveys the respondents were randomly chosen. This was especially true of the survey I made in 1985 when euthanasia was not the hot topic it is now and many of those selected were hearing the term "euthanasia" for the first time.

However, would those who favored euthanasia in the survey actually withhold or withdraw the treatment? Perhaps not. Certainly the following two factors would influence his or her decision:

Economic If the cost of medical care were to be paid by the patient, he or she and his or her family would be more likely to ask the physician to withhold or withdraw treatment. If the patient were receiving free medical care, he or she and his or her family would be more likely to ask the physician to continue the treatment.

Cultural There have been cases in which the patient, his or her children, and the physician all said that the treatment was meaningless and suggested withdrawing it, but nobody took action. The children feared that other relatives would blame them for violating the principle of filial piety, and the physician feared that he or she could be accused of malpractice or murder.

The attitude towards newborns and towards the elderly is different from that in the United States. It is very difficult to withdraw treatment from the elderly person who is terminally ill, whereas treatment for seriously defective newborns and very low birth weight infants is easily stopped. Due to the fact that some parents even give up on babies such as those with only a hare lip or seal fin deformity, we feel it necessary to take measures to protect them. The reasons are:

Historical   Infanticide has been a traditional practice in China. As early as 300 BC, an ancient philosopher Han Fei criticized female infanticide in the book Han Fei Zi compiled by his disciples.

Economic   It is considered an unbearable burden for a young couple to raise a seriously defective newborn or a very low birth weight infant.

Cultural   Newborns with a serious deformity have been considered monsters and were labelled "monster fetuses." These babies were not accepted by the community.

Political   Under the policy of "one couple, one child," the parents tend to withdraw treatment from the child so that the one child they may raise will be healthy.

There seems to be a paradox in China: severe measures for birth control on the one hand, and arduous efforts to solve the problem of infertility on the other. Perhaps nobody in China would deny that overpopulation is one of the biggest problems and that, to solve this problem, some measures have to be taken to control the rate of population growth. A seemingly reasonable goal set by the government is to maintain the population at a level no higher than two billion by the year 2000. In China nobody has argued against the need to control the growth rate. If this cannot be done, it will create a great burden not only upon China itself but also upon its neighbors and the other countries of the world. Many people, even though they wish to have more than one child, are nevertheless content with that one because they feel they have a commitment to the welfare of the society at large.

The issue which can be argued is whether the policy of "one couple, one child" is optimal for controlling overpopulation. The optional alternatives which have been proposed are:

"One couple, one and a half children." This proposal was suggested by Professor Li, T-L, Beijing Medical University. It means that if a couple gives birth to a girl the first time, they may have the option of a second pregnancy.

"Stop after giving birth to a boy if the parents live in a rural area." This was suggested by Dr. Gu, Z-S, Shihezi Medical College Hospital, Xinjiang Autonomous Region. It means that a couple living in the countryside may continue to bear children until they have a boy.

"One couple, two and a half children if the parents live in a rural area." This was suggested by an official in the Office of Works in Rural Areas after negotiation with some peasants who want two or three children. It means that if a couple in the countryside have girls the first two times, or one girl and one boy, they may have the option of a third pregnancy.

All of these alternatives show that the issue is not whether or not repro-ductive rights should be limited, but rather what is the most acceptable and efficient way to affect such a limitation. However, none of these suggestions were accepted by policymakers, perhaps because they are a bit too complicated to be practical.

Recently, there was another suggestion to the effect that it would be better to take a *laissez faire* policy on the population problem. It has been argued that, following the examples of advanced countries, the people themselves will feel it necessary to limit family size in order to promote the development of the econ-omy and provide for compulsory education. But when will the Chinese people do that? At the time when China has a population of 4, or of 10 billion popula-tion? And even then, in view of the strong adherence to Confucian tradition in China, such a general practice is unlikely. It should not be forgotten that, when Westerners criticized the practice of limiting the right to reproduction and withdrew financial support for the population development program, they did not face the fact that we were left with the very serious problem of overpopula-tion in China. In many cases, because of the lack of efficient contraceptives and qualified medical personnel, abortion became a final resort. Withdrawal of assistance only worsens this situation.

There is a clear difference between the attitude towards abortion in the United States and that found in the People's Republic of China. The dominant Confucian view never treats the fetus as a human being. It values the dead body, teaching that, when dying, the body should be kept intact. In the Three Teachings (Confucianism, Taoism, and Buddhism) which shaped Chinese culture, only Chinese Buddhism put any restraints on abortion because it teaches that the fetus is a form of life. According to Buddhist doctrine, the Buddhist mission is to save all forms of life "from the bitter sea to the other shore—Western paradise." Modern doctors, however, question from a differ-ent ethical perspective, that is, whether a fetus older than 28 weeks should be treated as a human being.

In this tradition, there is no problem in using tissues and organs of the aborted fetus for transplantation. On the other hand, it is very difficult to procure dead bodies and organs for medical education and transplantation because, according to one of the Confucian classics, *Book of Filial Piety*, "skin and hair cannot be damaged because they are inherited from the parents." Although the Chinese now believe that the body will be destroyed after burial and cremation is becoming very popular in China, they still prefer keeping a body intact to using the crematorium. Medical professors have been known to ask workers or crematoria to send them corpses to dissect for educational purposes. In the capitol of Xinjiang Autonomous Region, Ulumuqi, the direc-tor of the crematorium was sued and arrested for selling corpses. Many profes-sors or other faculty members in the Xinjiang Medical College testified that the director had only sent them the bodies of those without relatives and that they were to be used for medical education. These educators claimed that if the director of the crematorium were found guilty and sentenced to prison, they would be willing to go to jail for him.

The infertility rate of newly-married couples and their consequent behavior might be similar in China to those in other countries. But the eagerness of infertile Chinese couples may be stronger than that of couples in other countries. Under the influence of Confucianism, a man or woman without a child would bear a heavy psychological burden. One of the requirements of filial piety is to extend the life of ancestors to future generations. According to Mencius (one of the greatest Confucianists, next only to Confucius), there are three vices which violate the principle of filial piety, and the biggest of these is to be without offspring. Traditional Chinese believe that barrenness is due to lack of virtue or to the lack of virtue of one's ancestors. The burden is especially heavy for women. Infertility is always blamed on wives who are stigmatized and abused by the family as a result of failure to conceive.

How, then, ought we to reconcile between the strong emphasis on birth control and the development of reproductive technologies? There are two interpretations of the policy "one couple, one child." One interpretation is "no child is better than one." The other is "one child is better than more than one and less than one." It seems that the latter has been widely accepted. Some officials and ethicists argue that solving the problem of infertility may decrease resistance to the family limitation policy, a policy which is only a limitation and not a deprivation of the right to reproduce. The development and use of reproductive technology will promote the infertile family's happiness by assisting them in their first exercise of the basic right to reproduce.

The Chinese are worried about overpopulation as well as quality of life. Even though they are spiritual individualists in the sense that they have always been taught to actualize self-development, self-perfection, and self-improvement, they have also been taught that they are members of the larger family— "descendants of the Red Emperor and the Yellow Emperor." They feel that they have commitments of duty to this family. Any programs which are supposed to improve the quality of life for the nation, including compulsory sterilization of the mentally retarded and negative eugenics, are acceptable to the Chinese. This might be accomplished by reducing the number of physically and mentally handicapped persons by means of genetic counseling and screening combined with administrative measures such as prohibiting marriages between close relatives. Laws might be adopted which prohibit some types of physically and mentally handicapped persons from conceiving naturally, allowing reproduction only by AID. These methods are aimed at eliminating societal burdens. They are different from Hitler's positive eugenics, which elicits a strong negative response in China as in the West.

A strong practice of paternalism has been handed down from ancient times to the present. Chinese doctors have seldom ever talked about the patient's autonomy or self-determination, except when treating powerful persons. One traditional doctor says in his book, "When the ailing themselves cannot make any decisions, I will make them in their place. I always put myself in their place."[4] Since 1949, there has been a gradual fading away of familial paternalism, and there has developed in its place a decisionmaking mechanism in hospitals which emphasizes consultation between physician and family members involving the competent patient, sometimes including the patient's close friends or coworkers and the chief of the unit in which the patient works. Roughly speaking, the medical decision is made by the family after consulting with the attending physician. In this mechanism the patient's opinion is taken under adequate consideration, but is not considered to be an exercise of his or her right to self-determination.

In the making of a medical decision, not only the patient's interest, but also the interest of her or his whole family is placed under consideration. In the case of the terminally ill, if the patient has a higher salary and enjoys free medical care, he or she may prefer lingering in bed as long as possible, even though he or she wishes to die more peacefully and painlessly. In some cases, the patient may refuse to be informed and ask the physician to provide the information only to her or his spouse or children. It means that Chinese patients traditionally do not make a strong effort to exercise the right to self-determination. But recently some changes have taken place. For example, the cases I mentioned in the beginning of this paper (that some terminally ill persons committed suicide after their request for withdrawal of treatment has been refused by their physicians) show the awakening of the sense of autonomy. In this negative way they claimed their right to self-determination. When there is a consensus on the medical decision after deliberate consideration and sufficient consultation between the patient, his or her family, and the physician, nobody intervenes if there is no financial or emotional conflict between them.

Legal intervention in medical cases has no tradition. In the premodern period, the legal system was never involved in purely medical cases unless there was some suspicion of murder. During the Nationalist regime before 1949, physicians could be sued for malpractice, but the Chinese preferred to resolve their disputes outside the legal system. They felt that presence in court was shameful. After the 1950s, the settlement of medical disputes was transferred to health administrations. But there are no laws or regulations concerning medical disputes. In addition, health administrations are so busy that the treatment of medical disputes has been extremely unsatisfactory, protecting the right of neither patient nor physician. There have been cases in which relatives of the patient thought there was malpractice and, after becoming impatient with the slow and inefficient process of dealing with their complaint by the health administration, went to the physician's office and attacked him physically to retaliate for the perceived injustice. Now, after the Cultural Revolution, the legal system is again involved in medical cases. In Shanghai there is a draft of a law concerning medical disputes which has been experimentally used in the legal system since 1988. Information on the result of this experiment has yet to be gathered.

Both legal and ethical constraints on medical malpractice are underdeveloped in China. Since 1937, there has been no medical ethical code adopted by the Chinese Medical Association. An interesting development is that of December, 1988, when the Chinese Ministry of Health drew up and promulgated a brief ethical code for medical personnel. This code instructs personnel to "heal the wounds, rescue the dying, practice socialist humanitarianism," to "respect the patient's personality and his or her rights, treat all equally without discrimination," and to "respect the patient's privacy and to keep his or her confidence."[6]

Section Three

Contemporary Chinese medical ethics has been developed in a country with a backward economy, a power-centralized political system, a population of 1 billion—one quarter of whom are illiterate and semi-illiterate, and a cultural tradition of thousands of years. Chinese culture was shaped by the Three Teachings: Confucianism, Taoism, and Buddhism. Moral intuition as well as moral attitudes towards medical ethical issues and resolution of ethical dilemmas (at lay, professional, and societal levels) are affected by the longstanding entrenched traditional values and the current dominant ideology. The Three Teachings provide a unique organic worldview as a conceptual framework for the explanation and treatment of disease and a unique ethics with strong virtue-oriented and deontological focus for dealing with the relationship between physicians and patients. In the final section, I will attempt to provide an explanation of these characteristics as introduced and described in Section Two. They can best be understood in terms of Chinese culture, particularly by noting the unique influence of Chinese culture upon contemporary medical ethics.

Conceptions of Life, Death, and Suffering

In approximately the third century BC, the great Confucianist Xun Kuang and the great legalist Han Fei were said to have argued that a human being begins with birth and ends with death. Since then, this view has become a conventional Chinese view. Traditionally, the mourning period after a person's death continued for seven weeks, but a dead fetus was never mourned. There is a contradiction, however, to this traditional belief and consequent practice: when a baby is born, it is considered to be one year old. One explanation is that the Chinese emphasize the continuity between the fetus before birth and the baby after birth but they do not necessarily hold that the fetus is a human being or a person. When the abortion, spontaneous or induced, took place, the Chinese never said that a person or human being died. One reason for this view may be, perhaps, that the premodern Chinese have never developed a technique which allowed them to understand fetal life and development; even contemporary Chinese know very little about this process.

What then is life or death? Both Confucianists and Taoists see life as the coordination of *Qi* (vital force), death as the dispersion of *Qi*. The life of a person is the product of interaction between *Yang* (light *Qi*) and *Yin* (heavy *Qi*). *Yang* comes from Heaven and father, and *Yin* from Earth and mother. After the death of a person, *Yang* is returned to Heaven and *Yin* to Earth. So a person comes from nature and returns to it. The least intelligent being an amoeba, and the most intelligent being a human being, each consists of *Qi*, and they are integral parts of a continuum—a chain of beings which is never broken because nothing is outside of it.

Birth and death are two of the greatest events in human life, because each person only has one chance to be born and one chance to die. So the Chinese have a grand ceremony to celebrate these occasions. Birth and death are called "red and white happy events." Birth is nothing but a new form of *Qi*, and so is death. For Confucianism, what is valued is not human life itself, but living in an ideal way. The great historian Sima Qian said that every person must die, and that a person's death is as heavy as the Tai Mountains and as light as a feather of the wild goose. Confucius once said: "A man of humanity will never seek to live at the expense of injuring humanity. He would rather sacrifice his life in order to realize humanity."[2] What is valued is a meaningful, not a meaningless life. The meaning of life for Confucianists is found by following Confucian ethical principles which teach people to be human—to be worthy members of the universal family. Moreover, for Confucianists, to live or to die is not a thing which can be controlled by human beings. Confucius once said: "Life and death are the chance of Heaven; wealth and honor depend on Heaven."[2]

For Taoists, one school emphasizes the preserving of life by means of breathing properly, exercise, diet, sex, and appropriate medicines. What Taoists want to preserve is a natural existence in which will be maintained a harmony or balance of *Yin* and *Yang* within the human body and between it and the universe.

For the major Taoists, an ideal spiritual sphere for a human being is to transcend all distinctions or dichotomies including life and death. Why should we be pleasant at birth and sad at death? And the great Taoist Zhuang Zhou once said that the most unhappy thing in the world is mind-death, because then a person becomes a walking corpse.

For Chinese Buddhists, the highest goal a person can reach is Nirvana in which life and death are transcended. In this state all things in their own nature are truly experienced as unreal and void. To reach Nirvana and save all forms of life, it is necessary for a person to get rid of *karmas* and return to the emptiness of original mind.

As for suffering Confucianists see it as the tempering of one's moral character. As Mencius said: "When Heaven is about to confer a great responsibility on any man, it will exercise his mind with sufferings, subject his sinews and bones to hard work, expose his body to hunger, put him to poverty, place obstacles in the paths of his deeds, so as to stimulate his mind, harden his nature, and improve wherever he is incompetent."[2]

The Three Teachings have developed a doctrine to help the Chinese release themselves from suffering. There are two elements in this doctrine. The one is "non-action" (*Wu Wei*) which does not mean "do nothing," but rather do nothing unnaturally or beyond nature. One source of suffering is that which one desires to be rather than that which nature permits. The other is attachment. One can pursue something, seek for something, but must not be attached to it. If one is non- or de-attached and something that has been gained is lost one day, it will not cause any suffering to her or him. When a patient is terminally ill, why do we prolong his or her dying unnaturally? Why do we attach to this existence which is going to cease naturally? Let nature take its course. For Chinese Buddhists especially, suffering is caused by failing to know the truth that all things in the universe are nothing more than the apparent phenomena of mental activities; by keeping the mind in a state of emptiness and calmness, all suffering can be avoided.

The Chinese conceptions of life, death, and suffering have led them to the following attitude: Treasure human life but do not attach to it. The suffering experienced by the Chinese has been, perhaps, much greater than that experienced by any other nation but, by this attitude, the Chinese have been able to cope with the burden of death and release themselves from it.

Holistic Socio-Political Philosophy

A quasi-holistic socio-political philosophy has been developed from Chinese cultural tradition. It is based on two thousand years of power-centralized, autocratic monarchy—one that has lacked any rights-oriented, individualistic, liberal democratic tradition. In recent decades, Marxism—rather, a mixture of Russian and Chinese versions of Marxism—has become the dominant ideology. The historicism and social holism of this system, interwoven with traditional ideas, puts the greatest emphasis on nation, society, and country rather than on individuals.

In ancient China there were two factors which exerted far-reaching influence upon Chinese socio-political philosophy. One was ancestor worship, the other was the patriarchal clan system. Both of these imply respect for the elderly. In the patriarchal clan system, all members of a community are looked upon as blood related or kin-related in one way or another. The consequence is that family is seen as the model of society or country. This is a duty-oriented model in which each member has his or her own role responsibilities: children have the duty of filial piety to their parents, parents have the duty of kindness to their children. There are also similar reciprocal duties between husband and wife, brothers and sisters, friends, ruler and subjects, superior and inferior, teacher and student, physician and patient, and so on.

Although the relationship between the members of each pair is reciprocal, they are not equal. The father, husband, and ruler always play a guiding role in their relationships with son, wife, and subject. The authority figure in a family or clan is the patriarch; in a country it is the ruler—the patriarch of the country. In this system all the decisions about family or state affairs are made by the patriarch, the head of the family, or the head of the country. In premodern China, a county magistrate was called "parental official of the county." Now, however, patriarchal authority is in decline. Decisions involving the family still need to be made by all members of the family after consultation, not by any one individual.

I have mentioned that the Chinese are spiritually individualistic in the sense that they always pay a considerable amount of attention to self-development and self-perfection. Mencius illustrated this in the solution he provided to a hypothesized dilemma presented by him to his disciples in a thought experiment. The dilemma is: "If the safe-king Shun's father, the Old Blind Man, had committed murder, and the honest man Gae Yao had been appointed as the Minister of Justice, what ought Shun to do?"

Mencius's solution is: "Shun ought to resign from the position of the Son of Heaven (king), take his father out of jail stealthily, escape with him to a mountain, and support him up to his end."

Mencius's solution to this dilemma shows that he gave the priority to the principle of filial piety which ought to be developed before all others. But in later periods, Confucianists advocated the meta-principle of "loyalty first, filial piety second." And since the Song Dynasty when neo-Confucianists upheld the preservation of heavenly principles and the elimination of human desires, the Chinese have gradually lost their atomistic character, and have become instead water droplets in an ocean.

Marx defined the essence of a human being as the sum of social relations. For Marxists, society is more than the sum of individuals and, consequently, societal institutions and their changes cannot be explained in terms of individual human actions. Chinese Marxists always describe the relationship between individuals, collectives, and country as that between leaves, branches, and root. Marxist social holism implies that individual interests should be subordinated to public interests. And Marxist historicism implies that it is necessary for human beings to sacrifice the not-so-happy present for the future happy life. When Chinese traditional quasi-holistic, socio-political philosophy is combined with Marxist holism, there is an exponential effect which leads to the strong statement: Rights-oriented individualism is essentially alien to the Chinese.

However, with the advance of modernization, the phenomenon I call "the awakening of the rights sense" can be observed: students and intellectuals are striving for civil rights, girls in villages are claiming the right to freely chosen marriages (as opposed to accepting arranged marriages), and patients are asserting the right to self-determination.

Chinese Ethics: A Unique Virtue-Oriented and Deontological Ethics with Weak Normative Aspects

Chinese ethics may be said to be the expression of the discovery of what it is to be a human being. We are born human in the biological sense, but we are badly in need of discovering what it means to be human in the moral sense. For a

Chinese, the statement: You are not human! is a very serious epithet. The uniqueness of being human cannot be reduced to biological, psychological or sociological structures and functions because a living person is far more complex and meaningful than a momentary instance of existence. Inherent in the structure of the human is the infinite potential for development. However, the actual process of this development or self-cultivation cannot be separated from ordinary human experience and daily life. For Confucianists, humaneness (ren) or loving others is what distinguishes humans from animals. This is the primary moral duty. For Confucianists, humaneness should be practiced from the near to the far, beginning with filial piety. They emphasize that the practice of humaneness arises in the agent's inner heart, and it is useless to impose ethical or legal constraints from outside without the cultivation of this virtue, in the heart. As Confucius said: "The achieving of humaneness depends upon oneself; how can (it depend) upon others? If a man is not humane, what is the use of knowing norms?"[18]

The basis of being human, as Mencius argues, is in the inner structure of human nature—human nature as good. A human being is born with four seeds: the heart of commiseration, the heart of shame and dislike, the heart of deference and compliance, and the heart of right and wrong. These are developed by self-cultivation into the four virtues of humaneness, righteousness, propriety, and wisdom, respectively. Why does a human being do evil? Because his or her original mind was obstructed by selfish desires and external forces. So self-cultivation consists of searching for the lost original mind. Much of the later work done by Chinese philosophers concentrated on how to find the original mind, that is, on self-cultivation.

This approach has had a far-reaching influence upon Chinese medical ethics. As I have explained in an article on traditional medicine,[10] Chinese medical ethicists have always emphasized that medicine is the art of humaneness. The focus of this art is the search for ways to cultivate the heart of humaneness in medical personnel by rectifying themselves. This emphasis has resulted in neglect of the social control of medical knowledge by ethical and legal constraints.

However, medical ethics has become one of the most flourishing disciplines in China at a time when China is changing from a monolithic country into a rather pluralistic one. We are now encountering the historical period of so-called modernization (a paradigm shift period indeed!) during which the Chinese want to condense the Renaissance, the Reformation, the Enlightenment and the Industrial Revolution in a matter of decades. There are, and will continue to be, conflicts and tensions between different, incompatible or even incommensurable values in all fields. This tends to make everything uncertain and changeable both in public life and the field of medical care. The only reasonable way of resolving these conflicts and tensions between different social and cultural groups is through continuing dialogue, consultation, and negotiation between different social and cultural groups.

Notes

1. Cai G.F, et al A preliminary approach to the problems of medical ethics. *Medicine and Philosophy*, 1980; 2:44–48.

2. Chan W.T. *A Source Book on Chinese Philosophy*. Princeton NJ: Princeton University Press 1963;43.

3. Guo Q.X., et al. A survey on euthanasia. *Medicine and Philosophy*, 1988;6:34–36.

4. Huai Yuan. *A Thorough Understanding of Medicine in Ancient and Modern Times*, 1936. The name and location of the publishing house are not mentioned in the book.

5. Ma, An, et al. A preliminary analysis of the present situation of China's population. *Population Research*, 1984;3:8.

6. People's Daily, 1988 December 12;1. See also *Chinese Hospital Management* 1989;9 (no.3):5.

7. Qiu R.Z. A report on the First National Conference on Social, Ethical, and Legal Issues in Euthanasia. *Studies in Dialectics of Nature*, 1988;6:61–63.

8. Qiu R.Z. AID confronts the law in China. *Hastings Center Report*, 1989;6: 3–4.

9. Qiu R.Z. Equity and public health care in China. *The Journal of Philosophy*, 1989;283–288.

10. Qiu R.Z. Medicine—the art of humaneness: On the ethics of traditional Chinese medicine. *The Journal of Medicine and Philosophy*, 1988; 13:277–300.

11. Qiu R.Z. Philosophy of medicine in the 1970's. In: *Studies in Philosophy of Science*, Beijing: The Knowledge Press, 1982;281–331.

12. Qiu R.Z. The concepts of death and euthanasia. *Medicine and Philosophy*, 1980;1:77–79.

13. Qiu R.Z., et al. A survey on bioethics. *Medicine and Philosophy*, 1988; 6:34–36.

14. Qiu R.Z., et al. Can late abortion be ethically justified? *The Journal Philosophy*, 1989;14:343– 350.

15. Sass H.M., ed. *Case Studies for Bioethical Diagnosis*. Zentrum fur Medizinishe Ethik: Ruhr-Universitat Bochum, 1989;1.

16. Sun Simiao. *The Important Prescriptions Worth a Thousand Pieces of Gold*. Printed in the period of Wanli's reign, Ming Dynasty. Volume 1;9–11.

17. Unschuld P. *Medical Ethics in Imperial China—A Study of Historical Anthropology*, Berkeley, CA: UC Press, 1979;102.

18. Wang J. The new document of medical ethics. *Chinese Journal of Medicine*, 1944;30:39–40.

19. Ware J.A., trans. *The Sayings of Confucius*. New York: Mentor Books, 1955;76,129. There is some change in the quoted English translation.

20. According to the estimate by participants of the First National Conference on Social, Ethical, and Legal Issues in Reproductive Technology held in Yueyang, Hunan Province in November 1989. The proceedings are not available.

21. Read at the First International Conference on the Future of Medicine: The Western and Eastern Perspectives 2000. Bad Homburg: Federal Republic of Germany 1989 (March). The proceedings have not yet been published.

22. At the First National Conference on Social, Ethical, and Legal Issues in Euthanasia, many papers were submitted which reported the results of these surveys.

Health Ethics in Chinese Law

———————————INTRODUCTION TO READING———————————

The current Chinese government has on a number of occasions promulgated positions on matters of direct relevance to their understandings of medical ethics. Some of these were published for Western readers in the *Journal of Medicine and Philosophy*. The excerpts reprinted here draw on the Constitution of The People's Republic of China, adopted at the 5th National People's Congress, December 4, 1982, and by the Chinese Ministry of Health earlier that same year. The second of these adopts the format of a series of maxims for medical workers as does the following document adopted by the Chinese Academy of Medical Sciences. The overtly social and political nature of these documents-which make clear that the health worker's duty extends beyond the individual-is reminiscent of the Oath of the Soviet Union.

The Constitution of the People's Republic of China

Adopted by the 5th Session of the 5th National People's Congress, December 4, 1982, it came into force upon promulgation by the announcement of the National People's Congress, December 4, 1982.

Chapter I: The General Principles . . .
Article 21. In order to protect people's health, the state shall develop health care undertakings, promote modern and traditional Chinese medicine, and encourage and support collective or state-owned enterprises and sub-district organizations to set up health care facilities and to develop health care activities for the masses . . .

Chapter II: The Fundamental Rights and Duties of Citizens . . .
Article 45. Every citizen of the People's Republic of China has the right to get material assistance from the state and society when he or she is aged, ill, or disabled. The state shall develop social insurance, social relief facilities and the delivery of health care that are needed for citizens to enjoy these rights.

The state and society shall guarantee the life of disabled servicemen, comfort and compensate martyrs' families, and give favored treatment to servicemen's families.

The state and society shall help to arrange the work, life, and education of blinded, deaf, mute, and other handicapped citizens . . .

Article 49. Marriage, family, mothers and children are under the state's protection.

Both husband and wife have the duty to put into practice family planning.

The parents have the duty to support their children until they are adult; adult sons and daughters have the duty to support their parents.

Violating the freedom of marriage and maltreating elderly, women, or children, shall be prohibited.

Maxims for Medical Workers in Hospitals

Laid down by China's Ministry of Health, February 1982
1. Ardently love the motherland, the Communist Party, socialism, and the thought of Marxism-Leninism and Mao Zedong.
2. Try hard to study politics and endeavor to gain professional proficiency; be both well-read and expert.
3. Display the spirit of 'healing the wounded, rescuing the dying, and practicing revolutionary humanitarianism'; have compassion and respect for patients; serve the people whole-heartedly.
4. Take the lead in observing the laws and decrees of the state; carry out health care regulations in an exemplary way.
5. Submit oneself to organizations, be concerned with the collective, be of fraternal unity, have the courage to carry out criticism and self-criticism.
6. Have a boundless sense of responsibility in one's work; rigorously enforce rules and regulations and operating instructions.
7. Be honest in performing one's duties; stand fast at one's post; conscientiously fulfill one's duties; consciously resist unhealthy tendencies.
8. Pay attention to politeness; actively take part in the patriotic health campaign; beautify the environment; keep the hospitals clean and tidy and quiet.

Maxims for Medical Workers

Laid down by the Chinese Academy of Medical Sciences.

Heal the wounded, rescue the dying.

Treat people equally, without discrimination.

Have a sense of responsibility.

Constantly improve one's skill.

Be honest and upright.

Seek no personal gain.

Words cordial and kind.

Be dignified and sedate.

Put patient's interest first.

Unite with one's colleagues.

Regulating Medical Ethics in China

Hans-Martin Sass

————————————INTRODUCTION TO READING————————————

The Chinese Ministry of Health issued further regulations in 1988 that are relevant to the ethics of medical practice in that country. The document is introduced for the Western reader by Professor Hans-Martin Sass.

———————————————————————————————————————

In December 1988, the Ministry of Health of the Peoples Republic of China issued regulations regarding medical ethics for health care professionals. The regulation was distributed to all hospitals through normal administrative channels (*see* Appendix) . . . and publicly discussed and published in part in the December 12, 1988, issue of *Ren-min-ri-bao*, the leading national daily newspaper. The English version has been translated by Shi Da-pu, vice president Xian Medical University, Xian, and president of the Chinese Society for Medical Ethics, founded in 1988.

The regulation, which requires further cross-cultural and ethical evaluation, is indicative of the challenges the developing countries face when traditional systems of value and historically established cultures of health care and patient-physician relationships are confronted with the introduction of modern medicine and the changes it brings to the efficacy, distribution, and administration of medical services.[1]

Among the most interesting aspects of the regulation are the following:

1. Supported by millenniums of Confucian administrative tradition and a few decades of Marxist party rule, the national health care administration[2] understands itself as the prime subject responsible for fiduciary paternalism in setting the rules for good professional moral conduct.

2. The regulation promotes three interrelated goals: a value-based society, the quality of medical ethics, and the promotion of health services (article 1). Medical ethics does not only cover traditional individual physician-patient relationships, but also the cooperation among health care professionals, including nurses and administrators, and the institutional ethics of hospitals (articles 2 and 5). No differences are mentioned in regard to specific moral obligations of physicians as compared to those of administrators or nurses: they all are health care "workers."

3. The "interest of the patient" has to be the prime interest of the health care worker. Good medical practice and ethics is understood as the practice of socialist humanitarianism, but no obligation toward the Chinese government is stated in this code; this is in contrast to the oath of the Soviet physician and of the solemn vows of medical school graduates in the German Democratic Republic, which expresses "the high responsibility I have to my people and to the Soviet government,"[3] responsibility "to the people and the socialist state;"[4] it is stated, however, that health care shall be administered "under the surveillance of the masses" (article 8).

4. The integration of moral expertise and technical expertise in the health care profession is within the Confucian tradition. The physician traditionally had to study philosophy extensively, while the patient's first obligation was to search for an "enlightened" physician.[5]

5. The performance standard of individual health care professionals as well as the standards of health care providing institutions will be of relevance for individual carrier promotion and for rating hospitals (articles 5, 7, 9, and 10). Promotion and punishment are part of professional life. Values or the absence of values have consequences; this is spelled out very clearly. As in any system of assessment and supervision, abuse in evaluating professionals on the basis of ethical or technical performance cannot be excluded; this might be the reason that the essential and concrete role of medical ethics in job promotion and in rating of hospitals is rarely addressed in American or European bioethics literature.

In a contribution for a Bochum research colloquium on medical ethics involving Chinese and German physicians and ethicists, Cao Zeyi, vice minister of health of the Peoples Republic of China, stated the prime role of political bodies in general and of health care administrations in particular is to promote values and professional moral conduct: "Social and cultural change, when resulting from legislation, is stable and lasting particularly when it meets with ethical consciousness. It is therefore of notable significance to promote the studies on medical ethics and health legislation simultaneously. . . . It is imperative to affirm, through health legislation, all moral and ethical codes commonly accepted and to turn them into the standard conduct of the society; whereas, to disseminate, through mass media, new medical technologies and new findings in the studies of medical ethics to change the outmoded medical ethics which are in conflict with social development."[6]

Cao Zeyi mentions the following topics as most challenging in actual administrative decision making and in academic research in China: (a) defining criteria for death and life in the presence of high-tech medicine; (b) moral judgment regarding the continuation or withholding of treatment of brain-dead or comatose patients; (c) protecting the physician's obligations toward the patient against those toward public interest; (d) balancing resource allocation of preventive and primary medicine against obligations in specialized medical and nursing care; (e) respect of personal preference, such as individual requests for euthanasia, which is strongly supported by Deng Yingchao, the widow of late Prime Minister Zhou En-lai; (f) educating the public in regard to the benefits of organ donation and autopsy (both have encountered strong resistance based on traditional Chinese value concepts).

According to Cao Zeyi, "medical ethics is a multi-disciplinary subject encompassing medicine, philosophy, demography, ethics, law, etc.; it is broad in its research areas and rich in its content."

References

1. Cf. also *Health Ethics in Chinese Law*, The Journal of Medicine and Philosophy 14(1989), pp. 361– 362.

2. Ren-Zong Qiu, *Equity and Public Health Care in China*, The Journal of Medicine and Philosophy 14 (1989), pp. 283–287.

3. *The Physician's Oath of the Soviet Union* (1983), The Journal of Medicine and Philosophy 14 (1989), p. 353; cf. the 1971 version for the same responsibility, Encyclopedia of Bioethics (New York: The Free Press, 1978), vol. 4, p. 1755.

4. 'Solemn Vow' of *Those Graduating in the Field of Medicine at the Martin Luther University Halle- Wittenberg*, The Journal of Medicine and Philosophy 14 (1989), p.351.

5. Ten maxims for physicians and ten maxims for patients, In Ren-zong Qiu, *Medicine— the Art of Humaneness*, The Journal of Medicine and Philosophy 14 (1989), pp.295–297.

6. Cao Zeyi, *Medical Ethics in China*. (Bochum: Zentrum fuer Medizinische Ethik, 1989).

Appendix

Regulations on Criteria
for Medical Ethics and Its Implementation
Ministry of Health, People's Republic of China

Article 1. The purpose of the criteria is to strengthen the development of a society based on socialist values, to improve the quality of professional ethics of health care workers and to promote health services.

Article 2. Medical ethics, which is also called professional ethics of health care workers, guides the value system the health care workers should have, covering all aspects from doctor-patient relationships to doctor-doctor relationships. The criteria for medical ethics form the code of conduct for health care workers in their medical practice.

Article 3. The criteria for medical ethics include the following:

1. Heal the wounded, rescue the dying, and practice socialist humanitarianism. Keep the interests of the patient in your mind and try every means possible to relieve patient suffering.

2. Show respect to the patient's dignity and rights and treat all patients alike, whatever their nationality, race, sex, occupation, social position and economic status is.

3. Services should be provided in a civil, dignified, amiable, sympathetic, kind-hearted and courteous way.

4. Be honest in performing medical practice and conscious in observing medical discipline and law. Do not seek personal benefits through medical practice.

5. Keep the secrets related to the patient's illness and practice protective health care service. In no case is one allowed to reveal the patient's health secret or compromise privacy.
6. Learn from other doctors and work together in cooperation. Handle professional relations between colleagues correctly.
7. Be rigorous in learning and practicing medicine and work hard to improve knowledge, ability, skills and service.

Article 4. Education in medical ethics is mandated for the implementation of these regulations and for supporting medical-ethical attitudes. Therefore good control and assessment of medical ethics has to be introduced.

Article 5. Education in medical ethics and the promotion of medical ethics must be part of managing and evaluating hospitals. Good and poor performances of working groups have to be judged and assessed according to these standards.

Article 6. Education in medical ethics should be conducted positively and unremittingly through linking theories with practice aiming to achieve actual and concrete results. It should be the rule to educate new health care workers in medical ethics before they start their service; in no case are they allowed to practice before they get such an education.

Article 7. Every hospital should work out rules and regulations for the evaluation of medical ethics and should have a particular department to carry out the evaluation, regularly and irregularly. The result of the evaluation should be kept in record files.

Article 8. The evaluation of medical ethics should include self-evaluation, social evaluation, department evaluation and higher-level evaluation. Social evaluation is of particular importance, and the opinions of the patients and public should be considered and health service should be offered under the surveillance of the masses.

Article 9. The result of the evaluation should be considered as an important standard in employment, promotion, payment and the hiring of health care workers.

Article 10. Practice the rewarding of the best and the punishment of the worst. Those who observe medical ethics criteria should be rewarded and those who fail to observe criteria of medical ethics should be criticized and punished accordingly.

Article 11. These criteria are suitable for all health care workers including doctors, nurses, technicians and health care administrators at all levels in all hospitals and clinics.

Article 12. Provincial health care offices may work out detailed rules for the implementation of these criteria.

Article 13. These criteria become valid on the date they are issued.

Reference

1. China Hospital Administration, no 3, vol 9, 1989, p. 5. Translated by Shi Da-pu, M.D.; vice president of Xian Medical University; president, Chinese Society for Medical Ethics.

6

African and African-American Perspectives

Introduction

Until recently, even those who were aware that not all medical ethical systems had the roots in the Hippocratic Oath tended to limit their vision of the alternatives to the major Western religious and secular philosophical traditions together with the historic Eastern religions. That was the extent of the scope of the first edition of this volume. It should be apparent, however, that the claim that any religious or cultural system of belief and value will have embedded within it an incipient medical ethic, should hold for all cultures including those of Africa and the Pre-Columbian Western Hemisphere. The only limit on the development of a medical ethic is the cultural differentiation of a medical sphere from the religious, shamanistic, and magical. To the extent that a culture recognizes a sphere of medical interventions, it should be able to derive a set of normative implications for these choices. This volume cannot survey every such culture. For one reason, the literature simply still does not exist. For another, as these cultures have contacted the world religions and philosophies, they have evolved so that they are constantly changing, incorporating new bits and pieces of belief and value as well as new beliefs about medical efficacy. Two major groups of traditions, however, have generated enough of a literature accessible to Western thought that they deserve our attention. This chapter will examine African cultures and the African-American biomedical ethics that is now being recognized as distinct from Western liberal political philosophy and Hippocratic professional ethics. The next chapter will do the same for Hispanic cultures.

It is a serious mistake to speak as if there were one homogeneous African culture. The ancient cultures of West Africa are themselves diverse, incorporating different religious and cultural belief systems and they, as a group, differ significantly from those of Eastern, Central, and Southern Africa. Someday the scholarship of anthropology, sociology, religious studies, and ethics will be sufficiently rich to permit formal, serious analysis of individual cultures and tribes within Africa in a way that is understandable to Western medical ethicists. A full volume of comparative African medical ethics would be a reasonable goal. But for now, we shall make do with a representative selection of one comparative article by an African scholar who understands the complexity of the African intellectual scene. That will be followed by a review article by the leading scholar on African American medical ethics. She too would certainly acknowledge that it is an oversimplification to discuss all African-American thought as if it were homogeneous. African Americans have interacted with other American thought as well as European and other systems throughout the world to the point that it is as rich and complex as either African thought or Anglo-American and other hyphenated American thought.

AFRICAN MEDICAL ETHICS

African Ethical Theory and the Four Principles

Peter Kasenene

—————————INTRODUCTION TO READING—————————

Author Peter Kasenene, Senior Lecturer and Head, Department of Theology and Religious Studies, at the University of Swaziland, Kwaluseni, Swaziland, helps Western students of medical ethics understand African thought in this area by presenting a perspective on African medical ethics within the context of some of the ethical principles that have come to dominate Anglo-American medical ethics: the principles of beneficence, nonmaleficence, autonomy, and justice. In doing so, he does an excellent job of relating an African world view to the field of bioethics as understood by Anglo-American readers.

Kasenene begins by emphasizing the difficulty in discussing an explicitly African world view. The vast diversity of African-ontology compounded by the variety of "non-traditional" influences (e.g. Christianity, Islam, and other Western influences) necessitates large generalizations. These generalizations however are, in his view, valid in so far as they describe real patterns of thought and behavior endemic to traditional African ontology.

Kasenene then identifies two additional ethical principles which underlie African life. The first was advanced by the controversial missionary Tempels who asserted that African society is based on the recognition of a "vital force" which individuals seek to acquire. The acquisition of "vital force" leads to a state of happiness whereas the diminution of "vital force" leads to a diseased state of evil.

The second principle Kasenene draws on was advanced by Mbiti who asserted the principle of Communalism in African ontology—the understanding that an individual exists corporately "in terms of family, clan, and whole ethnic group."

The remainder of the article is devoted to the incorporation of these two ethical concerns into the framework of more Western principles.

Introduction

The African world-view, in which people's ethics is rooted, is life-affirming, and societal activity centres on the promotion of vitality and fertility of human beings, livestock and the land on which their livelihood depends. Sickness and disease, which disrupt people's well-being, have always been unwelcome, and when they are experienced, attempts are made to restore a state of wholesomeness using both natural and supernatural means.

What is African?

It should be noted that writing about an aspect of life from an African perspective creates a number of problems. One of them, for example, is that Africans are not a monolithic society, Africa being home to a variety of between 800 and 1200 peoples, with different cultures.[1] It means, therefore, that generalization in this chapter is inevitable. This comment should not give an impression that one cannot speak of an African view or an African perspective. Despite variety, there is a common Africanness about the culture and world-view of Africans.

The second problem arises from the changes that are taking place in Africa. In recent years Africa has experienced profound and radical changes as a result of colonialism, foreign religions, western education and technology, contact with both the west and the east and the inevitable changes arising from within. The process of acculturation and general adaptation has undermined or even disrupted, to some degree, the traditional ethos. Thus there are remarkable differences in values among Africans; urban and rural, educated and illiterate, Christian or Muslim and traditionalist.

This does not, nevertheless, mean that the African traditional values, attitudes, ideas and norms have been completely abandoned. The traditional ethos still dominates and it is this ethos we shall discuss in relation to health care.

Ethics in Traditional Societies

In traditional societies moral authority is enshrined in custom, the basis of which is the belief in ancestors who, after their death, retain their authority over the living. Right actions are defined as those forms of conduct which are approved by the traditional standards or customary modes of behaviour of a society to which an individual belongs. Everyone is expected to conform to established norms and standards. An aspect of custom, however, is a people's philosophy of life. At this point it is pertinent to discuss briefly the basic philosophical principles underlying African ethics.

Two Basic Ethical Principles

In 1945 Placied Tempels, a Belgian missionary in the Congo (Zaire), published his celebrated work *Bantu philosophy*, based on his experience and knowledge of the Baluba people.[2] In this book Tempels discusses African ontology and ethics. Although the volume aroused great controversy, it was gradually endorsed by many African philosophers and theologians, though reservations were expressed regarding certain details. According to Tempels, 'life' or 'vital force' is central to African philosophy (ref. 2, p. 44).

The Vital Force Principle

According to Tempels, vital force is the meaning of 'to be'. The ultimate goal of anyone is to acquire life, strength or vital force; to live strongly. Everyone strives to make life stronger and to be protected from misfortune or from a diminution of life or of being (ref. 2, pp. 44–45). Supreme happiness is to possess the greatest vital force, and the worst misfortune is the diminution of this force which is brought about by illness, suffering, depression, fatigue, injustice, oppression and any other social or physical evil. This vital force is hierarchical, descending from God through ancestors and elders to the individual. Whatever increases life or vital force is good; whatever decreases it is bad. Human society is organized on the basis of vital force; life growth, life influence and life rank. This structure must be respected, and the individual is good in so far as he or she fulfils his or her duties to promote, support and protect the vital force within the community according to his or her rank.

The Communalism Principle

J. Mbiti discusses another aspect of African traditional ethics. According to him the key value in African societies is community (ref. 1, p. 205). This is influenced by the African understanding of being.

In African societies to be is to belong, and an individual exists corporately in terms of the family, clan and whole ethnic group. As Mbiti observes:

> Only in terms of other people does the individual become conscious of his own being, his own duties, his privileges and responsibilities towards himself and towards other people. When he suffers, he does not suffer alone but with his corporate group: when he rejoices, he rejoices not alone but with his kinsmen, his neighbours and his relatives whether dead or living. . . . Whatever happens to the individual happens to the whole group, and whatever happens to the whole group happens to the individual. The individual can only say 'I am, because we are; and since we are, therefore, I am' (ref. 1, pp. 108–109).

This is the key to understanding the African view of a person, in relation to the community. A person's identity and indeed his or her very life are through a group. Thus the Venda saying '*Muthu ndi muthu nga numwe*', meaning 'A person is person through another person'. The deeper meaning is that an individual by himself or herself is helpless and has little value. Another proverb of the same people expresses this idea clearly: '*Muthu u bebelwa nunwe*', meaning 'A person is born for the other'. This shows that, according to the Venda philosophy, which is similar to the philosophy of other African peoples, one cannot regard even one's own life as purely personal property or concern. It is the group which is the owner of life, a person being just a link in the chain uniting the present and future generations. For that reason one's health is a concern of the community, and a person is expected to preserve this life for the good of the group.

Implications for Health Care

African ethics based on the preservation and promotion of life or vital force and communitarian living present no problems in the application of the principles of beneficence and non-maleficence in health care. Respect for autonomy and justice and their applications, however, seem to create problems. It is upon these principles we shall focus in our discussion, but first let us examine health care in a traditional African setting.

Traditional Health Care

Health and disease are not universal concepts; they are shaped by a people's philosophy and culture. Health care, too, is determined by a people's view of a person and his or her relation to the environment. Health care attitudes and methods, therefore, have to take into account a people's philosophical and cultural concepts of health and disease.

Health, in traditional African societies, is all-inclusive, taking into account a whole person and his or her social environment. Briefly stated, health means personal integration, environmental equilibrium, and harmony between the integrated person and the environment. If any of those three factors is missing a person is not regarded as being healthy. Personal integration is achieved when all the major aspects of a person, namely the physical, mental and social, are sound and operating normally and successfully. On the other hand, environmental equilibrium means a harmonious natural and social surrounding. Health, therefore, does not mean only the faultless mechanical functioning of the body, but also prosperity and mutual coexistence and contentment. Even when one is physically well, for example, in an environment of war, famine, drought, envy, hatred, poverty and similar social or natural calamities, there is no state of health. Health means wholesomeness in a harmonious environment.

This is similar to the World Health Organization (WHO) understanding of health as 'a state of complete physical, mental, and social well-being and not merely the absence of disease or infirmity.³ Following from the above understanding, health care touches a very broad range of personal experience. Over and above the malfunctioning of the biological mechanism, the whole person and his or her social environment call for health care.

In a modern setting it may not be possible to regard health care in such an all-encompassing way. Nevertheless, this African holistic approach provides a challenge we cannot ignore completely. In health care it is not adequate to concentrate exclusively on the body. The psychological, social and environmental aspects of the person also need to be attended to.

The introduction into Africa of western medical institutions, medicines and technology has complicated and introduced ethical problems in health care. One case will be related to show some of the issues that are raised by medical care in an African setting.

The Maze Case

This is a real case the names having been altered to preserve confidentiality and a few additions having been made to make the issues clearer.

Mrs Maze, five months pregnant, went to hospital with swollen legs and hands. She also complained of severe headache, drowsiness and vomiting. On examination the doctor diagnosed her problem to be pre-eclampsia. He admitted her for constant and expert care and ordered complete bed rest for her. Mrs Maze asked the doctor not to reveal the nature of her sickness to her husband because if he knew he would think of marrying another wife. In fact she told the doctor to tell her husband a lie about her condition. In the evening Mr Maze came to visit his wife and wanted to know what she was suffering from. The doctor did not want to tell a lie; at the same time he did not want to violate the rule of confidentiality and so he told Mr Maze that he could not disclose the nature of Mrs Maze's sickness.

Three days later, Mr Maze and his relatives went to the hospital to collect Mrs Maze, arguing that an *inyanga* (traditional healer) would heal her faster. The doctor who had admitted her was called in by the medical staff and he pleaded with them to leave her in the hospital. According to the doctor, what Mrs Maze needed was sleep and rest. Mrs Maze's husband and in-laws insisted on taking her. The doctor explained to Mrs Maze the seriousness of her condition and advised her to stay in the hospital, but Mrs Maze said that she wanted to go. The doctor tried to persuade her to stay, but she refused. In the end the doctor gave her a form to sign confirming that she was leaving against medical orders. She did, and her in-laws took her to the traditional healer.

Two weeks later Mrs Maze was returned to the hospital in a coma and having continuous convulsions. At the hospital the medical staff were divided as to whether she should be attended to or not, having brought herself to that condition. The doctor who had admitted her was called and immediately started giving her treatment, which annoyed those hospital staff members who had wanted her to be sent away. She died three hours later.

The four ethical principles are called into play in this case.

Autonomy

In African traditional ethics, autonomy, the ability to think and act independently and freely, is limited by the emphasis put on communalism. African societies emphasize interdependence and an individual's obligations to the community. An individual who disregards the family or the community and does what he or she thinks to be right, is regarded as anti-social. Thus, excessive individual autonomy is regarded as being a denial of one's corporate existence.

This should not be misunderstood to mean that a person does not have an individual existence, personality and a certain degree of autonomy. Communalism permits a degree of personal independence. In fact a person, in African ethical thinking, has to think and act independently. This is what distinguishes one person from another. A person who becomes famous and respected in the community as a hero or heroine, or as a virtuous person, is one who has proved to be superior to the ordinary person in some way, and has evolved a life plan of his or her own, achieving through his or her own efforts and ingenuity what is admired by the community. This life plan, however, is moulded in agreement with the traditional norms of the community. An individual has to strike a balance between creativity, originality and independence on the one hand, and conformity on the other.

Some members, however, must remain under the control, guidance and protection of the community, especially the mentally deformed, the insane, the senile, children and those who are temporarily unable to depend on themselves. Traditionally, women too were expected to be dependent on their husbands or fathers. This, however, has changed and women, especially those living in urban areas and working in the professions, have regained their independence and can act autonomously in many respects. The problem which remains, apart from male attitudes, seems to lie in the basic differentiation of male and female biological and social roles, and how to respect these without subordination. Mrs Maze was from a rural community where a woman still has to listen to and obey her husband and in-laws.

Quite apart from the dependent members of the community, African societies practise a high degree of paternalism. Although we have stated that African societies respect individual autonomy, and that a person is free to think and act independently, as long as his or her actions do not harm others or restrict their rights, this autonomy is not respected when the community believes that the person is acting against himself or herself. The community will restrict the free action of that individual for his or her own good. The good of the individual and of the group is more important than personal freedom or autonomy.

We need to keep in mind that, in the African concept of corporate existence, what harms an individual is considered harmful to the community. Thus it is accepted that it is right to interfere with a person's actions to prevent harm to others. Paternalistic intervention is justified on the grounds that the experience and knowledge of the elders should benefit the younger or less wise members of the community who might not understand the implications of their decisions or actions. Thus the communalistic value of mutual responsibility and caring often leads to paternalism.

One of the issues raised by the Mrs Maze case is confidentiality. A person's autonomy includes the right to privacy. In the hospital the health care worker has an obligation of confidentiality with regard to information about the diagnosis, treatment and prognosis of the patient's illness unless the patient has given permission to him or her to disclose them. Yet, because of the communal nature of African societies, relatives often want the doctor or nurse to let them know what the patient is suffering from, what treatment he or she is receiving and what the possible outcome of the treatment will be. Failure of the doctor or nurse to cooperate and reveal information sought by relatives can lead to the patient being 'stolen' from the ward by the relatives. This is perhaps the reason why Mr Maze and his relatives decided to take Mrs Maze out of the hospital to a traditional healer.

The second problem raised by this case is the freedom of the patient to choose the nature of medical care to be received. It was clear to the medical staff in the hospital that the traditional healers were not able to treat this case of pre-eclampsia. Many cases of this nature were known which, in the past, had been handled by traditional healers, leading to the death of the patient. All the patients with this disease who had been taken to traditional healers had either died or been returned to the hospital in a worse condition.

On the basis of respect for the autonomy of a patient to decide what treatment to receive, and from whom to receive it, Mrs Maze was allowed to go to a traditional healer and was accepted back by her doctor when she was returned. The cultural factor in respect for autonomy, however, is the group or communal influence on the patient. It may be argued, in relation to respect for autonomy as understood in western culture that insofar as an autonomous agent's actions do not infringe upon the autonomous actions of others, that person should be free to perform whatever action he or she wishes, even if it involves serious risk for the agent and even if others consider it to be foolish.[4] This is not the case in African thinking. In African societies which emphasize corporate existence, a person is expected to conform to communal decisions.

It is debatable whether the decision of a patient should be respected when he or she 'decides' under the pressure of the family. Many people would say that a patient who decides or acts under the influence or pressure of his or her family is not acting autonomously. In Africa, however, autonomy, as we have noted, is both individual and communal.

In traditional health care usually it is the person providing the care, not the patient, who makes decisions on what action is to be taken. In this case Mrs Maze was given a chance to decide; a decision which cost her her life. The question is who should decide on the course of action in health care? Should it be the patient, the relatives or the doctor or nurse giving the care? The obvious answer is that there should be cooperation, and when possible, agreement, among all the parties involved. The problem which still remains is, what happens when there is no agreement among them? This introduces the issue of competence in decision-making during health care.

In traditional health care it is common for the traditional healer or the family to decide for the patient. They may do something against his or her wishes or for his or her care without consulting him or her, if it is believed that what they are doing is for his or her good. Beneficence is a higher value than autonomy. However, health care is now complicated, especially when modern technology is involved. In many cases the patient and even the family do not have a minimal required knowledge of the problem and how to deal with it. Should the doctor, in such cases, not act without consulting the patient or the family or ignore their views for the good of the patient?

Beneficence

Following from the vital force principle, everyone has a duty to do good to his or her neighbour, especially to friends, relatives and clansmen, in order to promote the vital force. Generosity, kindness, hospitality, sharing and charity, all of which promote vital force, are basic values. In African ethics these beneficent qualities are not mere virtues, but duties. When one is in a position to do so, for example, one is duty-bound to give food to a stranger, unless doing so will mean someone else in the family going hungry. Not to do so is regarded as immoral. This is based on the conception of community as one family, with mutual obligations. It is done in order to preserve and enhance vital force, or to restore it when it has been disrupted.

One also has an obligation to prevent harm from happening, when one can. Members of the community must oppose any action which diminishes vital force or must apply remedies if the event has already occurred. Thus, in terms of health care, mutual obligation extends to preventive and curative medicine.

In order to promote or restore vital force, health care is highly valued. It should be emphasized, however, that when care is being administered the interests and needs of the patient are weighed against the good of the whole community. It is for this reason that people suffering from contagious diseases are traditionally isolated, or even helped to die, if they threaten the health of the community. The good of the patient is considered in the context of the good of all parties concerned, especially the good of the patient's immediate family.

As noted above, the concept of a person's wholeness underlies the African understanding of health and health care. The challenge to modern health care is that beneficence should not be directed only to the elimination of the disease, but rather it should be concerned with the patient's whole person and his or her social involvement in the community, in order to promote and enhance his or her ability to play his or her social role.

Non-Maleficence

The vital force principle establishes the duty not to cause harm, injure or do anything that reduces the vital force of the individual members of the community or threatens its collective existence. One should not even refrain from doing what would stop harm being done to others. However, the vital force philosophy also recognizes the existence of abnormal and yet potentially powerful influences from minerals, plants, and animals, which can be manipulated as forces for evil or good. There are also human beings who are believed to harm others although unaware of their own power and unable to stop themselves. These are witches who, according to the traditional ethos, must be neutralized by rituals or even eliminated. Other people are harmful voluntarily; these include sorcerers and murderers, who are regarded as anti-social because they are anti-life and are therefore hated. In the past such people could openly be killed by the community in order to save the rest. These days, because of modern laws, their power is either 'neutralized' with Christian rituals or, when this fails, they are secretly killed. All anti-life forces, substances and people must be neutralized or even be eliminated in order to preserve and promote the vital force in the community. In terms of health care the traditional healer and the community are required never to do harm to the patient unless it is in his or her best interests or for the good of the community. In modern health care this is a principle worth following; never to do harm to a patient unless the nurse or doctor, after serious consideration, believes that it is in the interests of the patient or it is necessary for the protection of other patients. According to African ethics, harm should be allowed only as a lesser evil or when all means to stop it have failed. In doing so, justice, if possible, must be done.

Justice

Justice is highly valued in communal existence in order to maintain social order, peace and solidarity and to avoid disintegration of the community. Because of the communal nature of African societies, justice is first and foremost a social affair. An offence against an individual is an offence against the community, and for the good of the community everyone's needs must be attended to without discrimination. Health care is, consequently, made available to everyone according to his or her needs. Since health care, in a traditional setting, is simple and inexpensive, this is easy to do.

African societies, however, emphasize a social hierarchy, consisting of, in descending order of prestige, kings, chiefs, religious specialists, grandparents and parents, older brothers and sisters down to the youngest member of the family and community. Justice, like any other aspect of society, is understood in hierarchical terms. It is giving or receiving what one deserves according to one's status in the community. No one has rights other than those given him by membership in the community. Justice in African societies is based on each according to his or her needs and status in society.

In medical care, faced with patients whose interests or needs conflict, the doctor or nurse is faced with the dilemma of whose needs or interests should be attended to first. In the case of Mrs Maze, she was readmitted to the hospital in a critical condition requiring immediate attention, yet humanly speaking she was responsible for her own state, having refused to follow the doctor's advice. Was it fair for the doctor to leave the other patients in order to attend to her?

Was it fair that more expensive and intensive care, at the expense of bona fide patients, should have been afforded her, whereas if she had listened to the doctor probably all she would have needed was bed rest and probably occasional mild sedatives? However, the principle of justice had to be weighed against beneficence.

Availability of health care services is another moral challenge. The state has an obligation to provide at least a minimum standard of health care available to those in need of it. According to African ethical principles, once health care facilities are provided, accessibility should not be based on need alone, but also on status. Since ethical rules and principles often change with time and circumstances, this view is changing and emphasis is put on need more than on status. This, it is believed, is a more just and objective approach.

Conclusion

From the above discussion it is apparent that cultural and individual ethics influence people's understanding of health and health care activities. In providing health care these factors have to be taken into account so that the care given is adequate and relevant to the situations in which people live. In the African context, and in accordance with the traditional ethical values, health care should extend to the whole person, seriously taking into account the interdependence of the various aspects of a person. A patient should be helped, for example, to heal his fears, misunderstandings, quarrels, jealousies, hatreds and other factors which militate against health. Secondly, both the patient and the whole family should be involved in health care. This approach is extremely important in the application of the four principles if we are to avoid health care turning into a mechanical exercise, but instead want it to be a personal relationship with its part to play in the attempt to bring about wholesomeness for the person.

On the subject of autonomy, it is important that the patient's independence is respected in deciding the nature of health care to be provided, especially if he or she is competent to take a rational decision in the matter. However, unless the patient objects, his or her relatives, especially the close ones, should be regarded as part of the team which is involved in the patient's care; therefore they deserve to know about the patient's sickness and treatment, and should have a say in the whole healing process.

In some societies autonomy may be regarded as of higher value than beneficence, non-maleficence and justice. In general this should be respected. In African culture, however, beneficence has a higher value, which justifies paternalistic interventions either by the doctor, who is supposedly more knowledgeable than the patient in the matter, or by the family, who may be in better condition or position than the patient to judge wisely what is best for him or her.

In health care it is important to help those in need in order to enhance their vital force. In doing so, however, it is important to consider the social nature of a person and to balance the patient's needs, rights and interests with those of other patients, the family and the community as a whole.

It is also important to avoid any action or non-action which weakens the vital force and harms the patient. In African ethical thinking, however, harm may be done to avoid greater harm either to the patient or to the community as a whole.

In doing all this justice must prevail. Those in need of health care should receive it according to their respective needs. There are situations when social status, which is an important consideration in Africa, is not a relevant factor, i.e. when people's lives are threatened. In such cases it should not be a deter-mining factor in the provision of health care. As elsewhere, in the matter of healing, those with equal needs should be treated equally and those with unequal needs should be treated unequally.[4] Again this should be balanced with the general good of the community.

It should be emphasized, finally, that in African ethical thinking, of supreme and simultaneous importance is the good of the patient and the welfare of the community. Principles are secondary, and only a means to an end.

References

1. Mbiti, J. 1969. *African religions and philosophy*, p. 101. Heinemann, Oxford.
2. Tempels, P. 1959. *Bantu philosophy*. Presence Africaine, Paris.
3. Gillon, R. 1985. (quoted). *Philosophical medical ethics*, p. 148. John Wiley & Sons, Chichester.
4. Beauchamp, T. L. and Childress, F. J. 1979. *Principles of biomedical ethics*, pp. 59, 174. Oxford University Press, New York.

AFRICAN-AMERICAN MEDICAL ETHICS

Toward an African-American Perspective on Bioethics

Annette Dula

──────────────INTRODUCTION TO READING──────────────

In the following reading, Annette Dula, of the University of Colorado, offers a comprehensive perspective on biomedical ethics from an African-American perspective. In the first section she suggests that the African-American perspective on bioethics stems from two bases—blacks' health and medical experiences and a legacy of black activist philosophy, which differs from mainstream philosophy in its attention to action and social justice.

In her next section, Dula examines mainstream issues in bioethics rele-vant to African Americans: the history of medical abuse against African

Americans, particularly with reproductive issues; the birth control movement; the issue of informed consent and the Tuskegee experiments as the
ultimate symbol of informed consent violations which have plagued the
African-American community.

Dula concludes by assessing how a "professional" African-American
view on bioethics is important not only to the African-American community but to the entire discipline. Through the analogy of the Black psychology and Women's movements, she argues that the professional
perspective can "voice the concerns of those not in the power circle."

Over the last twenty years, the field of bioethics has assumed major importance, as advances in medical technology and rising costs of health care have
forced society to come to terms with difficult ethical choices surrounding life
and death, allocation of resources, and doctor/patient relationships. Today, one
finds university departments and academic programs, hospital ethics committees, bioethics think tanks, and Presidential task forces devoted to medical
ethics policy and decision-making. Furthermore, numerous conferences, journals, and books disseminate information and knowledge generated by the new
profession.

However, the mainstream literature emerging from this influential new
field rarely includes discussions of race, class, and gender. Influential ethics
centers, such as the Hastings Center in Briarcliff Manor, New York, do address
cultural issues, but primarily from an international perspective. One reason for
the dearth of critical discussion of cultural and social issues here in the United
States may be the demographic makeup of bioethicists. Although feminist
bioethicists are beginning to have a louder voice, the field is dominated by
white, male, middle-class professionals and academics. These men decide what
is important, they frame questions, and they make policy recommendations.
The voices of those outside of the power circle—racial minorities, the poor,
women—have been excluded from ongoing debates on ethics and health care
policy. At best, such exclusion from decision-making results in paternalistic
decisions made for the "good" of the powerless. At worst, it victimizes the
powerless. For example, as Fox points out in her discussion of the sociology of
bioethics, "relatively little attention has been paid [by bioethicists] to the fact
that a disproportionately high number of the extremely premature, very low
birthweight infants, many with severe congenital abnormalities, [who are]
cared for in NICU [neonatal intensive care units,] are babies born to poor,
disadvantaged mothers, many of whom are single, nonwhite teenagers."[1]

I aim to show that the articulation and development of professional
bioethics perspectives by minority academics is necessary to expand the narrow
margins of debate. Without representation by every sector of society, the
powerful and powerless alike, the discipline of bioethics is missing the opportunity to be enriched by the inclusion of a broader range of perspectives.

Although I use African-American perspectives as an example, these points apply to other racial and ethnic groups—Hispanics, Native Americans, Asians—who have suffered similar health care experiences.

In the first section of this paper, I suggest that an African-American perspective on bioethics has two bases: (1) our health and medical experiences, and (2) our tradition of black activist philosophy. In the second section, I show through examples that an unequal power relationship has led to unethical medical behavior toward blacks, especially regarding reproductive issues. In the third section, I argue that developing a professional perspective not only gives voice to the concerns of those not in the power circle, but enriches the entire field of bioethics.

Medical and Health Experiences

The health of a people and the quality of health care they receive reflect their status in society. It should come as little surprise, then, that African-Americans' health experiences differ vastly from those of white people. These differences are well documented. Compared to whites, more than twice as many black babies are born with low birthweight[2] and twice as many die before their first birthday.[3] Fifty percent more blacks than whites are likely to regard themselves as being in fair or poor health.[4] Blacks are included in fewer trials of new drugs[5]—an inequity of particular importance for AIDS patients, who are disproportionately black and Hispanic. The mortality rate for heart disease in black males is twice that for white males; recent research has shown that blacks tend to receive less aggressive treatment for this condition.[6] More blacks die from cancer, which, unlike in whites, is likely to be systemic by the time it is detected.[2] African Americans live five fewer years than do whites;[7] indeed, if blacks had the same death rate as whites, 59,000 black deaths a year would not occur.[8] McCord and Freeman, who reported that black men in Harlem are less likely to reach the age of 65 than are men in Bangladesh, conclude that the mortality rates of inner cities with largely black populations "justify special consideration analogous to that given to natural-disaster areas."[9]

These health disparities are the result of at least three forces: institutional racism, economic inequality, and attitudinal barriers to access.[10] Institutional racism has roots in the historically unequal power relations between blacks and the medical profession, and between blacks and the larger society. It has worked effectively to keep blacks out of the profession, even though a large percentage of those who manage to enter medicine return to practice in minority communities—where the need for medical professionals is greatest. Today, institutional racism in health care is manifested in the way African Americans and poor people are treated. They experience long waits, are unable to shop for services, and often receive poor quality and discontinuous health care. Moreover, many government programs do not target African Americans as a group. Instead, the government targets populations such as the poor or pregnant women. As a result, benefits to racially defined populations are diffused.

Black philosopher W.E.B. DuBois summed up the economic plight of African Americans: "To be poor is hard, but to be a poor race in a land of dollars is the very bottom of hardships."[11] Poor people are more likely to have poor health, and a disproportionate number of poor people are black. African Americans tend to have lower-paying jobs and fewer income-producing sources such as investments. Indeed, whites on average accumulate 11 times more wealth than do blacks.[12] Less money also leads to substandard housing—housing that may contain unacceptable levels of lead paint, asbestos insulation, or other environmental hazards. Thus both inadequate employment and subpar housing available to poor African Americans present health problems that wealthier people are able to avoid. In addition, going to the doctor may entail finding and paying for a babysitter and transportation, and taking time off from work at the risk of being fired, all of which the poor can ill afford.

Attitudinal barriers—perceived racism, different cultural perspectives on health and sickness, and beliefs about the health care system—are a third force which brings unequal health care. Seeking medical help may not have the same priority for poor people as it has for middle-class people. One study in the *Journal of the American Medical Association* revealed that, compared to whites, blacks are less likely to be satisfied with how their physicians treat them, more dissatisfied with their hospital care, and more likely to believe that their hospital stay was too short.[4] Also, many blacks, like people of other racial and ethnic groups, use home remedies and adhere to traditional theories of illness and healing that lie outside of the mainstream medical model.[13] Institutional racism, economic inequality, and attitudinal barriers, then, contribute to inadequate access to health care for poor and minority peoples. These factors must be seen as bioethical concerns. Bioethics cannot be exclusively medical or even ethical. Rather, it must also deal with beliefs, values and cultural traditions, and the economic, political, and social order. Medical sociologists have severely criticized bioethicists for ignoring cultural and societal particularities that limit access to health care.[1,14]

This inattention to cultural and societal aspects of health care may be attributed in part to the mainstream Western philosophy on which the field of bioethics is built. For example, renowned academic bioethicists such as Veatch, Beauchamp, and MacIntyre rely on the philosophical works of Rawls, Kant, and Aristotle.[15–17] In addition, the mainstream Western philosophic method is presented primarily as a thinking enterprise, rarely advocating for change or societal transformation. Thus for the most part, Western philosophers have either gingerly approached or neglected altogether to comment on such social injustices as slavery, poverty, racism, sexism, and classism. As pointed out in a recent article in *Black Issues in Higher Education*, mainstream philosophy until recently was seen as above questions of history and culture.[18]

Black Activist Philosophy

The second basis for an African-American perspective on bioethics is black activist philosophy. Black philosophy differs from mainstream philosophy in its emphasis on action and social justice.[19] African-American philosophers view the world through a cultural and societal context of being an unequal partner. Many black philosophers believe that academic philosophy devoid of societal context is a luxury that black scholars can ill afford. Moreover, African-American philosophers have purposely elected to use philosophy as a tool not only for naming, defining, and analyzing social situations, but also for recommending, advocating, and sometimes harassing for political and social empowerment—a stance contrary to mainstream philosophic methods.[20] Even though all bioethicists would do well to examine the thinking of such philosophers as Alain Locke, Lucius Outlaw, Anita Allen, Leonard Harris, W.E.B. DuBois, Bernard Boxill, Angela Davis, and Cornel West, references to the work of these African-Americans are rarely seen in the bioethics literature.[19-21]

Although the professionalization of bioethics has frequently bypassed African-American voices, there are a few notable exceptions. Mark Siegler, director of the Center for Clinical Medical Ethics at the University of Chicago, included three African-American fellows in the 1990–91 medical ethics training program; Edmund Pellegrino of the Kennedy Institute for Advanced Ethics co-sponsored three national conferences on African-American perspectives on bioethics; and Howard Brody at Michigan State University is attempting to diversify his medical ethics program. Additionally, a number of current publications offer important information. For example, the National Research Council's *A Common Destiny: Blacks and American Society* provides a comprehensive analysis of the status of black Americans, including discussions on health, education, employment, and economic factors; Marlene Gerber Fried's *From Abortion to Reproductive Freedom* presents many ideas of women of color concerning abortion; and several new journals (e.g., *Ethnicity and Disease*, published by the Loyola University School of Medicine, and the *Journal of Health Care for the Poor and Underserved*) call particular attention to the health experiences of poor and underserved people.

Clearly, bioethics and African-American philosophy overlap. Both are concerned with distributive justice and fairness, with autonomy and paternalism in unequal relationships, and with addressing both individual and societal ills. African-American philosophy, therefore, may have much to offer bioethics in general and African-American bioethics in particular.

Mainstream Issues Relevant to African Americans

A shocking history of medical abuse against unprotected people is also grounds for an African-American perspective in bioethics. In particular, reproductive rights issues—questions of family planning, sterilization, and genetic screening—are of special interest to black women who have been singularly exploited in each of these areas.[22] (Therefore, black women may view these issues differently from white women—which argues for including black women's perspectives in bioethics.) The history of the birth control movement and the Tuskegee experiment illustrate concretely the need for African Americans to become invested in the bioethics debate.

The Birth Control Movement

A critical examination of the American birth control movement reveals fundamental differences in perspectives, experiences, and interests between the white women who founded the movement and African-American women who were affected by it. Within each of three phases, the goals of the movement implicitly or explicitly served to exploit and subordinate African-American as well as poor white women.[23]

The middle of the 19th century marked the beginning of the first phase of the birth control movement, characterized by the rallying cry, "Voluntary Motherhood!" Advocates of voluntary motherhood asserted that women ought to say "no" to their husbands' sexual demands as a means of limiting the number of their children. This concept was irrelevant to African-American women; refusing a man's sexual demands was not an option for these women, especially during slavery. The irony, of course, was that while early white feminists were refusing their husbands' sexual demands, most black women did not have the same right to say "no" to these white women's husbands. Indeed, African-American women were exploited as breeding wenches in order to produce stocks of enslaved people for plantation owners. Meier and Rudwick comment on slave-rearing as a major source of profit for nearly all slave-holding farmers and planters: "Though most Southern whites were scarcely likely to admit it, the rearing of slaves for profit was a common practice. [A] slave woman's proved or anticipated fecundity was an important factor in determining her market value; fertile females were often referred to as 'good breeders.'"[24]

The second phase of the birth control movement gave rise to the actual phrase "birth control," coined by Margaret Sanger in 1915.[23] Initially, this stage of the movement led to the recognition that reproductive rights and political rights were intertwined; birth control would give white women the freedom to pursue new opportunities made possible by the vote.[22] This freedom allowed white women to go to work while black women cared for their children and did their housework.

Eventually, the second stage of the birth control movement coincided with the eugenics movement, which advocated improvement of the human race through selective breeding. When the white birth rate began to decline, eugenists chastised middle-class white women for contributing to the suicide of the white race:

> Continued limitation of offspring in the white race simply invites the black, brown, and yellow races to finish work already begun by birth

control, and reduce the whites to a subject race preserved merely for the sake of its skill.[25]

Eugenists proposed a two-fold approach for curbing "race suicide": imposing moral obligations on middle-class white women to have large families, and on poor immigrant women and black women to restrict the size of theirs. For the latter, Guy Irving Burch of the American Eugenics Society advocated birth control.[18]

The women's movement adopted the ideals of the eugenists regarding poor, immigrant, and minority women, and it even surpassed the rhetoric of the eugenists. Margaret Sanger described the relationship between the two groups: "The eugenists wanted to shift the birth-control emphasis from less children for the poor to more children for the rich. We went back of that [*sic*] and sought first to stop the multiplication of the unfit."[26] Thus, while black women have historically practiced birth control,[27, 28] they learned to distrust the birth control movement as espoused by white feminists—a distrust that continues to the present day.[29]

The third stage of the birth control movement began in 1942 with the establishment of the Planned Parenthood Federation of America. Although Planned Parenthood made valuable contributions to the independence, self-esteem, and aspirations of many women, it accepted existing power relations, continuing the eugenic tradition by defining undesirable "stock" by class or income level.[23] Many blacks were suspicious of Planned Parenthood; men, particularly, viewed its policies as designed to weaken the black community politically or to wipe it out genetically.[38]

From the beginning of this century, both public and private institutions attempted to control the breeding of those deemed "undesirable." The first sterilization law was passed in Indiana in 1907, setting the stage for not only eugenic, but punitive sterilization of criminals, the feeble-minded, rapists, robbers, chicken thieves, drunkards, and drug addicts. By 1931, states had passed sterilization laws, allowing more than 12,145 sterilizations. By the end of 1958, the sterilization total had risen to 60,926. In the 1950s, several states attempted to extend sterilization laws to include compulsory sterilization of mothers of "illegitimate" children.[33] Sterilization laws are still in force in 27 states, but are seldom enforced, and where they have been, their eugenic significance has been negligible.[29]

Numerous federal and state measures perpetuated a focus on poor women and women of color. Throughout the United States in the 1960s, the federal government began subsidizing family planning clinics designed to reduce the number of people on welfare by checking the transmission of poverty from generation to generation. The number of family planning clinics in a given geographical area was proportional to the number of black and Hispanic residents.[34] In Puerto Rico, a massive federal birth control campaign introduced in 1937 was so successful that by the 1950s, the demand for sterilization exceeded facilities,[31] and by 1965, one-third of the women in Puerto Rico had been sterilized.[32]

In 1972, Los Angeles County Hospital, a hospital catering to large numbers of women of color reported a seven-fold rise in hysterectomies.[34] Between 1973 and 1976, almost 3,500 Native American women were sterilized at *one* Indian Health Service hospital in Oklahoma.[35] In 1973, two black sisters from Montgomery, Alabama, 12-year-old Mary Alice Relf and 14-year-old Minnie Lee Relf, were reported to have been surgically sterilized without their parents' consent. An investigation revealed that in the same town, 11 other young girls of about the same age as the Relf sisters had also been sterilized; 10 of them were black. During the early 1970s in Aiken, South Carolina, of 34 Medicaid-funded deliveries, 18 included sterilizations, and all 18 involved young black women.[36] In 1972, Carl Schultz, Director of the U.S. Dept. of Health, Education, and Welfare's Population Affairs Office, acknowledged that the government had funded between 100,000 and 200,000 sterilizations.[37] These policies aroused black suspicions that family planning efforts were inspired by racist and eugenist motives.

The first phase of the birth control movement, then, completely ignored black women's sexual subjugation to white masters. In the second phase, the movement adopted the racist policies of the eugenics movement. The third stage saw a number of government-supported coercive measures to contain the population of poor people and people of color. While blacks perceive birth control *per se* as beneficial, blacks have historically objected to birth control as a method of dealing with poverty. Rather, most blacks believe that poverty can be remedied only by creating meaningful jobs, raising the minimum wage so that a worker can support a family, providing health care to working and nonworking people through their jobs or through universal coverage, instituting a high-quality day care system for low-or no-income people, and improving educational opportunities.[39]

Informed consent

Informed consent is a key ethical issue in bioethics. In an unequal patient/provider relationship, informed consent may not be possible. The weaker partner may consent because he or she is powerless, poor, or does not understand the implications of consent. And when members of subordinate groups are not awarded full respect as persons, those in positions of power then consider it unnecessary to obtain consent. The infamous Tuskegee experiment is a classic example. Starting in 1932, over 400 poor and poorly educated syphilitic black men in Alabama were unwitting subjects in a U.S. Public Health Service experiment, condoned by the Surgeon General, to study the course of untreated syphilis. Physicians told the men that they were going to receive special treatment, concealing the fact that the medical procedures were diagnostic rather than therapeutic. Although the effects of untreated syphilis were already known by 1936, the experiment continued for 40 years. In 1969, a committee appointed by the Public Health Service to review the Tuskegee study decided to continue it. The Tuskegee experiment did not come to widespread public attention until 1972, when the *Washington Star* documented this breach of medical ethics. As a result, the experiment was halted.[40]

It may be tempting to assume that such medical abuses are part of the distant past. However, there is evidence that violations of informed consent persist. For example, of 52,000 Maryland women screened annually for sickle cell anemia between 1978 and 1980, 25 percent were screened without their consent, thus denying these women the benefit of prescreening education or follow-up counseling, or the opportunity to decline screening.[41] A national survey conducted in 1986 found that 81 percent of women subjected to court-ordered obstetrical interventions (Caesarean section, hospital detention, or intrauterine transfusion) were black, Hispanic, or Asian; nearly half were unmarried; one-fourth did not speak English; and none were private patients.[31] The role of the medical profession in such cases is an open question.

How a Professional Perspective Makes a Difference

Thus far, I have shown some grounds for African-American perspectives on bioethics, based on black activist philosophy and the unequal health status of African-Americans. I have also argued that a history of medical abuse and neglect towards people in an unequal power relationship commands our attention to African-American perspectives on bioethics issues. In this final section, I will argue that a professional perspective can voice the concerns of those not in the power circle. Two examples—black psychology and the white women's movement—illustrate that professional perspectives can make a difference in changing society's perceptions and, ultimately, policies regarding a particular population.

Black Psychology

Until recently, mainstream psychology judged blacks as genetically and mentally inferior, incapable of abstract reasoning, culturally deprived, passive, ugly, lazy, childishly happy, dishonest, and emotionally immature or disturbed. Mainstream psychology owned these definitions and viewed African-Americans through a deficit-deficiency model—a model it had constructed to explain African-American behavior.[43-46]

When blacks entered the profession of psychology, they challenged that deficit model by presenting an African-American perspective[46] that addressed the dominant group's assessments and changed, to a certain extent, the way society views blacks. Real consequences of black psychologists' efforts to encourage self-definition, consciousness, and self-worth have been felt across many areas: professional training, intelligence and ability testing, criminal justice, family counseling. Black psychologists have presented their findings before professional conferences, legislative hearings, and policymaking task forces. For example, black psychologists are responsible for the ban in California on using standardized intelligence tests as a criterion for placing black and other minority students in classes for the mentally retarded. The Association of Black Psychologists publishes the *Journal of Black Psychology*, and black psychologists contribute to a variety of other professional journals.[45] As a result of these and other efforts, most respected psychologists no longer advocate the deficit-deficiency model.

The Women's Movement

The women's movement is another example where members of a subordinated group are defining their own perspectives. The perspectives of white women have historically been defined for the most part by white men; white women's voices, like black voices, have traditionally been ignored or trivialized. A mere 20 years ago, the question, "Should there be a woman's perspective on health?" was emotionally debated. Although the question is still asked, a respected discipline of women's studies has emerged, with several journals devoted to women's health. Women in increasing numbers have been drawn to the field of applied ethics, specifically to bioethics,[48,49] and debate over issues such as maternal and child health, rights of women vs. the rights of the fetus, unnecessary hysterectomies and Caesareans, the doctor/patient relationship, and the absence of women in clinical trials of new drugs.

Unfortunately, however, the mainstream women's movement is largely the domain of white women. This, of course, does not mean that black women have not been activists for women's rights; on the contrary, African-American women historically have been deeply involved in fighting both racism and sexism, believing that the two are inseparable. Many black women distrust the movement, criticizing it as racist and self-serving, concerned only with white middle-class women's issues.[28,29,50] Black feminists working within the abortion rights movement and with the National Black Women's Health Project, an Atlanta-based self-help and health advocacy organization, are raising their voices to identify issues relevant to African-American women and men in general, and reproductive and health issues in particular.[35] Like black psychologists, these black feminists are articulating a perspective that is effectively promoting pluralism.

Conclusion

The disturbing health inequities between blacks and whites—differences in infant mortality, average lifespan, chronic illnesses, and aggressiveness of treatment—suggest that minority access to health care should be recognized and accepted as a *bona fide* concern of bioethics. Opening the debate can only enrich this new field, thereby avoiding the moral difficulties of exclusion. Surely the serious and underaddressed health concerns of a large and increasing segment of American society is an ethical issue at least as important as such esoteric, high-visibility issues as the morality of gestational surrogacy. The front page of the August 5, 1991, *New York Times* headlined an article, "When

Grandmother is Mother, Until Birth." Although interesting and worthy of ethical comment, such sensational headlines undermine the moral seriousness of a situation where over 31 million poor people do not have access to health care.

There is a basis for developing African-American perspectives on bioethics, and I have presented examples of medical abuse and neglect that suggest particular issues for consideration. Valuable as our advocacy has been, our perspectives have not gained full prominence in bioethics debates. Thus, it is necessary to form a community of scholars to conduct research and articulate the perspectives of African Americans and other poor and underserved peoples in this important field.

References

1. Fox R. The sociology of medicine. Englewood Cliffs, NJ. Prentice Hall, 1989.

2. Rene, AA. Racial differences in mortality: Blacks and whites. In: Jones W, Rice MF, eds. *Health care issues in black America: Policies, problems, and prospects.* New York: Greenwood Press, 1987:20–41.

3. Howze, DC. Closing the gap between black and white infant mortality rates. An analysis of policy options. In: Jones W, Rice MF, eds. *Health care issues in Black America; Policies,* Problems, and Prospects. New York: Greenwood Press, 1987: 119–39.

4. Blendon, R. Aiken L, Freeman H, et al. *Access to medical care for black and white Americans: A matter of continuing concern.* JAMA 1989 Jan 13;26(2):278–81.

5. Svensson CK. *Representation of American blacks in clinical trials of new drugs.* JAMA 1989. Jan. 13;261(2):263–265.

6. Wenneker MB, Epstein AM. *Racial inequalities in the use of procedures for patients with ischemic heart disease in Massachusetts.* JAMA 1989 Jan 13;261(2):253–7.

7. Report of the Secretary's Task Force on Black and Minority Health. Executive Summary. Vol. 1. Washington, DC: U.S. Department of Health and Human Services, August, 1985.

8. Miller SM. *Race in the health of America.* Milbank Q 1987;65 (Suppl. 2):500–28.

9. McCord C, Freeman, HP. *Excess mortality in Harlem.* New England Journal of Medicine, 1990 Jan 18; 322(3):173–177.

10. Jones W, Rice MF. "Black health care" In: Jones W, Rice, MF, eds. *Health care issues in black America: Policies, problems, and prospects.* New York: Greenwood Press, 1987.

11. DuBois WEB. *The souls of black folk: Essays and sketches.* Greenwich, CT: Fawcett Publications, Inc., 1961

12. Jaynes, GD, Williams, RM. *A common destiny: Blacks and American society.* Washington, DC: National Academy Press, 1989.

13. Watson WH. *Black folk medicine: The therapeutic significance of faith and trust.* New Brunswick: Transaction Books, 1984.

14. Keyserlingk, E. Ethical guidelines and codes—Can they be universally applicable in a multi-cultural society? In: Allenbeck P, Jansson B, eds. *Ethics in medicine: Individual integrity versus demands of society.* Karolinska Institute Nobel Conference Series. New York: Raven Press, 1990.

15. Veatch RM. *A theory of medical ethics.* New York: Basic Books, 1981.

16. Beauchamp T, Childress, J. *Principles in biomedical ethics,* Second ed. New York: Oxford University Press, 1983.

17. MacIntyre A. *After virtue: A study in moral theory.* Notre Dame, IN: University of Notre Dame Press, 1981.

18. Brodie M. In Locke's footsteps: *Black philosophers search for wisdom and validation.* Black Issues Higher Ed 1990 Dec 20;7(21):1.

19. Boxill B. *Blacks and social justice.* Totowa, NJ: Rowman and Allenheld, 1984.

20. Harris L. *Philosophy born of a struggle.* Dubuque, IA: Kendall Hunt, 1983.

21. West C. *American evasion of philosophy. A genealogy of pragmatism.* Madison: University of Wisconsin Press, 1989.

22. Davis, A. *Women, race, and class.* New York: Vintage Books, 1981.

23. Gordon L. *Woman's body, woman's right: Birth control In America.* Revised ed. New York: Penguin Books, 1990.

24. Meier A, Rudwick E. *From plantation to ghetto.* New York: Hill and Wang, 1970.

25. Popenoe P. *The conservation of family.* Baltimore: Williams & Wilkins, 1926.

26. Sanger M. *Autobiography.* New York: W.W. Norton, 1938.

27. Rodrique J. *The black community and the birth-control movement.* In: DuBois EC, Ruiz VL, eds. Unequal sisters: A multi-cultural reader in U.S. women's history. New York: Routledge, 1990.

28. Giddings P. *When and where I enter: The impact of black women on race and sex in America.* Toronto: Bantam Books, 1984.

29. Collins PH. *Black feminist thought: Knowledge, consciousness, and the politics of empowerment.* Boston: Unwin Hyman, 1990.

30. Haller MH. *Eugenics: Hereditarian attitudes in American thought.* New Brunswick: Rutgers University Press, 1984.

31. Presser HB. *Sterilization and fertility: Decline in Puerto Rico.* Berkeley: Institute of International Studies, 1973.

32. Gould, KH. *Black women in double jeopardy: A perspective on birth control.* Health Soc Work 1984; 96–105.

33. Morrison, JL *Illegitimacy, sterilization and racism: A North Carolina case history.* Soc Sci Rev 1965 Mar39:1–10.

34. Mass B. *Population target: The political economy of population control in Latin America.* Toronto: Women's Press, 1976.

35. Fried MG, *From abortion to reproductive freedom.* Boston: South End Press, 1990.

36. Aptheker H. *Sterilization, experimentation, and imperialism.* Political Aff. 1974 Jan;53(1):37–48.

37. Payne L. *Forced sterilization for the poor.* San Francisco Chronicle, 1974 Feb 26.

38. Littlewood TB. *The politics of population control.* Notre Dame, IN: University of Notre Dame, 1977.

39. Edelman MW. *Families in peril: An agenda for social change.* Cambridge: Harvard University Press, 1987.

40. Jones JH. Bad Blood: *The Tuskegee Syphilis Experiment: A tragedy of race and medicine.* New York: The Free Press: 1981.

41. Farfel MR, Holtzman, NA. *Education, consent, and counseling in sickle cell screening programs: Report of a survey.* Am J Public H 1984 Apr;74(4):373–5.

42. Kolder V, Gallagher J, Parson MT. *Court-ordered obstetrical interventions.* New Eng J Med 1987 May 7;316(19):1192–6.

43. Billingsley A. *Black families in white America.* Englewood Cliffs, NJ: Prentice Hall, 1968.

44. Jones R. *Black Psychology.* New York: Harper & Row, 1980.

45. White JL. *The psychology of blacks: An Afro-American perspective.* Englewood Cliffs, NJ: Prentice Hall, Inc., 1984.

46. Zinn MB. *Family, race, and poverty in the eighties.* Signs 1989 Summer;14(4):856–74.

47. Jenkins AH. *The psychology of the Afro-American: A humanistic approach.* New York: Pergamon Press, 1982.

48. Holmes HB. *Special issue: Feminist ethics and medicine.* Hypatia 1989 Summer;4(2).

49. Griffiths M, Whitford M. *Feminist perspectives in philosophy.* Bloomington: Indiana University Press, 1988.

50. Davis A. "Racism, birth control, and reproductive rights." In: Fried MG, ed. *From abortion to reproductive freedom: Transforming a movement.* Boston: South End Press, 1990.

INDEX

in Patient's Bill of Rights, 194–197
philanthropy in, 121–124
in political liberalism, 143–144
Protestant attitudes toward, 99–104
in Russian health care, 224–225, 230–232
Sun Simiao on, 311, 312–315
in traditional Chinese medicine, 301–302
Physician-physician relationship, in traditional Chinese medicine, 302–303
Physicians
in Ayurveda, 250–251
choosing of, 31
as contractors, 124–126
dominance and discipline of, 132–134
ethical principles for, 29–39, 39–41
God as, 65
laws controlling, 182–184
substitute, 35
Planned Parenthood, African Americans and, 363
Plato, 9, 12, 14, 16, 19
Platonists
on justice, 14
suicide and, 7
Pluralism, in Russian health care, 220–222
Poison, Hippocratic Oath proscription of, 4–5
Political liberalism. *See* Liberal political philosophy
Politics, rights and, 179–181, 182–184
Population control, in China, 328–329, 330
Positive freedom, 138, 139, 146
Positive rights, 136
Possessions, negative freedom and, 139
Poverty
and African-American health care, 360
in Catholic medical ethics, 81
medical ethics and, 31–32, 61
Prana
the Hindu self and, 246–247
persistent vegetative state and, 279
Precepts, Buddhist, 265–267
Precepts, 44, 47
ethical principles within, 43
Pregnancy

in Buddhist medical ethics, 267–268
in Catholic medical ethics, 88–91
in Hindu medical ethics, 253–255
Prescriptions, in medical ethics, 32
President's Commission for the Study of Ethical Problems in Medicine and Biomedical and Behavioral Research, report on equitable health-care access by, 187–194
Priests, in Catholic health care institutions, 83–85
Primary goods, 167
Primum non nocere principle, 46, 49
Principles of Medical Ethics, 39–41, 53–54
Privacy. *See also* Confidentiality; Silence
in African medical ethics, 352–353
in Bioethics Convention, 201
in Catholic health care institutions, 88
in Consumer Bill of Rights and Responsibilities, 213
in Hindu medical ethics, 251
in Islamic medical ethics, 236
Private property, as fundamental right, 170, 180
Professional conduct
dominance and discipline in, 132–134
medical ethics relative to, 30–33, 33–38, 116–134
Professional Dominance (Freidson), 132–133
Professional incompetence. *See also* Malpractice
in Chinese medical ethics, 331–332
dealing with, 132–134
Professional medical groups, ethics within, 116–134
Professional medicine, Confucianism against, 301
Professional misconduct, dealing with, 50–52
"Professional standard," in medical ethics, 156–157
Property rights, of individual in his own person, 170
Proportionate means of preserving life, 92–93
Proportionate reason, 112–113

Proprietary medicines, ethical use of, 36
Protestantism
covenants in medical ethics of, 116–134
Hippocratic Oath and, 117–118
medical ethics of, 56, 99–114
Roman Catholic medical ethics versus, 104–115
Psychiatry
African-American medical ethics and, 365–366
in Russian health care, 225–226
Purity
Hippocratic Oath and, 7
surgery and, 12–13
Pythagoras, 9, 16
Pythagoreans
Hippocratic Oath and, 8–9, 19–20, 21
on injustice and mischief, 14–15
on medical education, 17–18, 18–19
medical philosophies of, 9–15
on silence, 15
on surgery, 11–13
Qi, life and death and, 333
Qiu, Ren-Zong, 292, 318–319
on defective newborns, 285
Quack medicines, 49
in Ayurveda, 250–251
proscriptions against, 36
Quebec Bill 41, 184
Quran, Islamic medical ethics and, 234–239
Rabbinic decisions, on life prolongation, 74–75
Racism, African-American medical ethics and, 359–360
Ramsey, Paul, 99, 131
Richard McCormick and, 104–115
Rational collective choice, in justice, 167–168
Rational deliberation
in autonomy, 152–155
in justice, 167–170
Rawls, John, 110, 142, 163
on health care rights, 175–177
on justice, 166–170
"Reasonable person standard," in medical ethics, 156–157
Reasonable values, in medical ethics, 112–114